INTERVENTIONAL TECHNIQUES IN CARDIOVASCULAR MEDICINE

Developments in
Cardiovascular Medicine

VOLUME 119

The titles published in this series are listed at the end of this volume.

Interventional Techniques in Cardiovascular Medicine

edited by

V. Hombach
Department of Cardiology/Angiology/Pneumonology, University Hospital of Ulm, Ulm, F.R.G.

M. Kochs
Department of Cardiology/Angiology/Pneumonology, University Hospital of Ulm, Ulm, F.R.G.

and

A. J. Camm
Department of Cardiology, St. George's Hospital, London, U.K.

Springer Science+Business Media, B.V.

Library of Congress Cataloging-in-Publication Data

Interventional techniques in cardiovascular medicine / edited by
  V. Hombach, M. Kochs, and A. J. Camm.
      p.   cm. — (Developments in cardiovascular medicine: v. 119)
      Based on a symposium held at the University of Ulm in 1989.
      ISBN 978-0-7923-0956-7   ISBN 978-94-011-3802-4 (eBook)
      DOI 10.1007/978-94-011-3802-4
      1. Transluminal angioplasty – Congresses.   2. Tachycardia – Treatment – Congresses.
  3. Coronory heart disease – Treatment – Congresses.   I. Hombach, V. (Vinzenz)
  II. Kochs, M.   III. Camm, A. John   IV. Series.
      [DNLM: 1. Angioplasty, Transluminal, Percutaneous Coronary – Congresses.
  2. Coronary Arteriosclerosis – therapy – congresses.   3. Electrocoagulation – congresses.
  4. Tachycardias – therapy – congresses. W1 DE997VME v. 119 / WG 166 I618 1989]
  RD598.5.I63   1991
  617.4' 1059 – dc20
  DNLM/DLC
  for Library of Congress   90–5216
                                                                             CIP

ISBN 978-0-7923-0956-7

Contents

Preface

Since the introduction of balloon angioplasty for the relief of coronary artery stenoses and of anginal symptoms in patients with coronary artery disease by Andreas Grüntzig in 1977, the field of interventional technology and treatment strategies has grown enormously. For the reduction of hemodynamically significant coronary artery stenoses balloon angioplasty is the standard and reference method with a high primary success and low complication rate. Because of the relatively high recurrence rates of 30–40% of balloon angioplasty a whole family of different angioplasty techniques has been developed since then. Among those are atherectomy devices, laser angioplasty, radiofrequency angioplasty, high and low speed rotational angioplasty and stenting of stenosed vessels. Balloon angioplasty has been extended to aortic and mitral valve stenoses, and supraventricular and ventricular tachycardias can now be treated by catherter ablation techniques.

In 1989 an International Symposium on standard and newer interventional techniques has been held at the University of Ulm. This volume contains the essential parts and presentations of the international faculty of experts in the field. In four chapters the principles, advantages, pitfalls and future developments of coronary angioplasty, angioplasty of peripheral arteries, balloon valvuloplasty and of catheter ablation of supraventricular and ventricular tachycardias are described in detail. We hope that this 'State-of-the-Art' representation will be of great value for both the non-expert reader and the active researcher in the fields addressed within the book.

V. Hombach, M. Kochs and A. J. Camm

List of contributors

U. U. BABIC
Cardiovascular Center, Dragisa Misovic, Stejpana Radica 1, YU-11000 Beograd, Yugoslavia
Chapter 23

Y. BASHIR
Department of Cardiological Sciences, St. George's Hospital, Medical School, Cranmer Terrace, London SW17 ORE, U.K.
Chapter 27 co-author: A. J. CAMM

M. BORGGREFE
Clinic of Internal Medicine C, Wilhelms University Münster, Albert-Schweitzer-Str. 33, D-4400 Münster, F.R.G.
Chapter 28 co-authors: G. HINDRICKS, W. HAVERKAMP, A. MARTINEZ-RUBIO, U. KARBENN, TH. BUDDE and G. BREITHARDT

G. BREITHARDT
Clinic of Internal Medicine C, Wilhelms University Münster, Albert-Schweitzer-Str. 33, D-4400 Münster, F.R.G.
Chapter 32 co-authors: G. HINDRICKS, W. HAVERKAMP, M. BORGGREFE, A. MARTINEZ-RUBIO and TH. BUDDE

A. BUCHWALD
Department of Cardiology, University Clinic, Robert-Koch-Str. 40, D-3400 Göttingen, F.R.G.
Chapter 10 co-authors: C. UNTERBERG, H. TILL, K. NEBENDAHL, P. GRÖNE and V. WIEGAND

A. J. CAMM
Department of Cardiovascular Sciences, St. George's Hospital, Cranmer Terrace, London SW17 ORE, U.K.
Chapter 36 co-authors: M. A. DE BELDER and G. A. HAYWOOD

A. CRIBIER
Service de Cardiologie, Hopital Charles-Nicolle, 1, Rue de Germong, F-76031 Rouen Cedex, France
Chapter 24 co-author: R. KONING

H. DALICHAU
University of Göttingen, Department of Thoracic and Cardiovascular Surgery, Robert-Koch-Str. 40, D-3400 Göttingen, F.R.G.
Chapter 25 co-authors: K. L. NEUHAUS and U. TEBBE

C. DÜBER
Institute of Clinical Radiology, University of Mainz, Langenbeckstr. 7, D-6500 Mainz, F.R.G.
Chapter 13 co-authors: K. -J. KLOSE, H. KOPP and W. SCHMIEDT

T. EGGELING
Department of Cardiology/Angiology/Pneumonology, Medical Clinic and Policlinic, University Hospital of Ulm, Robert-Koch-Str. 8, D-7900 Ulm / Donau, F.R.G.
Chapter 2 co-authors: M. KOCHS, M. HÖHER, W. HAERER and V. HOMBACH

R. ERBEL
II. Medical Clinic, Johannes Gutenberg University, Langenbeckstr. 1, D-6500 Mainz, F.R.G.
Chapter 9 co-authors: M. HAUDE, U. DIETZ, P. STÄHR, H.J. RUPPRECHT, R. ZOTZ and J. MEYER

A. HANNEKUM
Department of Thoracic and Cardiovascular Surgery, University of Ulm, Steinhövelstrasse 9, D-7900 Ulm / Donau, F.R.G.
Chapter 37

R. HIBST
Institute for Lasertechnology, University of Ulm, Robert-Koch-Str. 8, D-7900 Ulm / Donau, F.R.G.
Chapter 17 co-authors: T. KOLBE, B. WEINBRENNER and V. HOMBACH

B. HÖFLING
Clinic Grosshadern, Medical Clinic I, Marchioninistrasse 15, D-8000 München 70, F.R.G.
Chapter 14 co-author: A. VON PÖLNITZ

V. HOMBACH
Department of Cardiology/Angiology/Pneumonology, Medical Clinic and
Policlinic, University Hospital of Ulm, Robert-Koch-Str. 8, D-7900 Ulm /
Donau, F.R.G.
Chapter 4 co-authors: M. HÖHER, M. KOCHS, T. EGGELING, W.
HAERER, S. WIESHAMMER, A. SCHMIDT, H. W. HÖPP and H. H.
HILGER

K. R. KARSCH
Division of Internal Medicine III, Department of Cardiology, Eberhard-
Karls University, Otfried-Müller-Str. 10, D-7400 Tübingen, F.R.G.
Chapter 7 co-authors: K. K. HAASE, M. MAUSER, W. VOELKER and
L. SEIPEL

H. KLEIN
Medical University Hannover, Department of Cardiology, Konstanty-
Gutschow-Str. 8, D-3000 Hannover 61, F.R.G.
Chapter 31 co-authors: H. J. TRAPPE, J. TRÖSTER and A. AURICCHIO

H. KORB
Clinic and Policlinic of Cardiac Surgery, University of Cologne, Joseph-
Stelzmannstr. G, D-5000 Cologne 41, F.R.G.
Chapter 11 co-authors: A. HOEFT, U. TEBBE, A. BOROWSKI and E. R.
DE VIVIE

M. KOCHS
Department of Cardiology/Angiology/Pneumonology, University Hospital
of Ulm, Robert-Koch-Str. 8, D-7900 Ulm / Donau, F.R.G.
Chapter 6 co-authors: W. HAERER, T. EGGELING, A. SCHMIDT, M.
HÖHER, S. WIESHAMMER and V. HOMBACH

K. -H. KUCK
University Hospital Eppendort, II. Medical Clinic, Department of Cardio-
logy, Martinistr. 52, D-2000 Hamburg 20, F.R.G.
Chapter 30 co-authors: M. SCHLÜTER, K. -P. KUNZE and M. GEIGER

M. MANZ
Medical University Clinic, Department of Cardiology, Sigmund-Freud-Str.
25, D-5300 Bonn 1, F.R.G.
Chapter 35 co-author: B. LÜDERITZ

J. MEYER
II. Medical Clinic and Policlinic, Langenbeckstr. 1, University of Mainz, D-6500 Mainz, F.R.G.
Chapter 3 co-authors: H.-J. RUPPRECHT, R. BRENNECKE, M. KOTTMEYER, G. BERNHARD, R. ERBEL and T. POP

C. J. MURDOCK
University Hospital, Arrhythmia Unit, University of Western Ontario, P.O. Box 5339, Postal Station A, London, Ontario, Canada N6A 5A5
Chapter 29 co-authors: G. M. GUIRAUDON, G. J. KLEIN, R. W. YEE and A. D. SHARMA

A. W. NATHAN
Department of Cardiology, St. Bartholomew's Hospital, West Smithfield, London EC1A 7BE, U.K.
Chapter 33

H.-H. OSTERHUES
Department of Cardiology/Angiology/Pneumonology, University Hospital of Ulm, Robert-Koch-Str. 8, D-7900 Ulm / Donau, F.R.G.
Chapter 20 co-authors: M. VOGELPOHL, C. FELDER, M. KOCHS and V. HOMBACH

E.-I. RICHTER
Radiology Centre, Division of Diagnostics, Clinic Nürnberg, P.O. Box 91 01 60, D-8500 Nürnberg 91, F.R.G.
Chapter 12 co-author: E. ZEITLER

H. ROSKAMM
Benedikt-Kreuz-Rehabilitationszentrum für Herz- und Kreislaufkranke, Südring 15, D-7812 Bad Krozingen, F.R.G
Chapter 1

D. ROTH
Institute of Physiology I, University of Tübingen, Gmelinstr. 5, D-7400 Tübingen, F.R.G.
Chapter 16 co-authors: P. C. DARTSCH and E. BETZ

G. STEINBECK
Clinic Grosshadern, Medical Clinical I, University of München, Marchioninistr. 15, D-8000 München 70, F.R.G.
Chapter 26

R. STEINER
Institute for Medical Lasertechnology, Surgical Clinic II, University of Ulm,
P.O. Box 4066, Ulm / Donau, F.R.G.
Chapter 5 co-authors: R. HIBST, T. KOLBE, X. M. LIU, W. PRIES, T.
ZÖPF and S. CYBA-ALTUNBAY

B.E. STRAUER
Medical Clinic and Policlinic B, Heinrich-Heine-University, Moorenstr. 5,
D-4000 Düsseldorf, F.R.G.
Chapter 19 co-authors: M. P. HEINTZEN and T. NEUBAUR

M. TYNAN
Department of Pediatric Cardiology, Guy's Hospital, London SE1 9RT,
U.K.
Chapter 22 co-authors: S. ARAB, S. QURESHI, E. BAKER, R. DOS
ANJOS, J. PARSONS and A. HAYES

R. VOISARD
Department of Cardiology/Angiology/Pneumonology, University Hospital
of Ulm, Robert-Koch-Str. 8, D-7900 Ulm, F.R.G.
Chapter 15 co-authors: P. C. DARTSCH, G. BAURIEDEL, L.
LAUTERJUNG, B. HÖFLING and E. BETZ

J. F. VOLLMAR
Department of Vascular, Thoracic & Cardiac Surgery, University of Ulm,
Steinhoevelstr. 9, D-7900 Ulm / Donau, F.R.G.
Chapter 21 co-author: S. CYBA-ALTUNBAY

P. WEISMÜLLER
Department of Cardiology/Angiology/Pneumonology, University Hospital
of Ulm, Robert-Koch-Str. 8, D-7900 Ulm / Donau, F.R.G.
Chapter 34 co-authors: U. MAYER, P. RICHTER, F. HEIECK, M.
KOCHS, M. HÖHER, B. KUHNT and V. HOMBACH

G. S. WERNER
Department of Cardiology, University of Göttingen, Robert-Koch-Str. 40,
D-3400 Göttingen, F.R.G.
Chapter 8 co-authors: A. BUCHWALD, C. UNTERBERG, E. VOTH, H.
KREUZER and V. WIEGAND

S. WIESHAMMER
Department of Cardiology/Angiology/Pneumonology, University Hospital
of Ulm, Robert-Koch-Str. 8, D-7900 Ulm / Donau, F.R.G.
Chapter 18 co-authors: M. VOGELPOHL, M. KOCHS, W. HAERER, M.
HÖHER, T. EGGELING, M. SCHMIDT, H.-H. OSTERHUES, P.
WEISMÜLLER and V. HOMBACH

PART ONE

Coronary angioplasty

1. Medical interventions for regression of coronary atherosclerosis

H. ROSKAMM

Introduction

One of the main questions cardiologists will be confronted with in the coming 5 years, is regression or at least retarded progression of coronary arteriosclerosis. The drugs to be discussed in that context are calcium antagonists, platelet aggregation inihibitors and lipid lowering drugs. This paper will focus on lipid lowering drugs, which have been used in several studies already published and will be used in various studies recently initiated.

Progression and regression of coronary arteriosclerosis

From the pathologist's point of view the mechanisms responsible for progression are lipid deposition, mural thrombi and atheroma with edema, haemorrhage, necrosis and once more mural thrombi. Important mechanisms for regression are resoption, lysis, organisation and retraction of thrombi [6]. Comparing intravitally taken coronary angiograms with postmortem results, Stolte et al. [6] identified rupture of a plaque and thrombosis as the prevailing factors connected with progression, while embolisation, lysis, organisation and retraction of a thrombus play the leading role in the process of regression.

These mechanisms are apparently connected with really significant alterations, which happen in a stepwise manner. The more or less continuous type of progression or regression during the early stages of coronary arteriosclerosis can probably only be investigated by quantitative measures. At present evaluation of progression and regression of coronary arteriosclerosis in a living individual is only possible by repeated coronary angiographies.

Observational studies have shown that progression is common in patients with coronary heart disease; after a time interval of approximately 5 years almost every patient with coronary arteriosclerosis shows progression. Pro-

V. Hombach et al. (eds), Interventional Techniques in Cardiovascular Medicine, 3–7.
© 1991 *Kluwer Academic Publishers.*

gression will be less frequent and less marked in segments showing no or only little stenosis in the first angiogram [3].

It must be considered though, that in most clinical studies the second coronary angiogram had been performed because of clinical reasons, mostly deterioration of symptoms, and thus these studies were based on a negative selection of patients.

In our own study of 164 patients with myocardial infarction at young age, a second coronary angiogram was routinely obtained 3.4 years after the first which was performed weeks or months after the infarction. This second angiogram was a systematic diagnostic measure, independent of the presence of symptoms or signs [5]. We thus avoided a negative selection for the second angiogram and found regression in 15% of our 164 patients and progression in 30%. Progressions were mainly those from a small stenosis in the first angiogram to a medium or severe stenosis in the second angiogram.

The regressions were without exception those from a severe stenosis at the first angiogram to a medium degree of stenosis in the second angiogram.

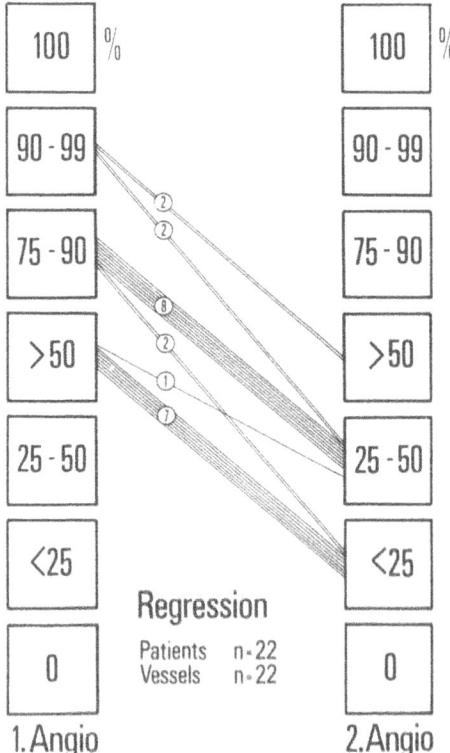

Figure 1.   Degree of stenosis at the first and second coronary angiography in 22 of 164 patients with myocardial infarction at an age under 40 who after 3.4 years on average showed a regression of stenosis of at least two grades, based on the AHA classification of stenoses [5].

All regressions occurred in infarction-related vessels (Figure 1). These regressions observed in infarction-related vessels of young patients are in our opinion due to late recanalisation and organisation of a thrombus. This type of regression is not what we are interested in if it comes to influences of lipid lowering drugs. With the exception of regression in infarction-related vessels of young patients, regressions of coronary arteriosclerotic lesions in the spontaneous development of coronary arteriosclerosis are rare.

Intervention trials with lipid lowering drugs

The influences of lipid lowering drugs have mainly been investigated in two large scale studies: the National Heart, Blood and Lung Institute's [2] and the CLAS-Study [1]. In the NHLBI-Study, 116 patients with hyperlipo-proteinemia type II and coronary artery disease received 24 g cholestyramine or diet alone. Total cholesterol decreased by 1% in the placebo group but up to 17% in the cholestyramine group. LDL decreased 5% in the placebo group and 26% in the cholestyramin group. There were no differences in HDL-cholesterol values between the two groups. Coronary artery disease had progressed in 49% of the placebo treated patients and 32% in the cholestyramin-treated patients. This was a significant difference. But not all angiographic parameters used for the evaluation of progression showed significant differences. There were only 3 patients with definite regression, one in the placebo group and two in the cholestyramin group. This is not surprising, because even in the cholestyramin group elevated cholesterol values were still present after treatment, average total cholesterol being 256 mg/dl, LDL-cholesterol 178 mg/dl. With such lipid values regression cannot be expected.

This was all different in the CLAS-Study [2]. One hundred and sixtytwo patients after bypass surgery, all nonsmokers, aged 40–59 years, with baseline cholesterol values between 185 to 350 mg/dl were randomized into a verum and a placebo group. The verum group was treated with 30 g colestipol and 3–12 g niacin, and showed a decrease of total cholesterol by 26% in relation to 5% in the placebo group, a decrease of LDL-cholesterol by 43% in relation to 5% in the placebo group, and 37% elevation of HDL-cholesterol in relation to 2% in the placebo group.

This dramatic improvement of cholesterol values was combined with a reduction in progression from 61 to 39%, and with regression in 16% versus 2% in the placebo group. Both differences were significant. In this study the end values for cholesterol (180 mg/dl total cholesterol, 97 mg/dl LDL-cholesterol) were far lower than in the first study and this made regression possible.

Even the subgroup with only slightly elevated cholesterol levels (total cholesterol 180–240 mg/dl) at baseline showed a significant reduction of progression. The total progression score in the placebo-treated subgroup

Table 1. Characteristics of the intervention studies planned with HMG-CoA reductase inhibitors, according to A. C. Arntzenius (personal communication).

Intervention Studies with HMG-CO-Reductase-Inhibitors

Authors	Country	Medication	Duration of treatment	n	Inclusion criteria
1. Barth et al.	NL	Pravastatin vs placebo	2 yrs	2 × 360	Chol. < 380 mg/dl
2. Blankenhorn et al.	USA	40 mg lovastatin vs placebo	2 + 4 yrs	2 × 130	Chol. 200–295 mg/dl
3. Brown et al.	USA	Lovastatin + colestipol vs placebo	2.5 yrs	2 × 55	90% perz. APO-B
4. Campeau et al.	Canada	Lovastatin vs warfarin	5 yrs	4 × 400	LDL 130–190 mg/dl
5. Kane et al.	USA	Resin + lovastatin + Niacin vs placebo	2 yrs	2 × 48	H. F. -hyperchol.
6. Hugenholtz et al.	Europe	20 mg simvastatin vs placebo	2 yrs	2 × 175	Chol. 213–309 mg/dl
7. Sacks et al.	USA	Pravastatin, niacin, resin vs fishoil + diet	2.5 yrs	90,60,40	Chol. 50–250 mg/dl HDL/LDL > 3
8. Roskamm et al.	Germ.	40 mg simvastatin vs placebo	2 yrs	2 × 125	Chol. 230–299 mg/dl after 2 weeks of diet

with high base-line cholesterol was 0.9, with individual progression scores between −3 and +3. It has been possible to reduce this figure to 0.3 in the placebo-treated group. In the subgroup with lower baseline cholesterol levels the progression score was 0.6 — as to be expected a bit smaller — but this figure has also been reduced to 0.3 in the verum group. Both treatment effects were significant.

Discussing the results of this important study we have to consider two points:

1. All patients were non-smokers, therefore hyperlipidemia will have been the leading risk factor for coronary arteriosclerosis in this study population.
2. Patients only qualified for randomization, if they had shown good compliance and good treatment effects in a prestudy with cholestyramin and niacin.

In a general population subjected to such an aggressive treatment this good complicance cannot be expected as, e.g., the Lipid Research Clinics Trial with cholestyramin has shown [4].

But with the new HMG-CoA-reductase-inhibitors, which promise simple treatment application with, e.g., one single tablet a day, there should be a chance. Recently 8 angiographic intervention studies with HMG-CoA-reductase inhibitors have been initiated or will be started in the near future.

Table 1 gives some characteristics of these studies. Important are the following points:

1. For the most part also patients with only slightly increased cholesterol values will be included in the study.
2. During the course of the study, the lipid values are being kept on a low or absolutely normal level.
3. Progression and regression will be evuluted with computer assisted quantitative coronary angiography.

If a delay of progression or even regression of coronary arteriosclerosis can be clearly shown in these studies, secondary prevention with diet and lipid lowering drugs will have a great future and might become a new part of interventional cardiology.

References

1. Blankenhorn DH, Nessim SA, Johnson RL, Sanmarco ME, Azen SP, Cashin-Hemphill L (1987) Beneficial effects of combined colestipol-niacin therapy on coronary atherosclerosis and coronary venous bypass graft. *J Am Med Ass* 257: 3233.
2. Brensike JF, Levy RI, Kelsey SF et al. (eds) (1984) Effects of therapy with cholestyramine on progression of coronary arteriosclerosis: results of the NHLBI type II coronary intervention study. *Circulation* 69: 313.
3. Kramer JR, Kitazume H, Proudfit WL, Matsuda Y, Williams GW, Sones jr, FM (1983) Progression of coronary atherosclerosis in nonoperated patients: relation to risk factors, in: Roskamm H (ed), *Prognosis of Coronary Heart Disease — Progression of Coronary Arteriosclerosis*, p. 137. Berlin, Heidelberg, New York: Springer.
4. The Lipid Research Clinics Coronary Primary Prevention Trial results (1984) II: The relationship of reduction in incidence of coronary heart disease to cholesterol lowering. *J Am Med Ass* 251: 365.
5. Roskamm H, Gohlke H, Stürzenhofecker P et al. (1983) Der Herzinfarkt im jugendlichen Alter (unter 40 Jahren): Koronarmorphologie, Risikofaktoren, Langzeitprognose der Erkrankung und Progression der Koronargefäßsklerose. *Z Kardiol* 72: 1.
6. Stolte M, Wittek D, Braun B (1983) Progression and regression of coronary arteriosclerosis — a pathologist's point of view, in: Roskamm H (ed), *Prognosis of Coronary Heart Disease — Progression of Coronary Arteriosclerosis*, p. 130. Berlin, Heidelberg, New York. Springer.

2. Digital coronary angiography

T. EGGELING, M. KOCHS, M. HÖHER, W. HAERER and
V. HOMBACH

Introduction

For more than 50 years investigators have been attempting to accurately describe the human coronary pathologic anatomy. The modern technique of coronary arteriography was introduced by Sones and Shirley [20] in 1959; they discovered that by selective transbrachial coronary cannulation one could safely opacify the left and right coronary artery in man. Other selective angiographic techniques such as the percutaneous transfemoral artery approach described by Judkins using different pre-formed catheters for specific procedures [11] quickly developed.

New interventional diagnostic and therapeutic techniques such as percutaneous coronary angioscopy, selective intracoronary thrombolysis, 'Percutaneuos Transluminal Coronary Angioplasty' (PTCA), 'High Frequency Coronary Angioplasty' (HFCA), 'Excimer Laser Coronary Angioplasty' (ELCA), Coronary Aterectomy and percutaneous transluminal coronary stenting have changed the requirements for selective coronary angiography. Today claims for coronary and cardiac angiographic imaging are the following:

- Improved resolution of coronary images.
- Reduction of x-ray dose.
- Automatic, observer independent, real-time quantitative angiography of coronary stenosis.
- Automatic, observer independent, determination of left ventricular function.
- Storage of images as road maps for interventional techniques.

Digital coronary arteriography

All over the world the 'gold standard' in cardiac imaging is still 35 mm cine film. For accurate interpretation of coronary anatomy images with sharp

9

V. Hombach et al. (eds), Interventional Techniques in Cardiovascular Medicine, 9–24.
© 1991 *Kluwer Academic Publishers.*

visualization of coronary artery edges and appropriate angiographic angulations are needed. If vessels overlap, foreshortening or incomplete opacification occur, significant stenoses could be missed completely.

Different attempts have been made to improve the image quality of conventional x-ray equipment for flouroscopy and 35 mm cine film acquisition.

The success of 'Digital Subtraction Angiography' (DSA) in non-cardiac angiography has led to a demand for a comparable technique in cardiac angiography. DSA uses the temporal subtraction method to enhance the vessel which is studied. As the non-cardiac vessels occupy a relatively fixed position, the acquisition frame rate (1–4 frames per second <fps>) is determined by the dynamics of the contrast bolus. Due to the high motility of the heart a fast acquisition capability of at least 25 fps is required. Some currently available versions of DSA equipment have the capability of fast

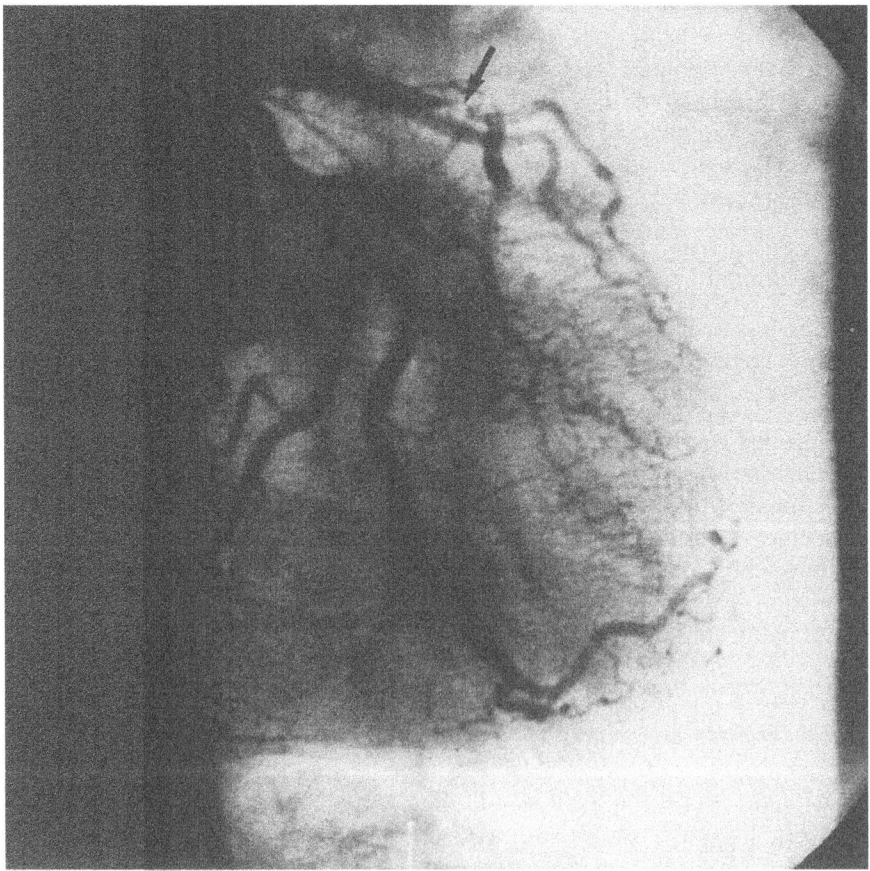

Figure 1.   30° RAO view of a significant left anterior descending (LAD) stenosis (arrow).

image acquisition (25 fps); but due to the post-processing subtraction method digitally processed images are not available on-line during fluoroscopy.

Cardiac imaging during the catheterization procedure requires immediate on-line digital processing [1,23]. This problem has been solved by image overframing and image processing in order to enhance small details (Digital Cardiac Imaging <DCI>, Philips, The Netherlands). The blurring effects of the x-ray system during flouroscopy are automatically counteracted by the use of a real-time unsharp masking algorithm. The result of this on-line processing is that the images displayed on the monitor have a sharp appearance and provide exact information of the coronary anatomy without applying longer fluoroscopy times or higher x-ray exposure to the patient. Parallel to digital fluoroscopy 35 mm cine film is exposed as film camera and TV camera receive their pulsed image information simultaneously from the output window of the image intensifier via a high-quality beam splitter.

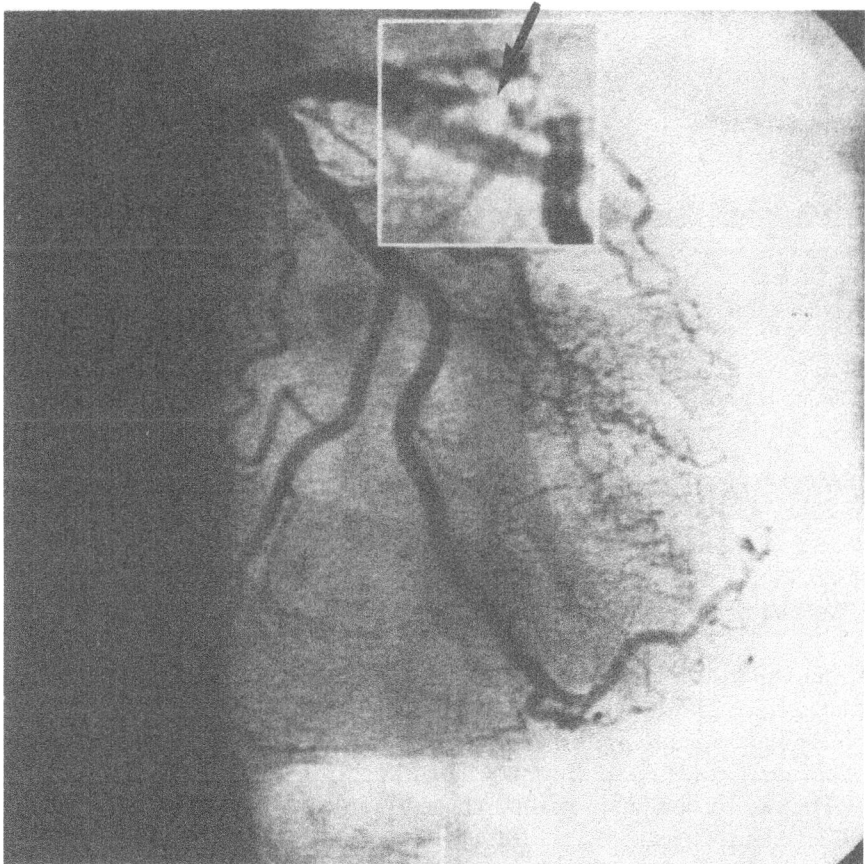

Figure 2. Magnified view of the LAD stenosis (arrow).

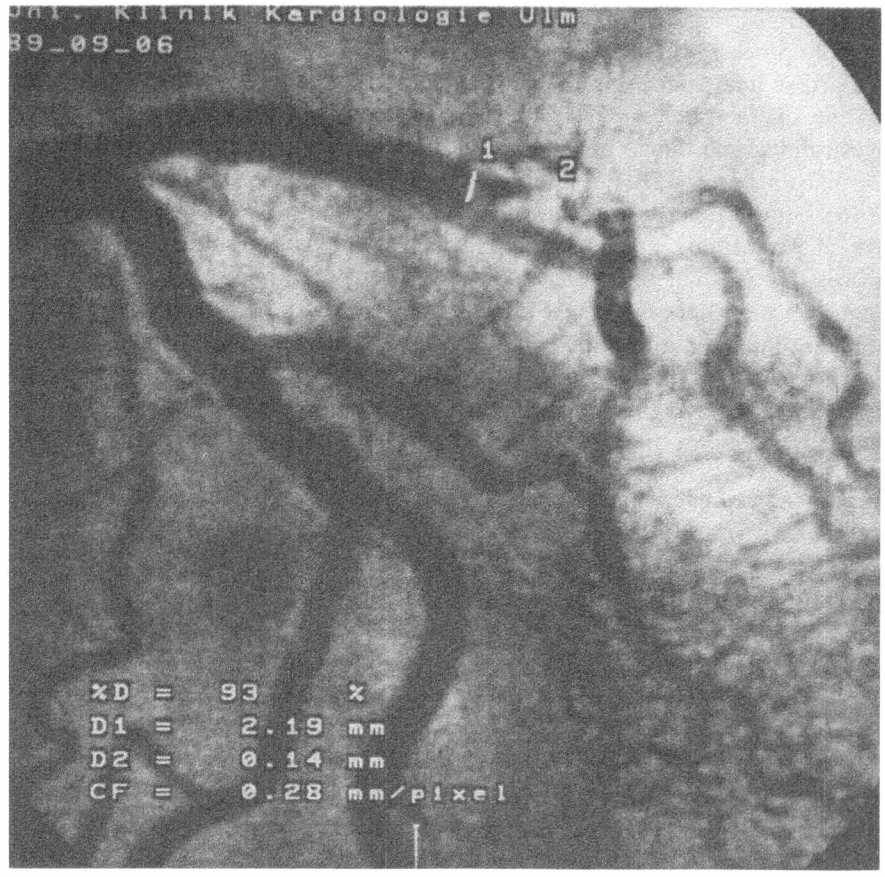

Figure 3.   Determination of vessel diameter (1) and stenosis diameter (2) of the LAD lesion indicating a diameter stenosis of 93%

Examples of coronary angiograms obtained using the DCI system are shown in Figures 1–11.

Quantitative coronary angiography

Visual interpretation of coronary lesions has certain limitations. Several studies have shown significant inter- and intraobserver variability in estimates of coronary stenosis [5,6,18] and poor correlation between visual estimates of coronary disease and coronary blood flow [13].

The era of computer-assisted coronary artery quantitation has begun in 1971, when Gensini et al. [8] introduced their system with a reported accuracy of $\pm$ 80 μm. All computer-assisted systems for automatic or operator-interactive determination of coronary lesions require accurate

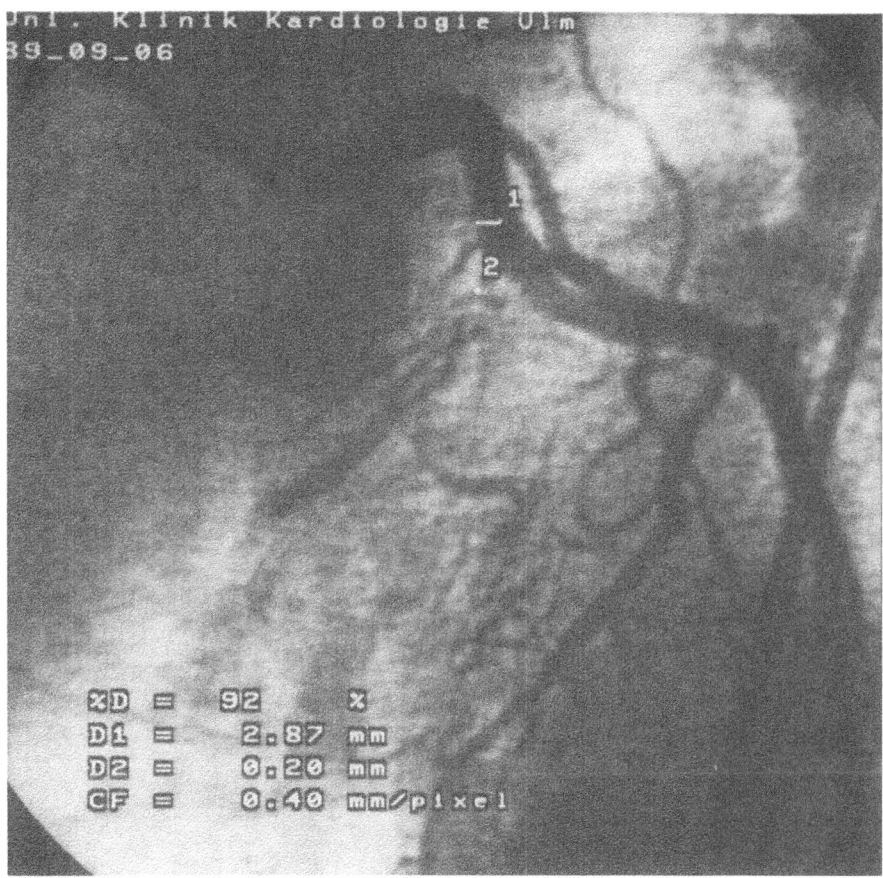

Figure 4. Determination of vessel diameter (1) and stenosis diameter (2) of the same LAD lesion in 45° left anterior oblique with 20° cranial angulation indicating a diameter stenosis of 92%

coronary images. Image formation is influenced by many factors. The quality of cardiac images depends on the variety of viewing angles used, the mechanism of contrast opacification of the coronary artery, x-ray energy absorption and the radiodensity of the background tissue. Different systems have been developed for computer assisted quantitation of coronary lesions.

The system developed by Reiber et al. [15] is an operator-interactive computer-assisted method for automatic edge detection of coronary vessels. The 35 mm cine-film is displayed on a video screen in different magnifications, and a video camera is centered to the region of interest. The video image is digitized using a 512 × 512 × 8 bit matrix. As calibration factor the contrast-filled coronary catheter is used. For vessel contour determination the user has to make centerline determinations at several locations. The computer performs edge detection with determination of absolute vessel

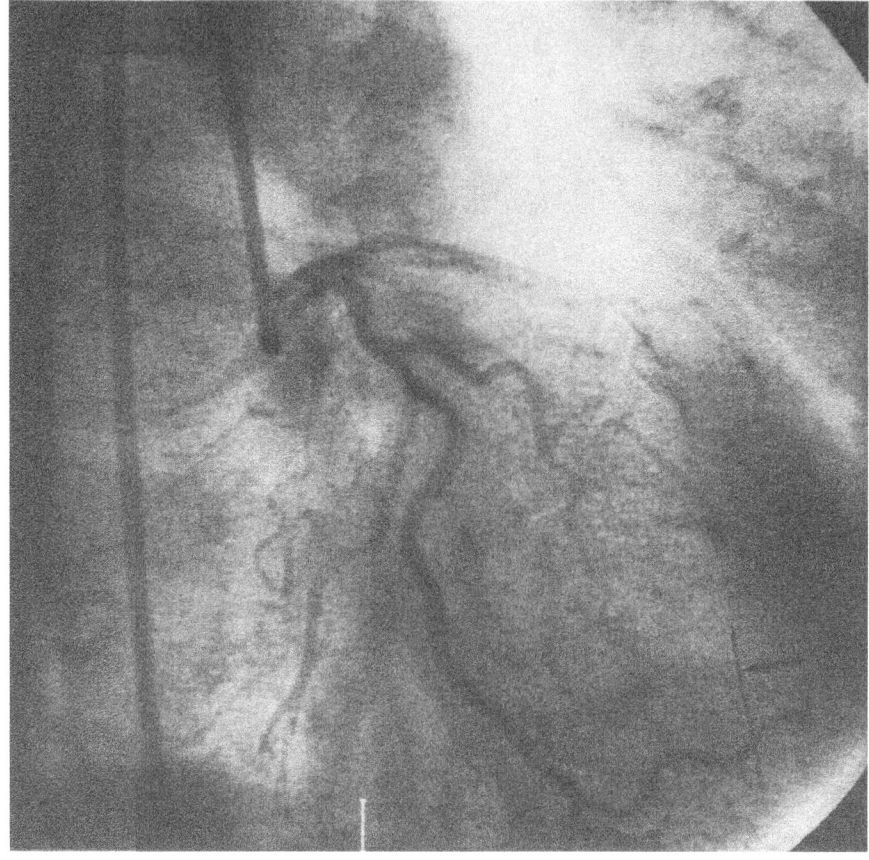

Figure 5.   Guide wire advanced into the distal part of LAD (arrow).

diameter, minimum diameter, mean diameter, and percent vessel diameter reduction. Measurement variabilities of less than 120 um are reported. The major disadvantage of this system is the non-availability of stenosis determination during the diagnostic or interventional study.

Sanders et al. [16] developed a system, which as well performs a digital post-processing of 35 mm cine-film images. The user has to determine the lumen border using a light pen on a video screen. The computer than calculates lumen diameter, segment lumen area and volume and percent diameter reduction. The reported variability in repeat dimensional estimates is low. The major disadvantages of this system are manual determination of lumen border by the user and the non-availability during the angiographic procedure in the catheterization laboratory.

A different system using digital subtraction angiographic (DSA) images was introduced by Tobis et al. [21,22]. The video signal is amplified and

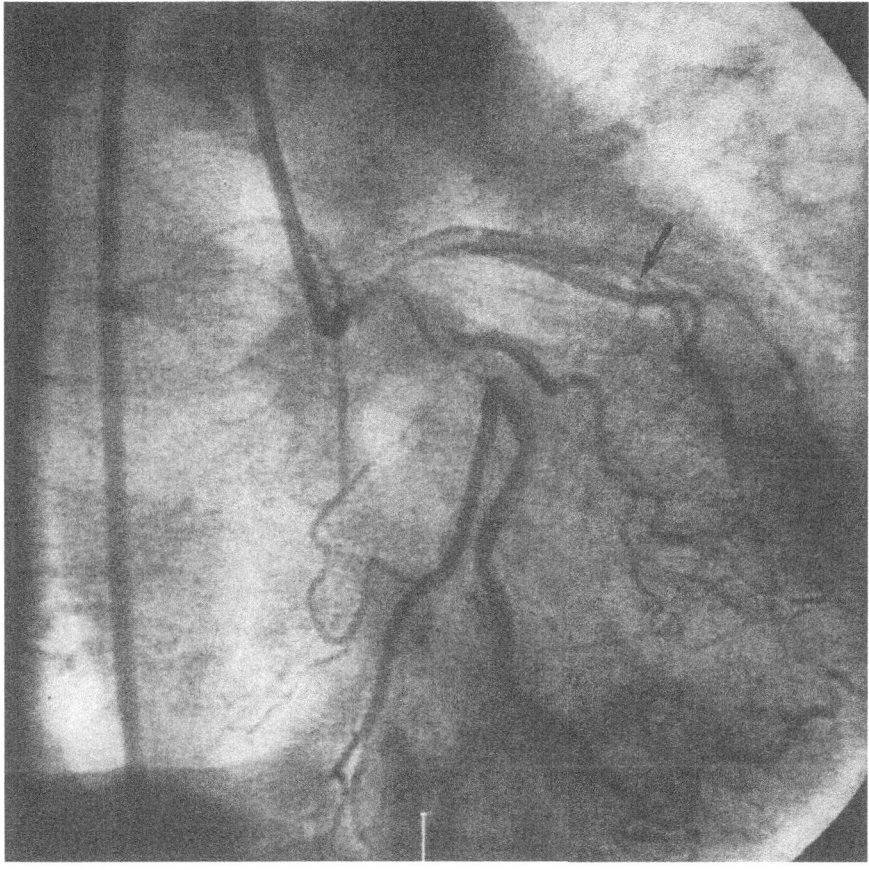

Figure 6.   Balloon catheter placed into the lesion (arrow indicating the middle of the balloon)

converted from an analog to a digital format using a 512 × 512 × 8 bit pixel matrix at 30 fps. The digital image may be processed immediately or stored on hard disk. The advantage of this system is the on-line availability during the angiographic study with improved contrast imaging due to the removal of overlying and interfering tissue densities by the digital subtraction process. The degree of stenosis is than determined using a conventional caliper. Misregistration artifact due to motion (respiration, body motion, cardiac arrhythmia) between the time of mask generation and vessel opacification is the major problem of this method.

The first computer-assisted system for quantitative coronary angiography was developed in 1975 by Brown et al. [2,3]. 35 mm cine-film is fivefold magnified, vessel borders of the diseased segment are traced manually from a proximal portion with 'normal diameter' through the stenotic area to a distal 'normal diameter'. These vessel borders are digitized and the computer

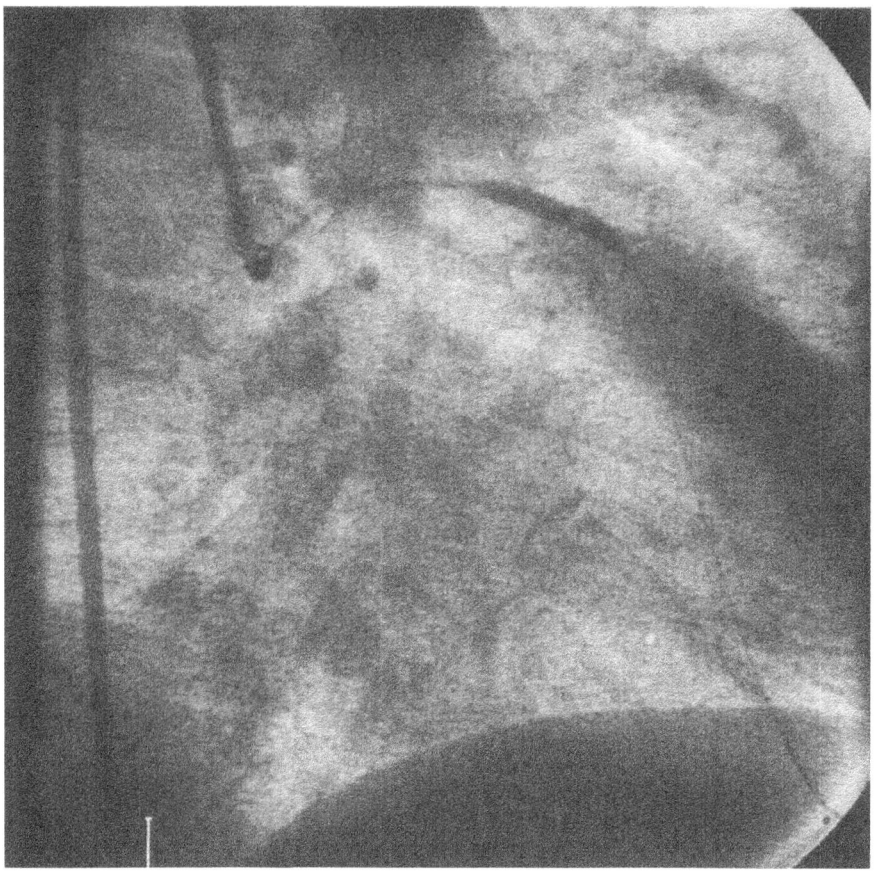

Figure 7.   Completely inflated balloon.

combines the two perpendicular images in a three-dimensional image of lumen geometry. From this computer approximation vessel diameters and cross-sectional areas are calculated. Disadvantages of this system are non-availability during the angiographic procedure and manual tracing of vessel borders.

The DCI system (Philips) offers the advantage of on-line processing of cardiac images during flouroscopy presenting excellent coronary images with enhanced vessel edges and removal of surrounding tissue. Additional use of the magnifying function allows exact visualization of coronary lesions. Nevertheless the system still has the disadvantage that manual determination of 'normal' and stenotic vessel diameter is required. A fully automatic computer program for vessel diameter determination will be soon available.

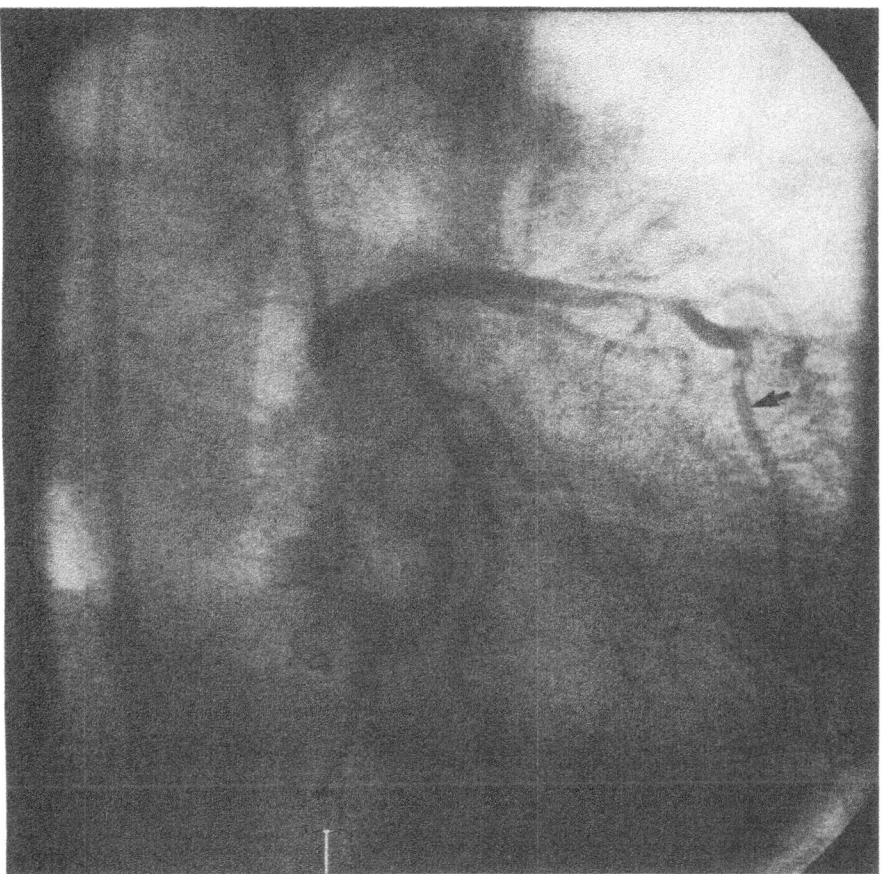

Figure 8. First angiographic control with guide wire still placed in the distal LAD showing complete filling of the LAD (arrows).

Determination of ventricular volumes, left ventricular ejection fraction and regional wall motion

In order to calculate left ventricular chamber volume the first step is to trace the left ventricular outline at the outermost margin. The aortic valve border is defined as a line connecting the inferior aspects of the sinuses. Calculation may be performed using biplane or single plane angiography. Biplane left ventricular angiography most often is performed in the 30° right anterior oblique (RAO) and 60° left anterior oblique (LAO) [24]. For mathematical calculation of ventricular volume the left ventricle can be approximated with considerably accuracy by an ellipsoid [7]. For use in single plane angiography the area-length ellipsoid method has been modified [9,12,17]. Images are

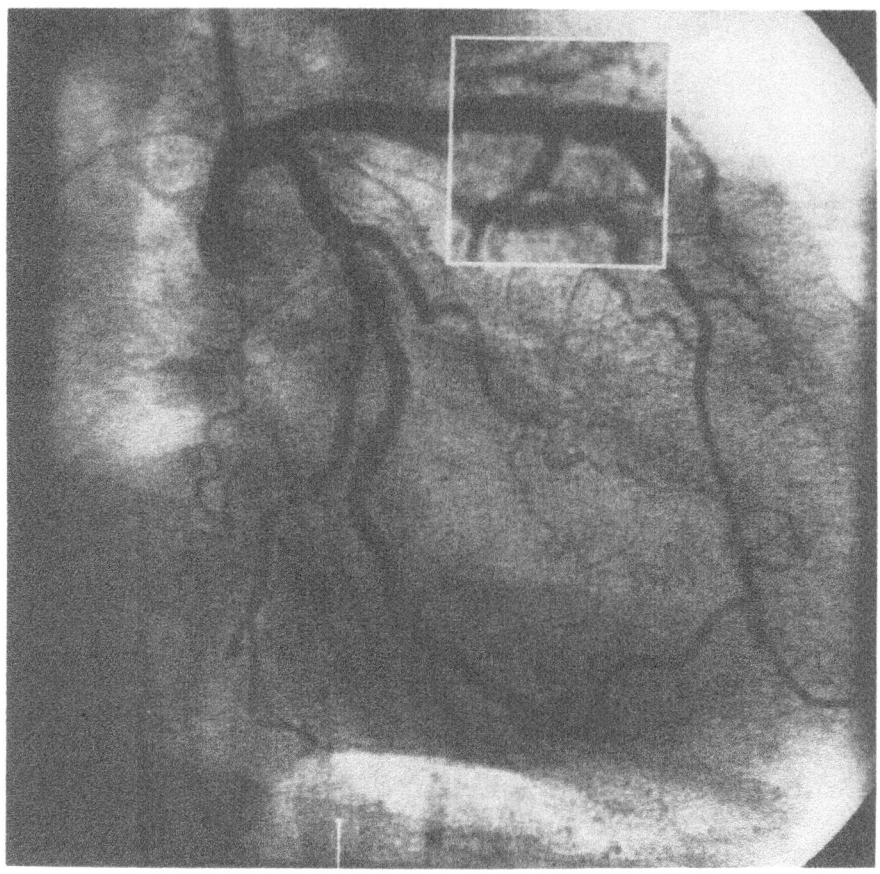

Figure 9.   Magnified result of the LAD-PTCA.

obtained in 30° RAO projection. Volumes determined by single plane technique tend to be significantly overestimated compared to biplane methods. Therefore special regression equations are performed.

The DCI system offers the potential for on-line quantification of left ventricular volume during the examination procedure. The program for calculation of left ventricular volume almost works automatically after calibration. The user determines the aortic valve border by connecting the inferior aspects of the sinuses valsalvae and marking the left ventricular apex on the TV monitor in enddiastolic and endsystolic frames. The computer automatically traces the ventricular borderline and offers the opportunity for observer interactive corrections. Endsystolic, enddiastolic left ventricular volumes, left ventricular ejection fraction and stroke volume are calculated (Figure 12). Furthermore the system allows for quantification of regional wall motion and centerline wall motion [4,14] (Figures 13, 14).

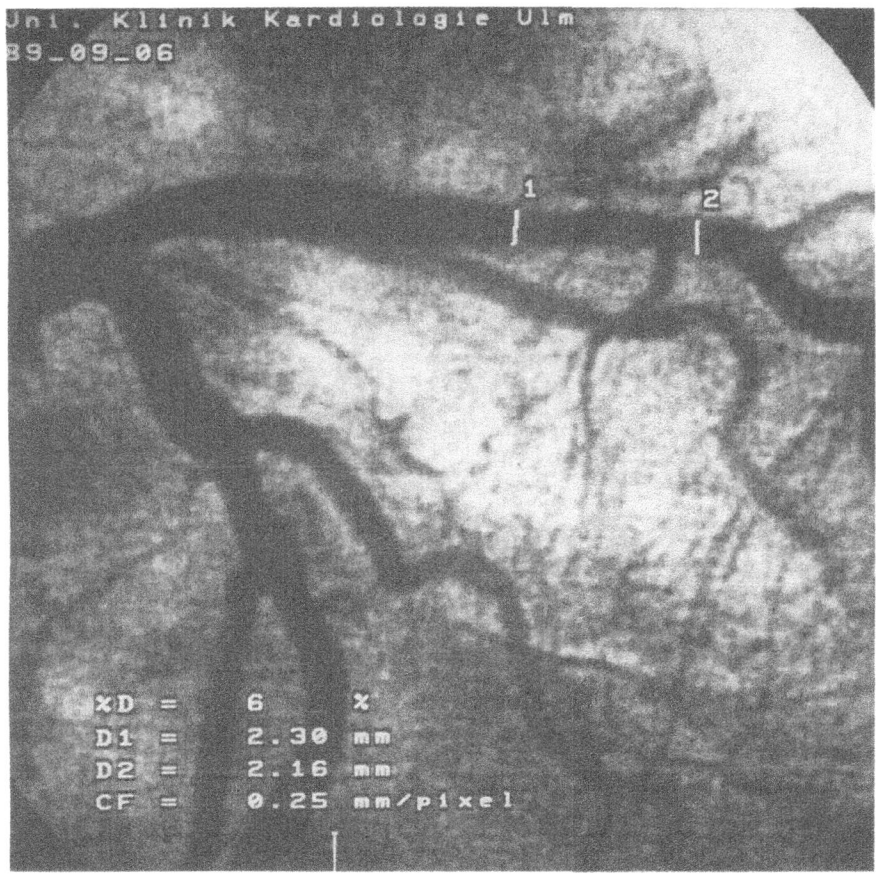

Figure 10. Determination of the residual LAD stenosis after PTCA indicating an excellent result in RAO view.

New techniques for the evaluation of coronary artery disease

Angiographic techniques have been improved during the past years to obtain sharper images of coronary lesions. Nevertheless angiography only provides for indirect visualization of vessel contours, but does not show the minute details of the coronary surface. Therefore several attempts have been made to directly visualize the coronary endothelial surface by percutaneous transluminal fiberoptic angioscopy (PTFA) [19]. Fiberoptic angioscopes with an external diameter from 0.5 to 1.8 mm are used. Images are relayed through a video coupler to a light-sensitive video camera and displayed on-line on a high-resolution video monitor [10]. Informations obtained from coronary angioscopy have shown that clinical coronary disease is caused by a cycle of events at the coronary endothelial surface. Atheroma

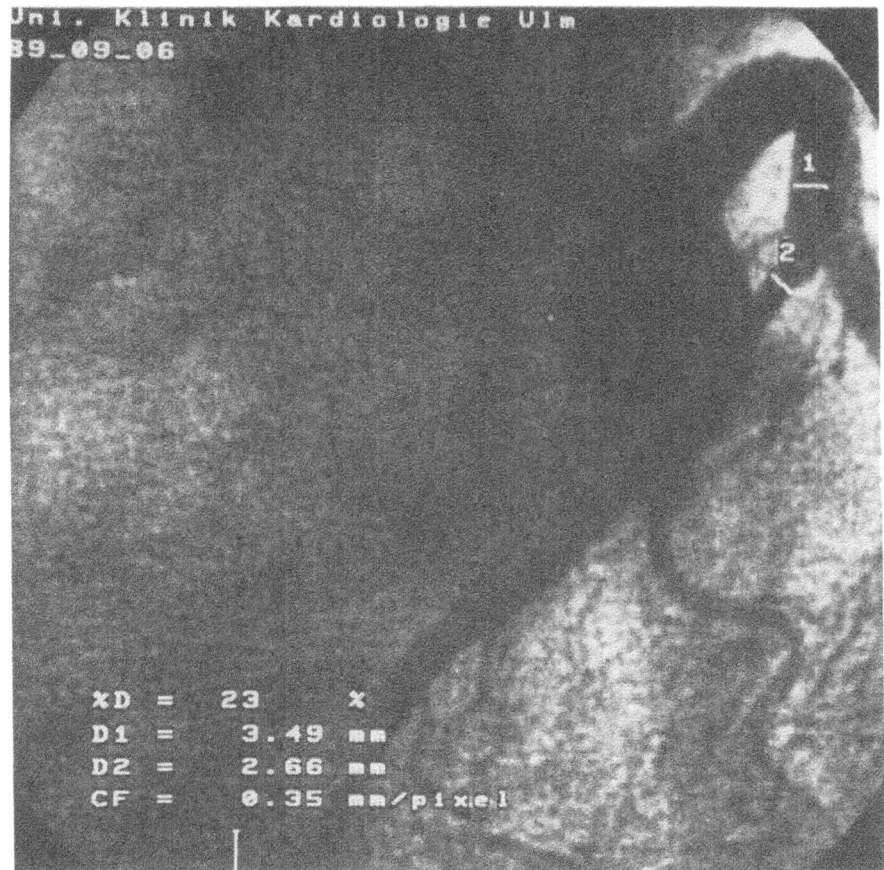

Figure 11.   23% residual LAD stenosis after PTCA in LAO view.

leads to coronary stenosis, a pre-existing atheroma may ulcerate and platelet aggregation leads to thrombus formation. The thrombus more or less occludes the coronary artery provoking unstable angina or myocardial infarction. After spontaneous or pharmacologically induced thrombolysis the coronary lesion heals until the next cycle begins.

Angiographic techniques with on-line computer processing of cardiac images will improve in the near future, offering excellent images of coronary arteries with immediate fully automatic determination of coronary lesions and left ventricular function. Further improvement of storage devices for digitized angiographic images may lead to a cine-film less catheterization laboratory in the future.

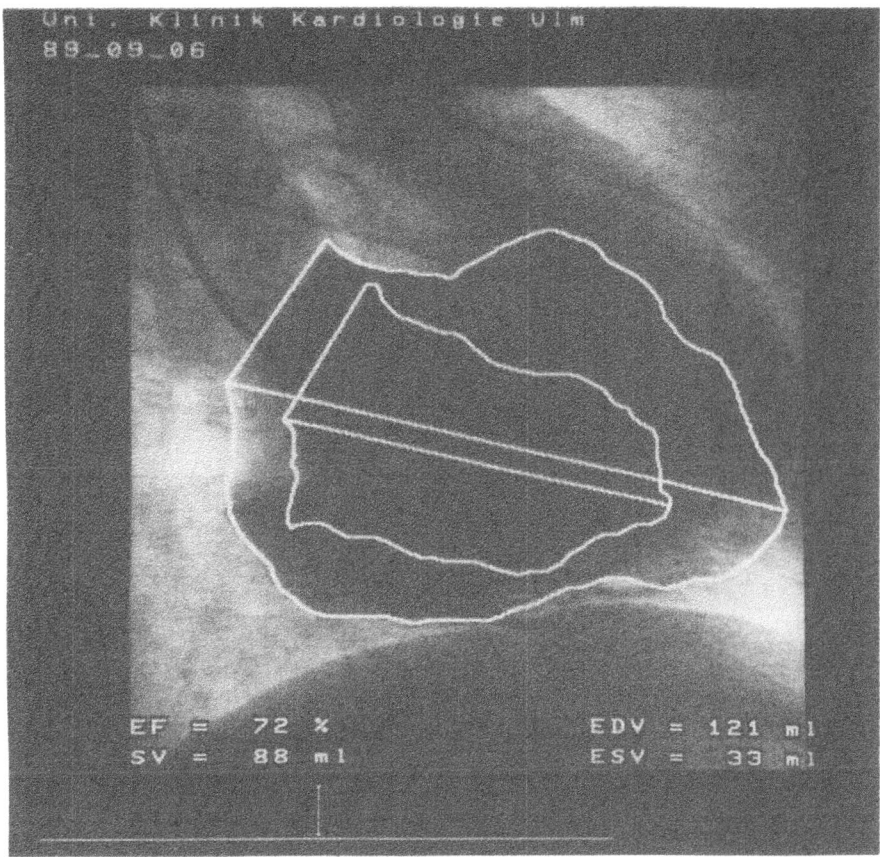

Figure 12. Determination of left ventricular endsystolic and enddiastolic volumes, stroke volume and ejection fraction using single plane angiography in RAO view.

References

1. Booth DC, Nissen SE, DeMaria AN (1986) The promise of digital cardiac angiography. *J Am Coll Cardiol* 8: 817.
2. Brown BG, Bolson E, Frimer M et al. (1977) Quantitative coronary arteriography: estimation of dimensions, hemodynamic resistance, and atheroma mass of coronary artery lesions using the arteriogram and digital computation. *Circulation* 55: 329.
3. Brown BG, Bolson EL, Dodge HT (1982) Arteriographic assessment of coronary atherosclerosis: review of current methods, their limitations, and clinical applications. *Arteriosclerosis* 2: 2.
4. Cole JS, Holland PA, Glaeser DH (1976) A semiautomated technique for the rapid evaluation of left ventricular regional wall motion. *Cathet Cardiovasc Diagn* 2: 185.

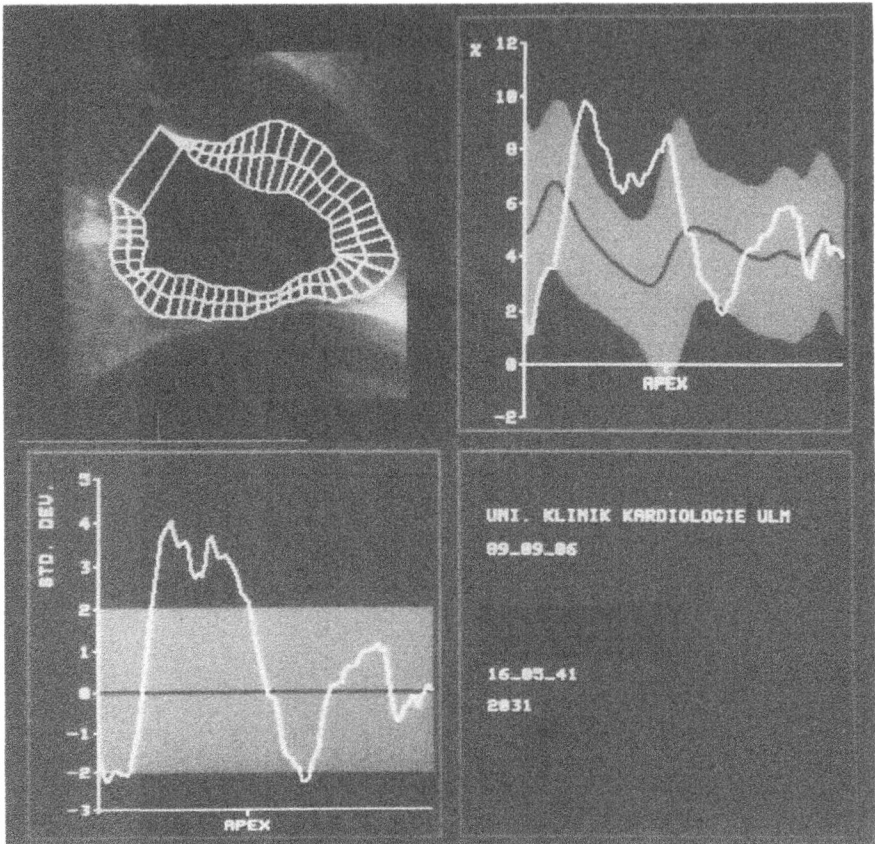

Figure 13.   Determination of left ventricular regional wall motion.

5. DeRouen TA, Murray JA, Owen W. (1977) Variability in the analysis of coronary arteriograms. *Circulation* 55: 324.
6. Detre KM, Wright E, Murphy ML et al. (1975) Observer agreement in evaluation coronary angiography. *Circulation* 52: 979.
7. Dodge HT, Sandler H, Ballew DW, Lord JD Jr (1960) The use of biplane angiocardiography for the measurement of left ventricular volume in man. *Am Heart J* 60: 762.
8. Gensini GG, Kelly AE, DaCosta BCB et al. (1971) Quantitative angiography: the measurement of coronary vasomobility in the intact animal and man. *Chest* 60: 522.
9. Greene DG, Carlisle R, Grant C, Bunnell IL (1967) Estimation of left ventricular volume by one-plane cineangiography. *Circulation* 35: 61.
10. Höher M, Hombach V, Höpp HW, Eggeling Th, Kochs M, Arnold G, Hannekum A, Hügel W (1988) Diagnostische Bedeutung der Angioskopie bei Patienten mit koronarer Herzkrankheit. *Z Kardiol* 77: 152.
11. Judkins MP (1967) Selective coronary arteriography: a percutaneous transfemoral technique. *Radiology* 89: 815.
12. Kennedy JW, Trenholme SE, Kasser IS (1970) Left ventricular volume and mass from single-plane cineangiocardiogram. A comparison of anteroposterior and right anterior oblique methods. *Am Heart J* 80: 343.

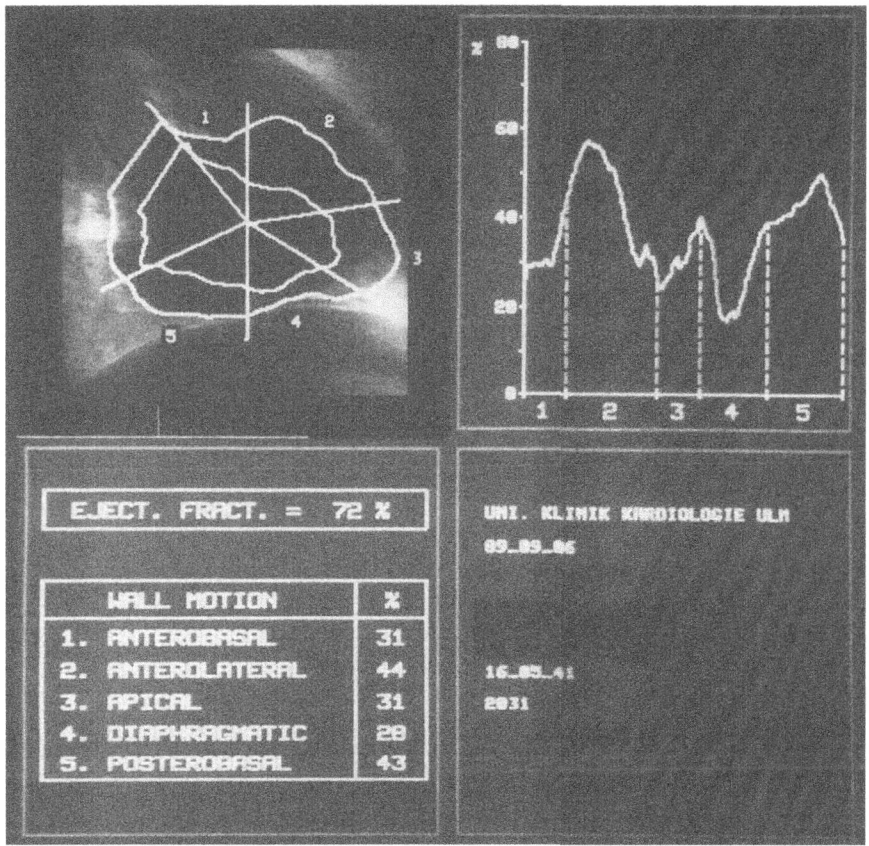

Figure 14. Determination of left ventricular wall motion using the centerline method.

13. Mates RE, Gupta ACB, Klocke FJ (1978) Fluid dynamics of coronary artery stenosis. *Circ Res* 42: 152.
14. Mathey DG, Sheehan FH, Schofer J, Dodge HT (1985) Time from onset of symptoms to throbolytic therapy: a major determinant of myocardial salvage in patients with acute transmural infarction. *J Am Coll Cardiol* 6: 518.
15. Reiber JHC, Serruys PW, Kooijman CJ et al. (1985) Assessment of short-, medium-, and long-term variations in arterial dimensions from computer-assisted quantitation of coronary cineangiograms. *Circulation* 71: 280.
16. Sanders WJ, Alderman EL, Harrison DC (1979) Coronary artery quantitation using digital image processing techniques. *IEEE Comput Cardiol* 7: 15.
17. Sandler H, Dodge HT (1968) The use of single plane angiocardiograms for the calculation of left ventricular volume in man. *Am Heart J* 75: 325.
18. Scoblionko DP, Brown BG, Mitten S et al. (1984) A new digital electronic caliper for measurement of coronary arterial stenosis: comparision with visual estimates and computer-assisted measurement. *Am J Cariol* 53: 689.
19. Sherman CT, Litvack R, Grundfest WS et al. (1986) Demonstration of thrombus and complex atheroma by in vivo angioscopy in patients with unstable angina pectoris. *N Engl J Med* 315: 913.

20. Sones FM, Shirley EK (1962) Cine coronary arteriography. *Mod Concepts CV Dis* 31: 735.
21. Tobis JM, Nalcioglu O, Henry WL (1983) Digital subtraction angiography. *Chest* 84: 68.
22. Tobis JM, Nalcioglu O, Iseri L et al. (1984) Detection and quantitation of coronary artery stenoses from digital subtraction angiograms compared with 35-millimeter film cineangiograms. *Am J Cardiol* 54: 489.
23. Vas R, Diamond GA, Foerster JS et al. (1982) Detection and assessment of severity of regional ischemic left ventricular dysfunction by digital fluoroscopy. *Am Heart J* 104: 732.
24. Wynne J et al. (1978) Estimation of left ventricular volumes in man from biplane cineangiograms filmed in oblique projections. *Am J Cardiol* 41: 726.

3. Balloon angioplasty for stable and unstable angina

J. MEYER, H.-J. RUPPRECHT, R. BRENNECKE,
M. KOTTMEYER, G. BERNHARD, R. ERBEL and T. POP

Introduction

In 1977 Andreas Grüntzig introduced percutaneous transluminal coronary angioplasty (PTCA) into the treatment of coronary artery stenoses [1]. He initially devoted his technique only to patients with stable angina pectoris. As early as 1978, however, Williams et al. [2] and our group [3] applied PTCA also to patients with unstable angina pectoris. Since then other groups have adopted the technique for unstable angina pectoris, verified the indication and contributed to the further success of the method [4–8].

In patients with unstable angina admitted to our hospital we always try to stabilize the situation under the conditions of the coronary care unit. Preferentially we schedule the coronary arteriography in cooperation with the cardiac surgeons, in order to perform both diagnostic arteriography and PTCA within the same cath-lab procedure. By this combined diagnostic-therapeutic approach we save time, avoid a second exposure of the patient to the cath-lab situation, save contrast material and other expenses, and we also lower the cost for personnel.

Methods

All patients with unstable angina had experienced either worsening in frequency, severity or duration of episodes of chest pain or presented with recent onset angina or pain at rest within the last two months. In all patients transient changes of the ST-segment and/or T-waves were documented. PTCA was performed in these patients after initial medical treatment including intravenous nitrates, beta blockers, calcium antagonists, acetylsalicylic acid, and intravenous heparin. Acute myocardial infarction was excluded by serial electrocardiograms and enzyme evaluations. Patients with left main stem stenosis and those with severe diffuse disease were not considered for PTCA. In patients with multivessel disease only the most severe lesion or in case of ST-segment changes the ischemia related lesions

25

V. Hombach et al. (eds), Interventional Techniques in Cardiovascular Medicine, 25–36.

were dilated initially. Further stenoses were taken care of in a later session. Informed consent was obtained in all patients. During the procedure a surgical team was always available in case of need. All patients received three times 20 mg nifedipine and 500 mg aspirin the day before the procedure. During the procedure, intravenous heparin in a dosage of 10,000–15,000 units as well as a continuous drip of low-molecular weight dextran was given. A Swan-Ganz-catheter was placed into the pulmonary artery. Immediately after the procedure, heparin (3000 units) and nitroglycerin (0.2 mg) was injected into the diseased coronary artery to prevent thrombus formation and coronary spasm. Control angiography was performed in multiple projections to confirm the result.

The angioplasty procedure was considered successful when it resulted in at least a 20% reduction of luminal diameter narrowing and luminal diameter narrowing of less than 50% without the patient undergoing major complications (death, myocardial infarction, emergency CABG). After the PTCA procedure, the femoral sheath was left in the groin and removed after 24 hours. During this period, all patients were on intravenous heparin. The patients were usually discharged three days after the procedure. They continued to receive treatment with nife dipine (60 mg daily) and aspirin (500 mg daily) for six months. Control arteriography was routinely recom-

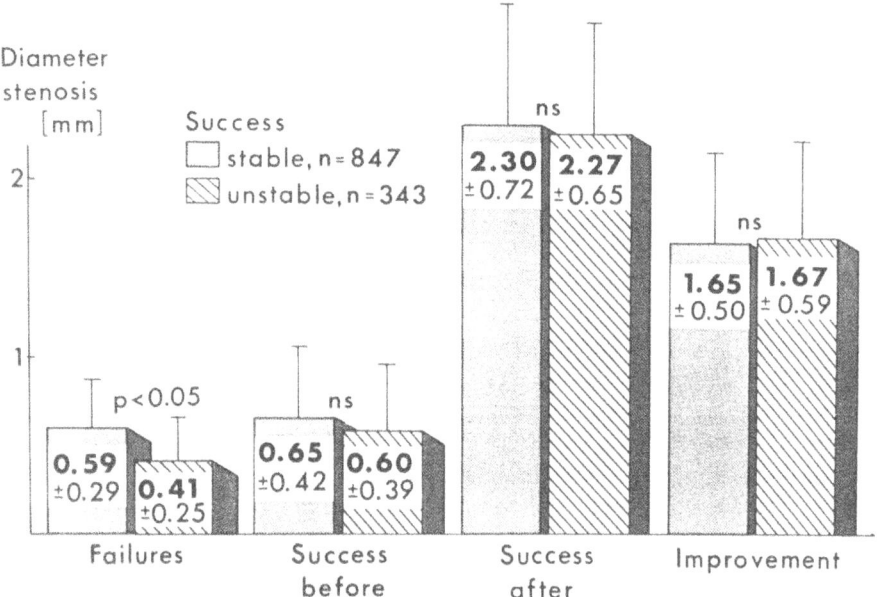

Figure 1.   Success rate of first dilatation in stable and unstable angina pectoris. Mainz 1982–1988. Comparison of the successful and the unsuccessful procedures.

mended and if indicated a second PTCA was performed six months after the initial PTCA procedure.

Early results

In the years 1978–1984 only balloons with a fixed guide wire at the tip of the balloon catheter were available. In those days the immediate results were not quite satisfying. By the advent of the steerable guide wires and the low-profile balloons the success rate rose and the complication rate dropped remarkably. Figure 1 shows the immediate results of dilatation in stable and unstable angina pectoris in the period 1982–1988. These numbers include those patients, in whom between 1982–1984 the old, very rigid catheter and balloon material was used.

In those patients, where we were not able to cross the lesion and inflate the balloon (failures) the stenosis diameter was remarkably lower than in those, where the PTCA procedure was successful. In successful and in unsuccessful procedures the residual vessel lumen in patients with unstable angina was smaller than in patients with the stable form. After successful dilatation the vessels could be enlarged to more than 2 mm. There was no significant difference between stable and unstable angina. The improvement of the vessel diameter was 1.65 mm in the average.

Complication rate

During the whole period of our experience between 1978–1988 we have treated a total of 1840 patients, 534 of them had unstable and 1306 stable angina pectoris. The number of serious events (death, emergency bypass operation and infarction) were 6% in the unstable and 1.5% in the stable form.

During the years 1986–1988 the numbers were in the same range (Table 1). Despite optimal medical treatment and very careful handling of the balloon material during the procedure, the complication rate in patients with

Table 1. Major PTCA complications. Time interval 1986–1988 (n = 1026)

Stable angina n = 733		Unstable angina n = 293
∅	Death	1 (0.3%)
6 (0.8%)	Emergency Op.	12 (4.1%)
4 (0.5%)	Infarction	5 (1.7%)
10 (1.4%)	Major events	18 (6.1%)
p < 0.01		

unstable angina is significantly higher than in those with the stable form (p
< 0.01)

Late results

A total of 685 patients with initially successful PTCA procedure had a
control coronary arteriography six months later (Figure 2). There were no
significant differences with respect to the lumen diameter before PTCA.
Immediately after the procedure patients with the unstable form had a
slightly but not significant smaller vessel lumen. At the six months follow up
in both diseased groups the treated coronary segment showed a remarkable
narrowing. In patients with initially stable angina, the vessel was significantly smaller than in those with the stable form (p < 0.05).

Since we knew the increased risk and the lower success rate of the
procedure and also the high recurrence rate of the stenoses, we performed a
long term follow up of our patients. In a consecutive series of patients we
followed not only those with successful PTCA but also those with a failed
procedure.

Patients and methods

Between January 1983 and June 1985 257 patients with stable angina and
147 patients with unstable underwent PTCA at our clinic. Since one patient
of each group was lost to follow up 256 versus 146 patients could be
followed over a long range. Information on long term outcome was obtained

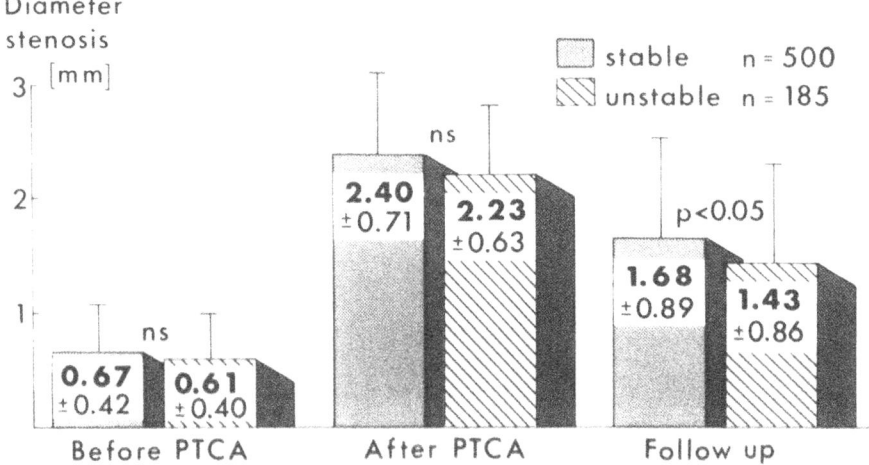

Figure 2.   Follow up control of successful PTCA procedures after six months in stable and
unstable angina pectoris (first dilatation procedure).

Table 2. Baseline characteristics of the long term follow up of patients treated between I/1983 and VI/1985

	Stable n = 256	Unstable n = 146 patients	
Mean age (yr)	51.0 ± 7.8	53.1 ± 8.7	ns
Sex (male)	219 (86%)	110 (75%)	$p < 0.05$
Risk factors			
History of smoking	198 (77%)	91 (62%)	$p < 0.01$
Hypertension	92 (36%)	69 (47%)	$p < 0.05$
Diabetes	28 (11%)	14 (10%)	ns
Hyperlipoproteinemia	106 (41%)	48 (33%)	ns
History of MI	83 (32%)	36 (25%)	ns
History of CABG	3 (1.2%)	2 (1.4%)	ns
Angina class (CCS)			
I	39 (15%)	—	
II	124 (48%)	—	
III	57 (22%)	45 (31%)	$p < 0.01$
IV	36 (14%)	101 (69%)	

MI (myocardial infarction); CCS (Canadian Cardiovascular Society).

by questionnaires and telephone interviews with the patient or his treating physician (Table 2).

The two groups with stable and unstable angina pectoris were comparable with respect to most baseline characteristics. The unstable group, however, contained a significantly higher percentage of females and hypertensive patients ($p < 0.05$), while smoking ($p < 0.01$) and history of acute myocardial infarction (ns) was more frequent in the stable group. As expected, patients with unstable angina were more symptomatic according to the classification of the Canadian Cardiovascular Society.

Coronary lesion

The location of coronary artery disease was similar in both groups. The majority of the stenoses were located in the LAD. The stenoses in the midportion of the vessels were more frequent than the proximal ones. Only a few patients showed a relatively distal stenosis (Table 3).

Before and after the procedure the mean diameter of the coronary stenosis between stable and unstable angina were not significantly different. Also the success rate was comparable. The relatively low success rate has to be contributed to the group of patients treated between 1982 and 1984, when the steerable guide wires and the low profile balloon were not yet available. In 1989 the success rates in both groups are 92%.

Control angiography was performed at the mean of six months in 75% of the lesions in the stable and in 70% of the lesions in the unstable group (ns). The restenosis rate was higher in the unstable cohort. The differences,

Table 3. Localisation and geometry of coronary lesions

	Stable n = 281	Unstable n = 162 lesions	
Dilated lesion			
LAD	174 (62%)	106 (66%)	
LCX	40 (14%)	25 (15%)	ns
RCA	67 (24%)	31 (19%)	
proximal	112 (40%)	61 (38%)	
mid	141 (50%)	86 (53%)	ns
distal	28 (10%)	15 (9%)	
Eccentric	156 (56%)	85 (52%)	ns

however, were not significant in this series. In the larger group of 685 patients (Figure 2) without complete follow up we were able to show significant differences between stable and unstable angina with respect to the relapse rate after six months. In the group of stable (n = 500) the restenosis rate was 28.2%, compared to 39.5% in 185 patients with unstable angina (p < 0.01).

Acute complication rate

Three patients (1.2%) in the stable angina and five patients in the unstable angina (3.4%) sufferend an acute myocardial infarction. There were two immediate bypass operations (0.8%) in the stable and two (1.4%) in the

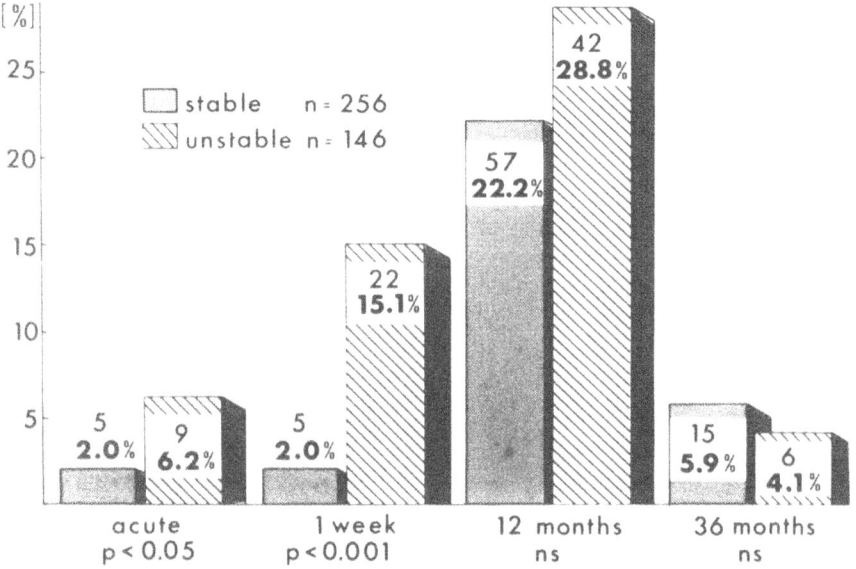

Figure 3. Time course of serious events after attempted PTCA. Comparison between stable and unstable angina.

unstable group. While in the unstable angina group two patients (1.4%) died immediately, there was no lethal outcome in the stable group. The total number of acute serious events were 2% in the stable and 6.2% in the unstable group (p < 0.05) (Figure 3).

Early follow up within one week

During the first week following the PTCA procedure an acute myocardial infarction occurred in three patients (1.2%) of the stable and eight patients (5.5%) of the unstable group. There was one bypass operation (0.5%) in the stable compared to 12 operations (8.2%) in the unstable group (p < 0.01). No patient died in the stable compared to two patients (1.4%) in the unstable group. The total number of serious events was five (2.0%) in the stable and 22 (15.1%) (p < 0.01) in the unstable group. (Figure 3).

Follow up within 12 months

Within the next 12 months another two patients (0.8%) died in the stable group (14th day and 10th month), three patients (1.2%) suffered from acute myocardial infarction, while a bypass graft was performed in 25 patients (9.8% and Re-PTCA in 27 patients (19.8%).

In the unstable group six patients (4.1%) died. Four patients (2.7%) developed an acute myocardial infarction and eight patients (5.5%) underwent surgery. The total number of serious events is outlined in Figure 4.

Mainly due to the results of the routinely scheduled control angiography six months later after PTCA, a second PTCA was performed in 27 patients (10.5%) of the stable group, compared to 24 patients (16.4%) in the

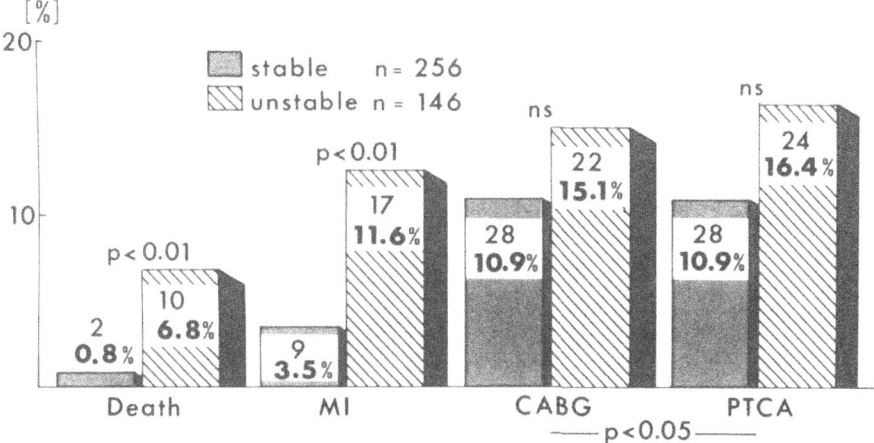

Figure 4.   Rate of serious events within 12 months after attempted PTCA procedure in stable and unstable agina.

unstable group. The overall event rate amounted to 57 (22.2%) in the stable and to 42 (28.8%) in the unstable group (ns).

Long term follow up within 36 months

Within the long term follow between the 12th up to the 36th month nine additional patients (3.5%) died in the stable group, one of them due to gastric cancer, the other from cardiac reasons. One patient (0.4%) suffered from acute myocardial infarction, while bypass surgery was performed in five patients (2%). In the unstable group three additional patients (2.1%) died, two patients (1.4%) had a new myocardial infarction and one (0.7%) underwent bypass surgery. During this long term interval, the total rate of cardiac events was 5.9% in the stable compared to 4.1% in the unstable group (ns).

During the whole period between the PTCA attempt and the 36th month the mortality rate in the stable group was higher during the late phase, whereas most of the lethal outcomes of the unstable group occurred within the first year after PTCA (Figure 3,5). A significantly higher percentage of patients suffered an acute myocardial infarction in the unstable group mainly within the first week after PTCA (19 patients (13.0%) compared to 10 patients (3.9%) (p. < 0.01)). The rate of bypass surgery was slightly higher in the unstable group. Most of the surgical procedures were performed within the first week following PTCA in the unstable group because of still persisting coronary symptoms.

Eventfree survivals

Survival without myocardial infarction, bypass surgery or repeat PTCA is outlined in Figure 6. The difference between the stable and the unstable

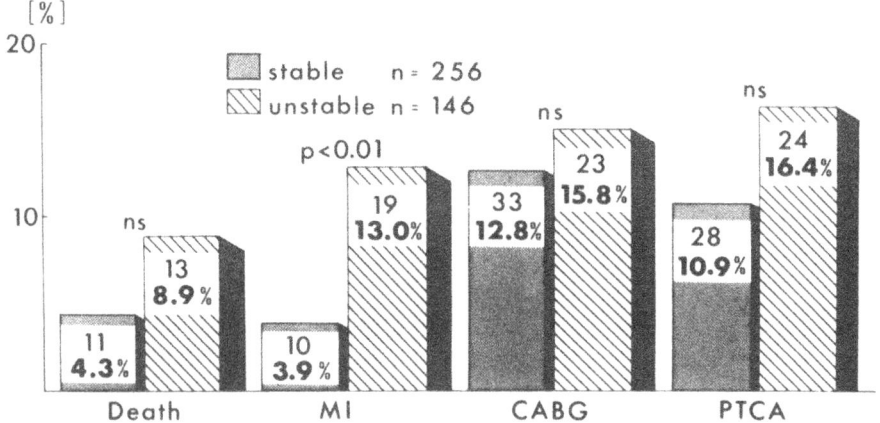

Figure 5.   Total event rate within 36 months after attempted PTCA procedure.

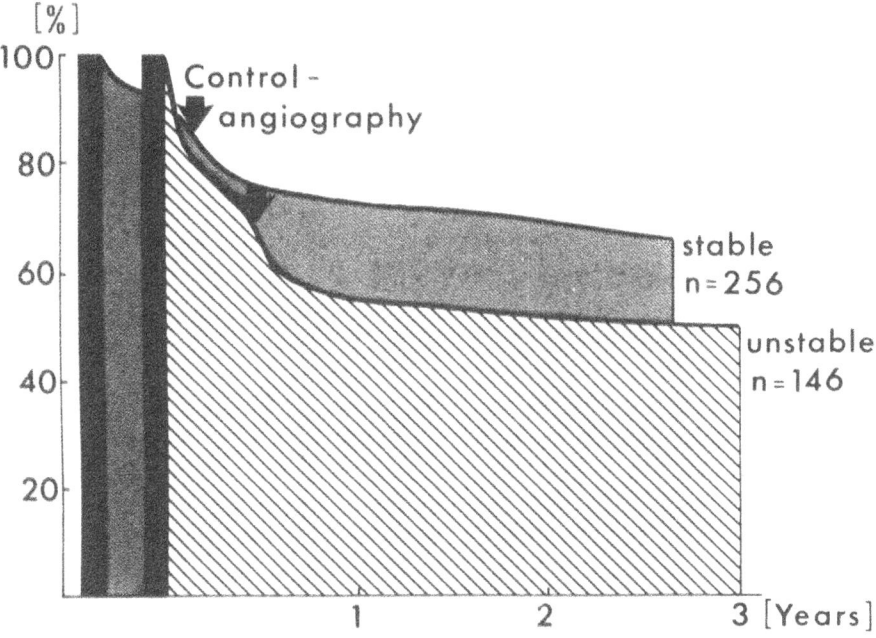

Figure 6. Eventfree survival curve after attempted PTCA in stable and unstable angina. Scheduled control angiography after six months.

patients occurs mainly within the first week after PTCA. A marked decline of the curve in both groups can be seen after six months, because of the high rate of re-PTCA at the time of the scheduled control angiography.

Quality of life

Quality of life was assessed in 240 surviving patients with former stable angina and 131 patients with primarily the unstable form (Table 4). Of the patients with previously stable angina 74% were asymptomatic compared to only 62% of the former unstable angina. Compared to the anginal class

Table 4. Quality of life: symptoms at the control questionnaire after 36 months (Canadian Cardiovascular Society Classification/CCS)

CCS	Stable angina n = 240	Unstable angina n = 131 patients
I	177 (74%)	81 (62%)[a]
II	40 (17%)	30 (23%)
III	13 (5%)	9 (7%)
Iv	10 (4%)	11 (8%)

[a]*p < 0.05

Table 5. Current medical treatment three years after PTCA

	Stable angina n = 240	Unstable angina n = 131
No antianginal therapy	105 (44%)	38 (29%) p < 0.01
Nitrates or β-blockers		
or Ca-Antagonists	96 (40%)	50 (38%)
Two substances	28 (12%)	39 (30%)
Three substances	11 (4%)	4 (3%)
Coumadine	11 (5%)	7 (5%)
Aspirin	75 (31%)	39 (30%)

before the PTCA procedure especially those in the unstable group had experienced an improvement of at least one class of the CCS classification.

Despite sometimes remarkably good angiographical results many patients were still on anginal treatment given by their home physician. On the other hand the rate of those patients taking anticoagulants and antiplatelet therapy was quite low and not different between both groups. Current medical treatment three years after PTCA is outlined in Table 5.

Discussion

Despite aggressive treatment with nitrates, beta-blockers, calcium antagonists, heparin, and acetylsalicylic acid many patients with unstable angina cannot be stabilized for a longer period of time [9, 10]. Therefore, early bypass surgery or PTCA is indicated in many of them. The initial angiographical result is not different between patients with stable and unstable angina. The complication rate, however, is higher in the unstable form. This is caused by mostly broken endothelium of the coronary vessel, where thrombotic material has the tendency to occlude the vessel [11–13]. Additional factors like elevated vasomotor tone and coronary spasm contribute to the unfavourable results [14–16]. PTCA in unstable angina has therefore to be considered as a method of higher risk. The standby of a cardiac surgeon is definitely necessary. In case of an artificial occlusion of the vessel these patients mostly show a very rapid deterioration. The collateral circulation is regularly much less developed than in patients with the stable form.

The higher complication rate in unstable angina has also been confirmed by Faxon et al. [4]. This joint study reported a higher in-hospital-mortality in those patients. The significantly enhanced rate of severe cardiac events during the first week following PTCA is caused by the complex unstable situation. The patients have a higher incidence to develop myocardial infarction so that urgent bypass surgery because of persistent ischemic symptoms is often indicated. Even if pharmacological studies have shown that some patients can be stabilized in the acute phase [9, 10], approximately 10% of patients ultimately receive bypass surgery (5, 7, 8, 15, 17].

The high event rate during the 12 months follow up in stable and unstable angina is mainly explained by a considerable number of repeat angioplasties or definite bypass graft operations, following the routine control six months after the initial procedure. The cumulative event rate is also higher in unstable than in the stable form [5, 7, 8]. Different results by the NHLBI-series may be caused by different criteria of instability and lack of ECG-criteria in this study [4].

The data show that PTCA can be performed in patients with unstable angina with a slightly lower success rate but a significantly higher rate of acute complications and cardiac events within the early follow up period.

The same group, however, has also a higher complication rate, when treated medically or with bypass surgery. In the long run those patients seem to have a poorer quality of life with respect to ischemic symptoms and current medical treatment. The cross-over rate to surgical treatment seems to be less pronounced after PTCA. To further clarify the role of PTCA in the management of unstable angina large randomized trials are needed to compare currently available PTCA techniques with advanced cardiovascular surgery and optimal medical treatment including fibrinolysis.

References

1. Grüntzig AR, Senning A, Siegenthaler WE (1979) Non-operative dilatation of coronary-artery stenosis: percutaneous transluminal coronary angioplasty. *N Engl J Med* 301: 61–67.
2. Williams DO, Riley RS, Singh AK, Gewirtz H, Most AS (1981) Evaluation of the role of coronary angioplasty in patients with unstable angina pectoris. *Am Heart J* 102: 1–9.
3. Meyer J, Böcker B, Erbel R, Bardos P, Messmer BJ, Effert S (1980) Treatment of unstable angina with percutaneous transluminal coronary angioplasty. *Circulation* 62: III-160.
4. Faxon DP, Detre KM, McGabe CH et al. (1983) Role of percutaneous transluminal coronary angioplasty in the treatment of unstable angina: report from the National Heart, Lung, and Blood Institute Percutaneous Transluminal Coronary Angioplasty and Coronary Artery Surgery Study Registries. *Am J Cardiol* 53: (12) 131C–135C.
5. De Feyter PJ, Serruys PW, van den Brand M, Soward AL, Hugenholtz PG (1985) Percutaneous transluminal coronary angioplasty in unstable angina pectoris: The Rotterdam Experience, in: Hugenholtz PG, Goldman BS (eds), *Unstable Angina—Current Concepts and Management*, pp. 229–237. New York: Schattauer Stuttgart.
6. Meyer J, Schmitz H, Erbel R, Kiesslich T, Böcker-Josephs B, Krebs W, Braun PC, Bardos P, Minale C, Messmer BJ, Effert S (1981) Treatment of unstable angina pectoris with percutaneous transluminal coronary angioplasty. *Cathet Cardiovasc Diagn* 7: 361.
7. Meyer J, Schmitz HJ, Kiesslich T, Erbel R, Krebs W, Schulz W, Bardos P, Minale C, Messmer PJ, Effert S (1983) Percutaneous transluminal coronary angioplasty in patients with stable and unstable angina pectoris. Analysis of early and late results. *Am Heart J* 106: 973.
8. Rupprecht HJ, Erbel R, Brennecke R, Pop T, Jung D, Kottmeyer M, Hering R, Meyer J (1988) Aktuelle Komplikations rate der perkutanen transluminalen Koronarangioplastie bei stabiler und unstabiler Angina. *Dtsch Med Wschr* 113: 409–413.

9. Lewis HD, Davis JW, Archibald DG et al. (1983) Protective effects of aspirin against acute myocardial infarction and death in men with unstable angina. *N Eng J Med* 309: 396–403.
10. Müller JE, Zoltan ZG, Pearle DL et al. (1984) Nifedipine and conventional therapy for unstable angina pectoris: a randomized, double-blind comparison. *Circulation* 69: 728–739.
11. Falk E (1985) Unstable angina with fatal outcome: dynamic coronary thrombosis leading to infarction and/or sudden death. *Circulation* 71: 699–708.
12. Davies MJ, Thomas AC (1985) Plaque fissuring—the cause of acute myocardial infarction, sudden ischemic death and crescendo angina. *Br Heart J* 53: 363–373.
13. Fitzgerald DJ, Roy L, Catelle F, Fitzgerald GA (1986) Platelet activation in unstable coronary disease. *New Engl J Med* 315: 913.
14. Epstein SE, Talbot TL (1981) Dynamic coronary tone in precipitation, exacerbation and relief of angina pectoris. *Am J Cardiol* 48: 797–803.
15. Maseri A, L'Abbate A, Baroldi G et al. (1978) Coronary vasospasm as a possible cause of myocardial infarction: a conclusion derived from the study of 'preinfarction' angina. *N Engl J Med* 299: 1271–1277.
16. Serruys PW, Steward R, Booman F, Michels R, Reiber JHC, Hugenholtz PG (1980) Can unstable angina pectoris be due to increased coronary vasomotor tone? *Eur Heart J* 1: B71–85.
17. Mulcahy R (1985) Natural history and prognosis of unstable angina. *Am Heart J* 109: 753–759.

4. Radiofrequency coronary angioplasty

V. HOMBACH, M. HÖHER, M. KOCHS, T. EGGELING, W.
HAERER, S. WIESHAMMER, A. SCHMIDT, H. W. HÖPP and
H. H. HILGER

Introduction

In 1977 Andreas Grüntzig performed the first balloon angioplasty in a
patient with a critical LAD stenosis [5]. Since that time considerable
improvements have been achieved both with the technique itself (steerable
guide wires, low profile and super low profile balloons with steerable or
fixed guide wires, monorail technique etc.) and the skills of the angio-
plasters. Therefore balloon angioplasty in the 1990s has become a standard
technique for reduction of significant coronary artery stenoses in patients
with coronary heart disease [1,5,9,14]. The acute and longterm results of
balloon angioplasty now seem to be standardized worldwide: acute success
rate: 80–90%, depending on the coronary artery to be treated and the type
of coronary artery lesion; rate of acute complications: about 10%, and that
of emergency bypass: 2–5% [1,2], recurrency rate at 3 months: 15–30%,
and at 6 months post-treatment about 40–50%.

Acute complications and recurrency rates [6] may be due to traumatization
of the vessel intima by balloon inflation, which among other factors may
cause the release of platelet aggregatory and coronary vasoconstrictor sub-
stances, as well as of proliferatory factors, that may result in growing of the
atheromata at the site of foregoing angioplasty. Moreover, with balloon
angioplasty the atheromatous material will be redistributed rather than
removed or condensed, as could be achieved by atherectomy or thermal
angioplasty. Therefore alternative methods of coronary angioplasty have
been designed or are under development, among which radiofrequency
angioplasty [7,8] and laser angioplasty [3,10–13] seem to be the most
effective and attractive methods for condensing or ablating atherosclerotic
plaques. Based on experiments with radiofrequency thermal recanalization
of thrombotically occluded arteries in domestic pigs [7] we have designed a
new catheter system for application of radiofrequency angioplasty in patients
with significant coronary artery stenoses.

37

V. Hombach et al. (eds), Interventional Techniques in Cardiovascular Medicine, 37–46.
© 1991 *Kluwer Academic Publishers.*

Methods

The high frequency electrical AC current is generated and released by the HAT 100 (Dr. Osypka GmbH, Grenzach-Wyhlen, FRG), the radiofrequency current is about 600 kHz, and the maximal energy delivered is 50 watts. In case of light arc production the frequency generator is automatically cut off by a special electronic circuitry (Figure 1).

The radiofrequency current is delivered to a specially designed RFCA-catheter, which either consists of a flexible helical wire similar to that used for pacemaker electrodes, or of a single thin straight wire, that is connected to a an electrode ring at the tip. The tip is formed like an olive with a conical shape at the distal end (Figure 2). The wire is coated by polyurethane tubing and the tip with ceramic coating so that the radiofrequency AC current is delivered perpendicularly to the front line of the tip. This prevents the vessel wall from local thermal damage due to radial energy delivery and heating, and therefore minimizes the risk of vessel wall perforation. The last goal is supported by the use of a conventional teflon coated guide wire, which can be advanced through the lumen of the RFCA-catheter, and placed distally to the targeted lesion, and thus, will stabilize the catheter tip within the central part of the vessel lumen (over-the-wire technique). The radiofrequency current is released via the monopolar tip electrode by forming the highest density of the electrical field in front of the atheromatous

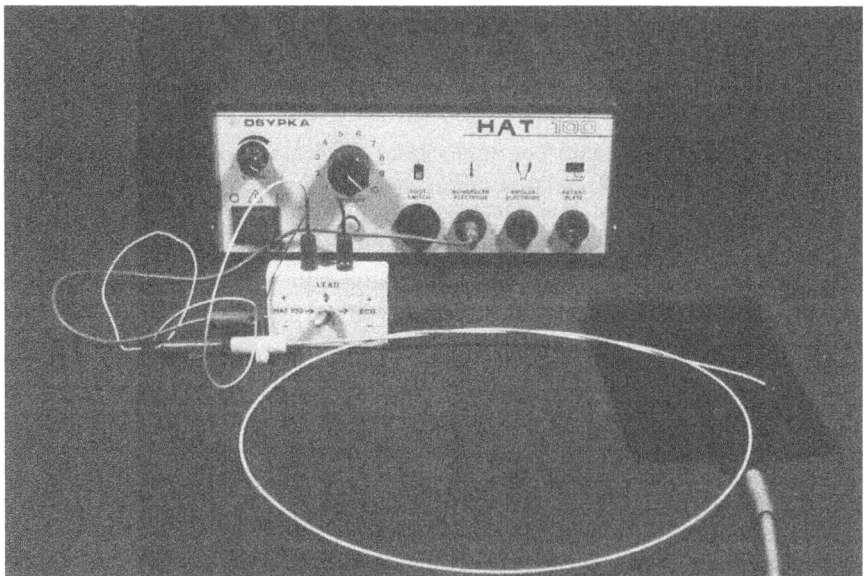

Figure 1.   Radiofrequency equipment used for radiofrequency coronary angioplasty (RFCA), which consists of the radiofrequency generator, the different electrode for delivery of radio-frequency AC-current, and the indifferent plate electrode placed in the back of the patient.

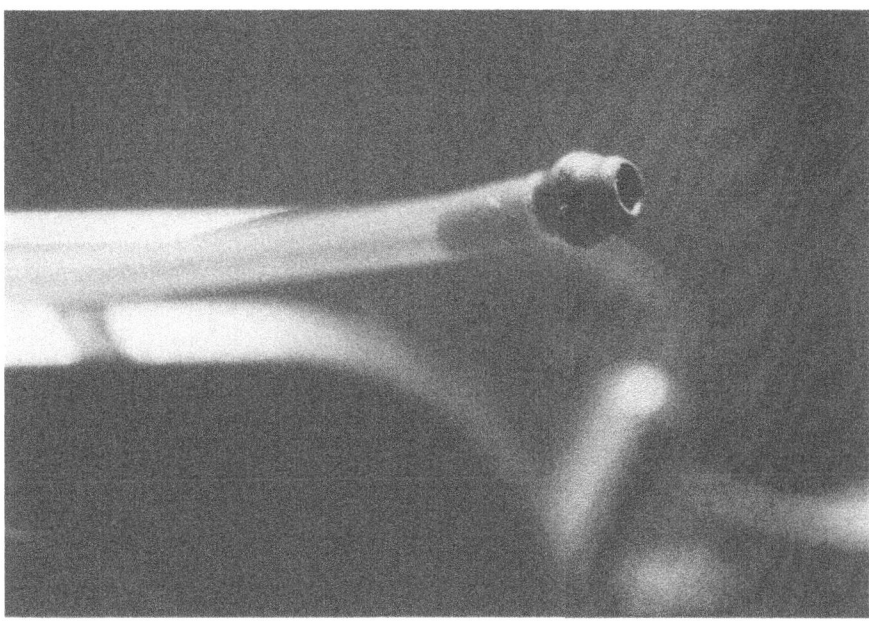

Figure 2. Most recent type of RFCA-catheter (tip). Note the conical shape of the olive-like tip, the different electrode for delivery of the RF-current just ahead the largest outer diameter of the tip, and the inner lumen for the flexible guide wire.

tissue, and running through the surrounding tissue to the indifferent plate electrode located on the back of the patient.

The angioplasty procedure is performed in the following manner. Following control coronary angiography the steerable guide wire is advanced over the stenotic part of the coronary artery and placed distally to the targeted lesion. Thereafter the RFCA-catheter is advanced over the guide wire, until the tip of the catheter faces the lesion to be treated. Then the radiofrequency current is delivered for a short period of 1–2 s, the catheter is slowly advanced over the stenotic area, and the radiofrequency current switched-off, when the tip of the catheter has passed the lesion. Then the RFCA-catheter is withdrawn to a position proximal to the lesion, a control coronary angiogram is performed, and the angioplasty procedure repeated if necessary. If there is resistance to advancing the catheter smoothly, the delivery of the radiofrequency current is immediately stopped in order to avoid vessel perforation. Following repeat angiography with a good anatomical result the catheter plus guide wire is withdrawn and a final coronary angiogram is taken. Pre- and post-angioplasty medication is identical to that used in patients undergoing balloon angioplasty (aspirin: 100–500 mg, nifedipine 20–30 mg, and long-acting nitrate 40–50 mg per day).

Patients

A total of 23 patients with coronary artery disease were treated by RFCA. Among those were 4 females and 19 males with ages from 35 to 77 years (Table 1). Most of these patients were suffering from stable angina pectoris due to hemodynamically significant coronary artery stenoses, and only a few had post-infarction angina. About ⅔ of the patients had a single vessel disease, 7 double and 2 triple vessel disease. The following stenotic arteries were treated: LAD: 11 patients, RCA: 5 patients, CFx: 6 patients, and a large first diagonal branch of the LAD: 1 patient.

Table 1. Clinical and angiographic data of the total group of patients treated with RFCA

Patients with CHD (males 19, females 4, age 35–77ys)	23
Stable angina	18
Unstable angina	1
Post-MI-angina	4
Single vessel disease	14
Double vessel disease	7
Triple vessel disease	2
Location: LAD	11
RCA	5
CFX	6
Diagonal	1

Abbreviations: CHD = coronary heart disease, ys = years, MI = myocardial infarction, LAD = left anterior descendent artery, RCA = right coronary artery, CFX = left circumflex artery, RFCA = radiofrequency coronary angioplasty.

In 18 patients angioplasty was performed first time, in 3 patients for repeat angioplasty, and in 2 patients a third angioplasty had to be performed because of re-restenosis. In 9 patients RFCA was solely applied, in another 10 patients followed by balloon angioplasty, and in 2 patients balloon angioplasty was performed first followed by RFCA because of a non-satisfactory primary result.

Results

In 14/23 patients (61%) a successful result with a reduction of diameter stenosis of equal or more than 20% (initial definition of success rate, given by Grüntzig) was achieved by RFCA alone (Figure 3). In the 14 patients with a success of RFCA, the per cent area stenosis was reduced from 93.8 +/− 2.9 % to 57.9 +/− 12.5 % as a mean, and to further 51.3 +/− 24.2 % by final PTCA. In the group with unsuccessful RFCA the per cent area

Radiofrequency Coronary Angioplasty

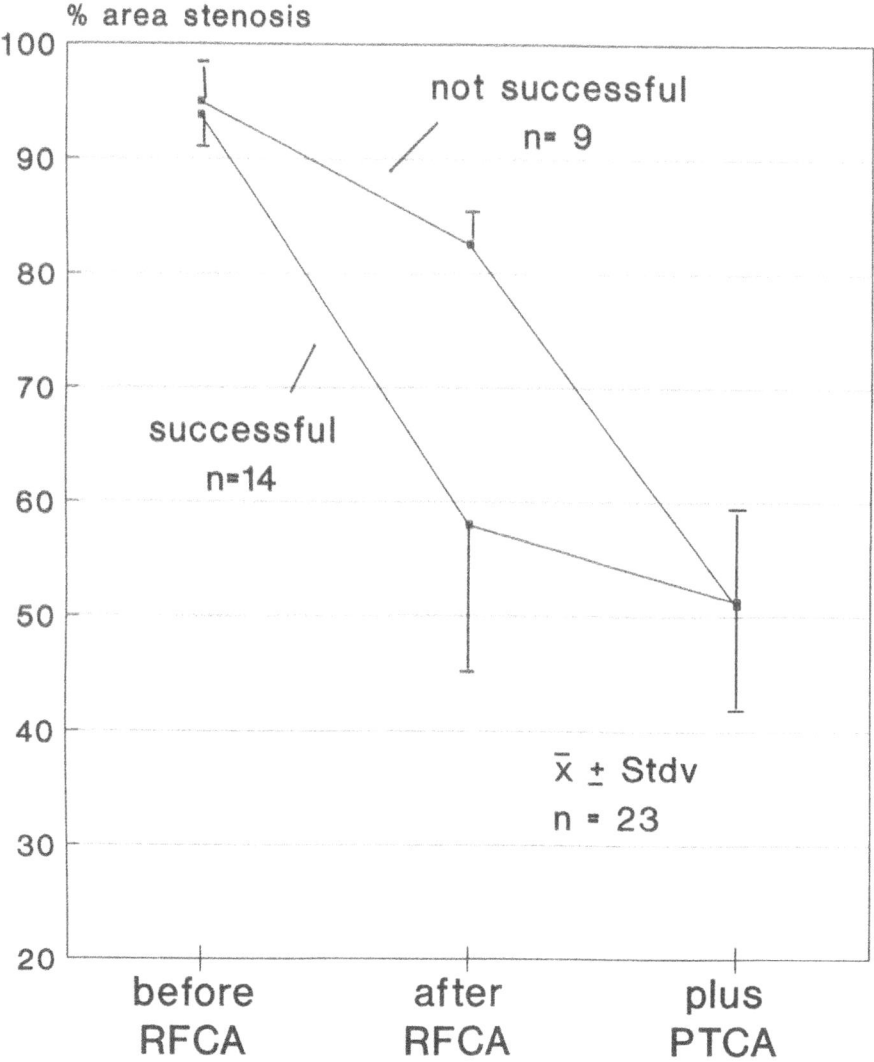

Figure 3. Results of primary RFCA in 9 patients with unsatisfactory and 14 patients with successful outcome and of additional PTCA. The results are given as per cent area stenosis, mean and standard deviation (Stdv).

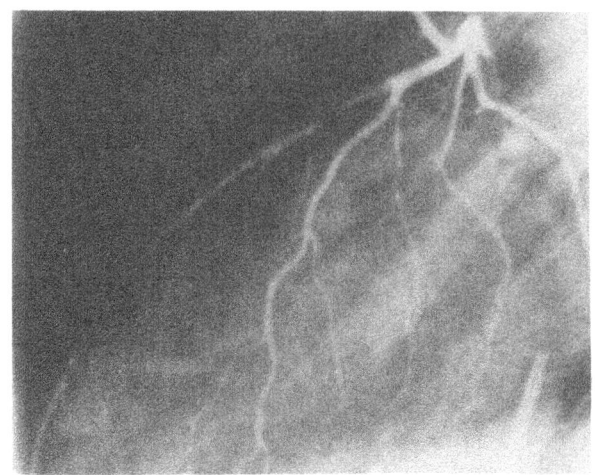

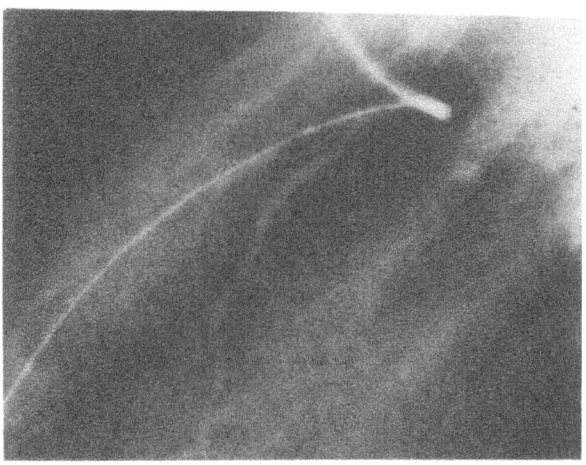

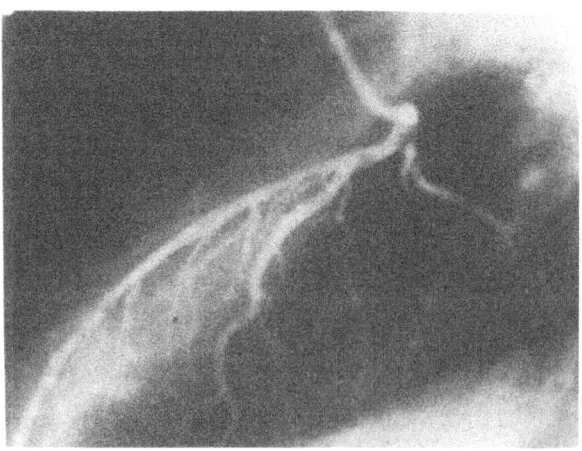

stenosis was reduced from initially 95.8 +/− 2.7 % to 82.5 +/− 2.5 % as a mean, and to further 50.9 +/− 30.4 % by PTCA (Figure 3). Thus, in all patients a successful result of angioplasty was finally achieved by both radiofrequency coronary angioplasty and balloon angioplasty (an example is shown in Figure 4).

A total of 3–12 episodes of radiofrequency current delivery were applied with a mean duration of 2.3 +/− 1.9 s, the total duration of RF-application was 8.1 +/− 6.9 s.

In 18/23 patients (78%) the RF-current delivery was uneventful. One patient experienced a short period of chest pain during and some minutes after RFCA, and only mild ST-segment elevations were seen at the end of the treatment of a tight LAD stenosis. Another patient developed a short episode of ventricular arrhythmia only during application of the RF-current, whereas the arrhythmia stopped immediately following cut-off of the RF-current delivery. In 1/23 patients (4%) a subtotal occlusion of the treated artery occurred, which could be relieved by subsequent balloon angioplasty. In a second patient (4%) a permanent occlusion of a smaller circumflex artery occurred due to intimal dissection following RFCA, and this problem could not be finally solved by PTCA.

As to now only a small cohort of 8 patients could be followed by repeat angiography. In one patient a restenosis and in a second one a repeat occlusion of a formerly recanalized and collateralized vessel occurred 3 months following angioplasty. Thus, the recurrency rate was 2/8 (25%). In 6/9 patients followed so far a significant improvement of the clinical status was observed.

Discussion

This pilot study demonstrates that hemodynamically relevant coronary artery stenoses can be successfully reduced by the new RFCA-technique. If one takes the initial (Grüntzig's) definition of success rates (reduction of equal or more than 20%) RFCA is effective to a similar degree as communicated for the PTCA success rates within the first series of NHLB-registry reports [1,2]. However, meanwhile the criteria of angioplasty success have been changed in that a reduction of the stenotic area should be achieved to equal or less than 50% [5]. Using this definition the success rates of presently 55–60% are lower than those recently reported for PTCA (80–90%), when performed by experienced angioplasty teams. Generally the mean reduction of stenotic areas is smaller with RFCA than with PTCA. The main reasons

Figure 4.   Radiofrequency coronary angioplasty in a patient with high grade LAD stenosis before (top) and after RFCA (bottom). The RFCA catheter is advanced in front of the stenosis over a conventional steerable guide wire (centre), and slowly moved through the stenotic area with continuous delivery of the radiofrequency AC-current until the distal part of the stenosis is reached (not shown) and a good angiographic result is obtained (bottom).

for this experience are technical peculiarities of the RFCA procedure as used in our present equipment. The RFCA-catheters have tips with fixed diameters (4,5,6 French), so that the active electrode ring cannot be expanded over a certain diameter. Therefore, the effect of the RFCA technique mainly depends on the diameter of the coronary artery in that the success rates will be higher in vessels with smaller calibre (1.5–2 mm diameter) than in those with larger diameters (2.5–4 mm). It would be of great advantage to have a multipurpose RFCA-catheter with a tip, that could be introduced into the coronary artery with its smallest diameter and then be expanded successively to its largest diameter. By this means one would need only one catheterization procedure for placing the catheter into the vessel to be treated without the need of several exchanges of catheters with different tip diameters. At present we are working on the development of such a multipurpose RFCA-catheter with variable tip size, in order simplify the angioplasty procedure and to improve the acute success rate of radiofrequency coronary angioplasty.

With respect to acute side effects we were happy that in none of the patients a perforation of the vessel wall was observed during application of RFCA. The reasons for this are that we have used relatively short exposure times of RF-current (up to 2–3 s) and that the catheterization was performed with the over-the-wire technique. Moreover, RFCA proved to be a nearly painless procedure without a significant number of ST-segment changes within the ECG. The explanation for this may be the fact that the tip of the RFCA-catheter did occlude the coronary artery only for a short time (seconds), when being advanced through the stenotic lesion. Whether traumatization of the coronary artery will be less with RFCA than with balloon angioplasty, as could theoretically be expected, has to be proven by further studies using coronary angioscopy. The most impressive experience was that this technique was so easy to handle, whereas balloon angioplasty seems to be more complicated and more advanced.

The rate of acute severe complications (2/23 = 8.6%) in our small series is higher than observed with PTCA, though one of this complication (vessel occlusion due to dissection) could be managed by subsequent balloon angioplasty. In our institution the rate of serious complications following PTCA, that require emergency bypass grafting, is 1%, compared to the 4% complication rate with radiofrequency angioplasty. Therefore the catheters have to be improved and refined in order to avoid gross or minor dissections of the vessel intima during the angioplasty procedure. Nevertheless, the rate of acute serious complications of the RFCA technique is considerably less than that reported so far for coronary excimer laser angioplasty [3, 10, 12], and also lower than the complication rate of hot tip radiofrequency angioplasty used for treatment of stenoses within peripheral arteries [4]. Future more extended studies will show, what the role of the new angioplasty technique will be, compared to the standard technique of balloon angioplasty. The differences of RFCA and PTCA, as shown in Table 2, may

Table 2. Comparison of the technologies of radiofrequency coronary angioplasty (RFCA) and coronary balloon angioplasty (PTCA).

	RFCA	PTCA
Mechanism	Coagulation Desiccation	Compression Intimal splitting
Performance	Easy and simple	More complicated
Vessel occlusion	None or short (sec)	During inflation
Pain	Very rare	Absent or present
St-segment changes	Negligible	Absent or present
Success rate	Lower (60–70%)	High (85–95%)
Complication rate	Higher (4–8%)	Lower (2–5%)
Recurrency rate	About 25%	About 20–40%
Improvements of Technology necessary	Major	Minor

indicate that both methods may be used as alternatives, but rather one may expect RFCA to be an adjunct to PTCA, so that the results of balloon angioplasty may be improved and the spectrum of CHD patients considered for angioplasty may be widened.

References

1. Cowley MJ, Block PC (1986) A review of the NHLB-PTCA registry data, in: Yang GD (ed), *Angioplasty*, p. 368. New York: Mc Graw Hill.
2. Detre KN, Myler RK, Kelsey SF, Raden van M, To T, Mitchell H (1984) Baseline characteristics of patients of the National Heart, Lung and Blood Institute Percutaneous Transluminal Coronary Angioplasty Registry. *Am J Cardiol* 53: 70.
3. Geschwind H, Boussignac G, Teisseive B, Vielledent C, Garton A, Becquemin JB, Mayiolini P (1984) Percutaneous transluminal laser angioplasty in man. *Lancet* 1: 844.
4. Grundfest W, Litvack F, Hickey A, Adler L, Foran R, Lewin P, Segalowitz J, Hestrin L, Forrester J (1989) Radiofrequency thermal angioplasty for the treatment of peripheral vascular occlusive disease: preliminary results of a clinical trial. *J Am Coll Cardiol* 13: Abstract: 14A.
5. Grüntzig AR, Senning A, Siegenthaler W (1979) Non-operative dilatation of coronary artery stenosis. *New Engl J Med* 301: 61.
6. Höher M, Hombach V, Kochs M, Haerer W, Schmidth A, Eggeling T (1990) Complications in conventional and new angioplasty techniques, in: Fleck E, Frantz E (eds), *Complications in PTCA*. Darmstadt: Steinkopff.
7. Hombach V, Höher M, Arnold G, Osypka P, Kochs M, Eggeling T, Höpp HW, Hirche Hj, Hilger HH (1987) Die Hochfrequenzangioplastie—eine neue Methode zur Rekanalisation verschlossener arterieller Gefäße. *Cor Vas* 1: 67.
8. Hombach V, Höher M, Kochs M, Wieshammer S, Haerer W, Eggeling T, Schmidt A, Höpp HW, Hilger HH (1989) Radiofrequency coronary angioplasty in patients with coronary artery disease—a new method for treatment of coronary artery stenoses, in:

Höfling B, v. Pölnitz A (eds), *Interventional Cardiology and Angiology*, p. 163. Darmstadt: Steinkopff.

9. Ischinger T, Meier B (1986) Outcome of coronary angioplasty, in: Ischinger T (ed), *Practice of Coronary Angioplasty*, p. 194. Berlin, Heidelberg, New York, Tokyo: Springer.

10. Karsch KR, Haase KK, Mauser M, Ickrath O, Voelker W, Duda S, Seipel L (1989) Perkutane transluminale koronare Eximer-Laserangioplastie. *Dtsch Med Wschr* 114: 1183.

11. Kochs M, Höher M, Haerer W, Eggeling T, Schmidt A, Hombach V (1991) Excimer laser coronary angioplasty-preliminary results, in: Hombach V, Kochs M, Camm AJ (eds), *Interventional Techniques in Cardiovascular Medicine*, p. 55. Dordrecht, Lancaster, Boston: Kluwer Academic Publishers.

12. Litvack F, Grundfest WS, Goldenberg T, Laudenslager J, Forrester JS (1989) Percutaneous excimer laser angioplasty of aortocoronary saphenous vein grafts. *J Am Coll Cardiol* 14: 803.

13. Margolis JR, Litvack F, Grundfest W, Eigler N, Goldenberg T, Laudenslager J, Tsoi D, Wong S, Segalowitz J, Hestrin L, Rothbaum D, Linnemeier T, Helfant R, Forrester J (1989) Excimer laser coronary angioplasty: Results of a multicenter study. *Circulation* 80: abstract: II–477.

14. Meyer J, Schmitz HJ, Kiessling R, Erbel R, Krebs W, Schulz W, Bardos P, Minale C, Messmer BJ, Effert S (1983) Percutaneous transluminal coronary angioplasty in patients with stable and unstable angina pectoris. Analysis of early and late results. *Am Heart J* 106: 973.

5. Laser angioplasty — technical aspects

R. STEINER, R. HIBST, T. KOLBE, X. M. LIU, W. PRIES,
T. ZÖPF and S. CYBA-ALTUNBAY

Introduction

In the early beginning of laser angioplasty the free laser beam of a continuous wave argon laser (488–514 nm) was used [1,2] for the recanalization of peripheral arteries. Uncontrollable thermal effects and the risk of damage and perforation of the vessel wall due to the penetration depth of the laser beam into the tissue stimulated further developments.

Ablative procedures

For removing biological materials such as plaques or tissue two types of laser tissue interactions can be used alternatively: thermal vaporization and

Table 1. Lasers used for angioplasty.

Tissue reaction			
Ablation		Thermal	
Excimer laser:	308 nm 17–200 ns	Argon laser:	488/514 nm, cw free laser beam
Er:YAG laser:	2.94 um 150 us	Nd:YAG laser:	1064 nm, cw – hot tip (metal) – sapphire tip – quartz tip
Holmium laser:	2.1 um 150 us		
Alexandrite laser: frequency doubled:	700–800 nm 350–400 nm 150–1000 ns	combined methods	
Pulsed dye laser:	400–800 nm 0.5–50 us		
Types of operation			
x-ray control endoscopically		x-ray control endoscopically	

47

V. Hombach et al. (eds), *Interventional Techniques in Cardiovascular Medicine*, 47–53.
© 1991 *Kluwer Academic Publishers.*

ablation (Table 1). Ablation is carried out by excimer lasers (308 nm) but pulsed IR-lasers (Ho, Er:YAG) are still under investigation. Procedures based on thermal reactions fail when plaques are calcified whereas ablation is not restricted to any type of material. The 308 nm UV-laser light, the visible and also the IR-laser light up to 2100 nm can be transmitted through quartz fibers of about 0.2 mm in diameter. These fibers may be bundled for flexible catheters with larger diameters. Commercially available metal coated fibers are detectable by x-ray control.

Using pulsed lasers for the ablative effect in angioplasty, three laser parameters can be independently varied: energy/pulse, pulse-width and the repetition rate of the pulses. Increasing radiant exposure (mJ/mm^2) the ablation rate goes up at moderate pulse repetition rate (Figure 1). The ablation process is purely energy dependent [7] and is not influenced by the pulse-width — at least up to 250 ns. Stretching the pulse is necessary to transmit more energy per pulse through the fibers because of the damage threshold of quartz of about 1 GW/cm^2. According to Figure 1 one would expect a more efficient laser ablation of plaques at the highest possible energies per pulse. The ablation process, however, due to the short laser pulses, is also connected with acoustic phenomena. Tissue damage is not only limited to thermal coagulation due to the laser reaction but also disruption must be taken into account. In Figure 2 the damage zones do not increase proportional with the energy density per pulse suggesting high

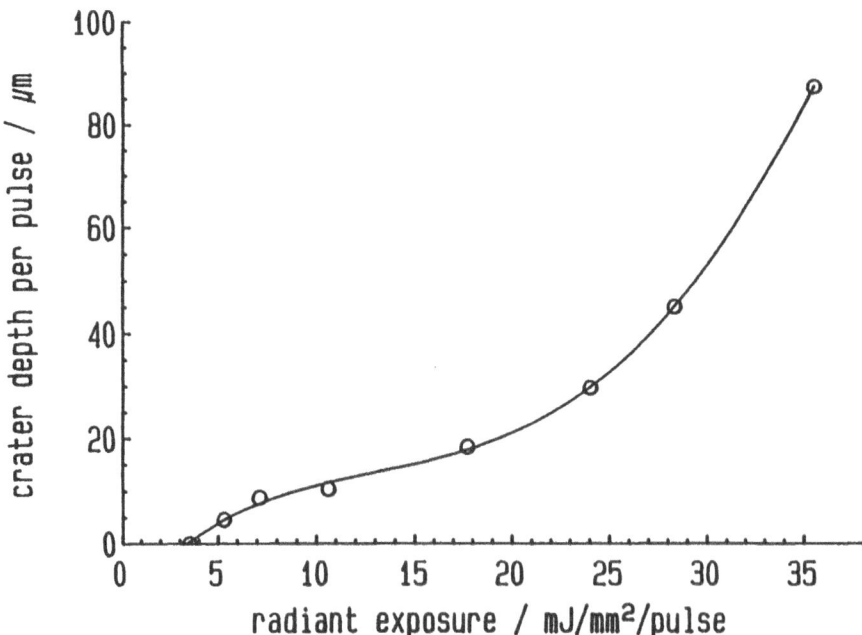

Figure 1.   Ablation rate of aorta with an excimer laser pulse at 308 nm.

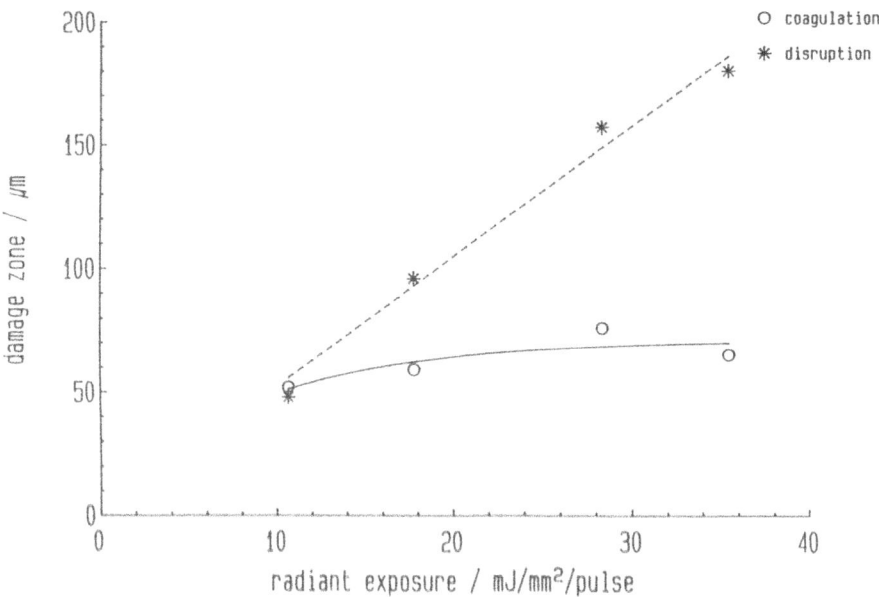

Figure 2.   Damage zones in relation to the energy density per pulse.

efficient ablation at large energies. Looking more carefully to the histologies, beside coagulation disruptions of the tissue can be seen. This starts at about 10 mJ/mm^2 and goes linearly with the energy per pulse augmenting the risk for producing larger fragments and ruptures during ablation. Therefore we would recommend to ablate at lower radiant exposures and higher repetition rates to minimize tissue damage. The increase of the coagulation zone with the pulse frequency is not so prominent in comparison with the danger of the acoustic effects.

Working with different fiber diameters the results indicate that the ablated tissue volume is purely energy dependent. This is demonstrated in Figure 3. The diagram shows the ablated channel depth for each fiber diameter. Normalizing these values to the cross-section of the fibers then equal ablation depths are the result.

It is interesting to see that the form of the fiber tip has a great influence on the damage zone. One would expect that a spherically rounded fiber tip ablates smoothly through the tissue but just the opposite occurs. Simply cleaved fiber ends (0.6 mm quartz fibers) with sharp edges show less damage than rounded fiber tips. Here the refocussing of the laser beam creates larger damage zones and the ablated channel wall is less smooth than using flat tips.

With single fibers, recanalization of arteries is only efficient in small arteries. The ablated channel has only the same diameter as the fiber. To increase the diameter it is possible to melt a small fiber piece of 600 μm to

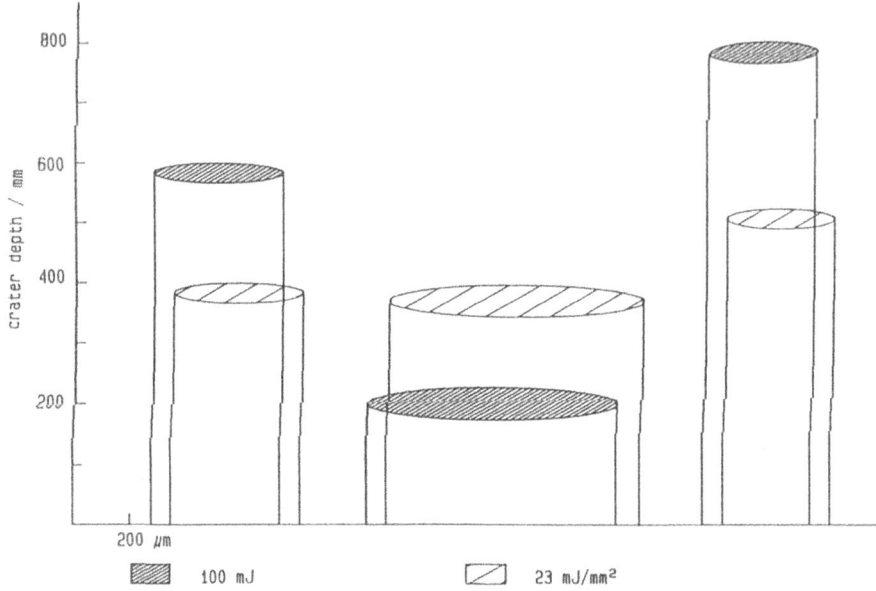

Figure 3.   Ablation depths in relation to the fiber diameter. Normalizing the data to the cross-section of the fiber result in equal ablation values indicating the energy dependence of the ablation process.

the end of a 200 μm fiber. This has the advantage of a highly flexible transmission system combined with a nearly 10 times higher ablation cross-section. Of course one is limited to the ablation threshold with the diameter of the fiber tip. Another approach are the multiple fiber catheters which are more flexible than a single fiber with the same cross-section. Working under visual control by inserting a thin optical fiber bundle would improve the

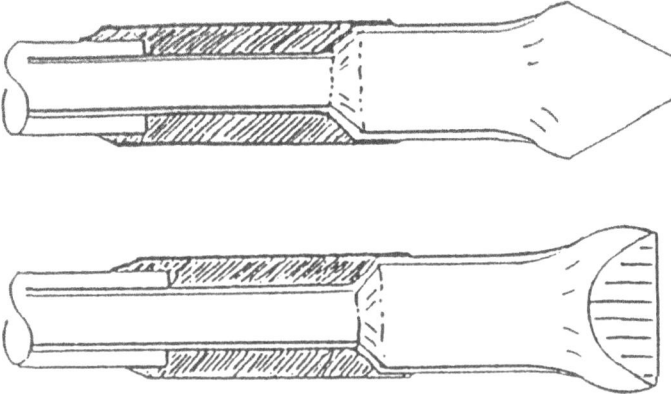

Figure 4.   Scheme of a wedge-shaped quartz tip for thermal catheters.

safety of the operation enormously, especially in partially closed arteries with calcified plaques.

Pulsed lasers in the visible spectral region as the alexandrite laser or the pulsed dye laser can provide much higher energies per pulse up to 1 Joule but the ablation threshold is increased as well. On the other hand it is still unknown whether the fragmented particles are still much larger than using the excimer laser and also acoustic affects may create even more damage. Going to the IR (holmium laser, Er:YAG laser), the ablation process becomes comparable with that of the excimer laser. Unfortunately, for the Er:YAG laser at 2.94 um the fiber technology (e.g., fluoride fibers) is still not so advanced that a fiber transmission system can be used in clinical routine work. In future, however, this laser can become an interesting alternative to the excimer laser.

Thermal reactions

There is already a large market for catheters with different types of thermal tips [3,4]. They are used for the recanalization of peripheral arteries in combination with conventional balloon dilatation. A low power Nd:YAG laser is normally sufficient to heat the simple metal or more sophisticated tips. These catheters are useful with soft and not calcified plaques [5,6].

The specific requirements for the tips are: (1) low heat capacity of the tip, (2) local heating of only the tip surface being in contact with the plaque so that the vessel wall itself is heat protected. For this reason a quartz catheter has been developed by melting a droplet of quartz at the fiber tip and shaping this catheter head as a wedge leaving a small ridge in between. The angle of the wedge is smaller than required for total reflection of the laser light (Figure 4). Therefore the light intensity is concentrated at the front of the tip where it also can leave the tip and penetrate into the plaque material. The part of the tip coming in contact with the vessel wall is much less heated to prevent from thermal damage. This shape has the advantage that it stabilizes itself when passing through the plaque. The diameter is limited to about 2.5 mm. This quartz tip has been tested in comparison with a Trimedyne laser probe (metal tip, PLR 775–2.5) with the same laser energy and also with a home-made tantalum tip as demonstrated in Figure 5. Heating with 40 Joules in 10 s of the tips in air show the temperature rise and decline over a time scale of 60 s. The highest temperature is reached by the quartz tip, where the energy is absorbed only at the blackened surface. The Trimedyne laser probe is heating very slowly and due to the high heat capacity the temperature also falls down relatively slowly. The temperature rise at the vessel wall has been tested with a micro thermocouple. In Figure 6 the temperature rise during angioplasty has been registered on a pen-recorder. There is no heating (two traces) higher than 50 degrees—except when the quartz tip directly touched the thermocouple. The advantage of

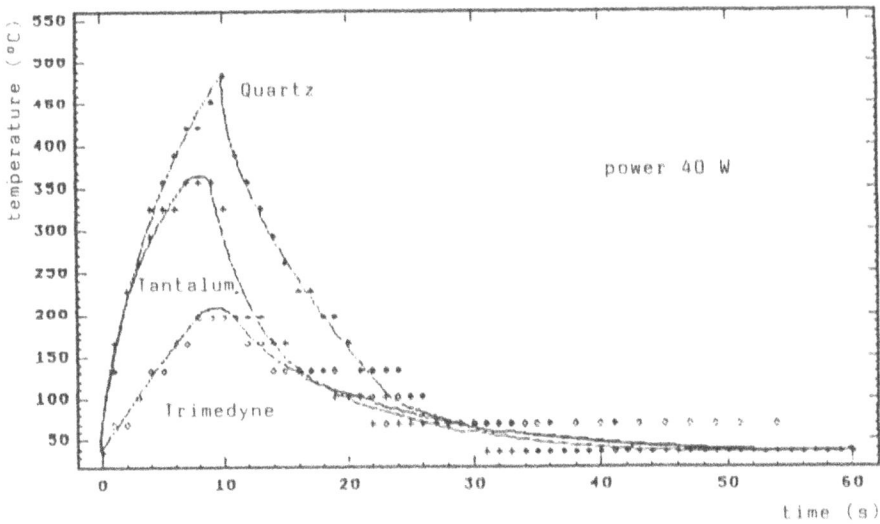

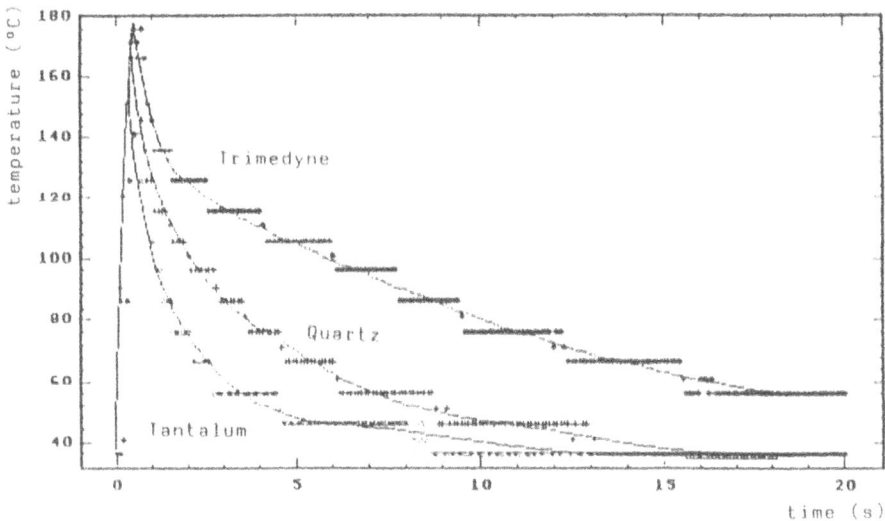

Figure 5.   Temperature rise of tips during heating (10 s, 4 W) in air (above). Decline of temperature after heating of the tips to the same temperature (below).

the quartz tip in comparison with the sapphire tip is that quartz fiber and tip are one single piece, whereas the sapphire tip needs a coupler to the fiber. Couplers may be heated up by the laser beam and the tip will be destroyed. The histology of angioplasty with the quartz tip shows nearly no carbonisation and very little thermal damage.

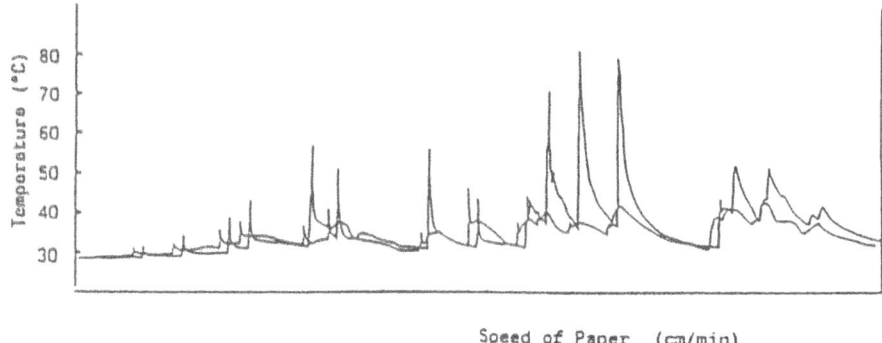

Speed of Paper (cm/min)

Figure 6. Temperature rise at the vessel wall during angioplasty (pulsed Nd-YAG laser; 40 W, 0.15 s) using a quartz tip.

Conclusion

Thermal catheters are only useful in larger peripheral arteries. Recanalization of small arteries should be performed by the ablative tissue reaction of the pulsed lasers. The excimer laser at 308 nm is state of the art but pulsed IR-lasers will become an interesting alternative. They both are capable to ablate calcified plaques. Working under visual control with flexible mini-scopes certainly will improve the application and the safety aspects. Also thermal catheters can be improved for more efficient recanalization at larger diameters.

References

1. Choy DSJ et al. (1985) Embolization and vessel wall perforation in argon laser recanalization. *Lasers Surg Med* 5: 297–308.
2. Choy DSJ (1986) Laser revascularization: state of the art. *Lasers Surg Med* 6: 408–411.
3. Welch AJ et al. (1987) Laser probe ablation of normal and atherosclerotic human aorta in vitro: a first thermographic and histologic analysis. *Circulation* 76: 1353–1363.
4. Labs JD et al. (1987) Thermodynamic correlates of hot tip laser angioplasty. *Invest Radiol* 22: 954–959.
5. McCowan TC et al. (1988) Laser thermal angioplasty for the treatment of obstruction of the distal superficial femoral or popliteal arteries. *Amer J Roentgenol* 150: 1169–1173.
6. Fleisher HL et al. (1987) Human percutaneous laser angioplasty. Patient selection criteria and early results. *Amer J Surg* 154: 666–670.
7. Wieshammer S et al. (1988) Ultraviolet laser ablation of biologic tissue. Quantitation of etch rate as a function of incident fluence. *Lasers Life Sci* 2: 125–135.

6. Excimer laser coronary angioplasty: preliminary clinical experience

M. KOCHS, W. HAERER, T. EGGELING, A. SCHMIDT, M. HÖHER, S. WIESHAMMER and V. HOMBACH

Introduction

At time, balloon angioplasty is the well established standard procedure for nonsurgical treatment of coronary stenosis with a success rate of about 90 to 95%. The major limitations of balloon angioplasty such as poor results in recanalisation of chronic obstructed arteries, in the treatment of diffuse atherosclerotic vessels and the high incidence of restenosis [1, 3, 13] are the reasons for the development of alternative techniques like atherectomy, rotational atherectomy and other methods of mechanical revascularisation [4, 12, 18], radiofrequency angioplasty [8], hot balloon angioplasty [19] and different methods of laser applications in peripheral and coronary arteries [6, 19, 20, 21].

Based on its mechanism of action especially laser seems to be a most promising tool in the treatment of vascular obstructions [1, 17]. Unlike balloon angioplasty, which dissects and rearranges the plaque material to increase the vascular lumen, laser energy reduces obstructive lesions by vaporisation or by thermal compression of vacuolated tissue. The surface left behind by this procedure usually is smooth. Hypothetically this may lead to a reduced recurrence rate of obstruction at this site [1, 15].

Because of the availability of several lasers at different wave-lengths, the choice of a laser for intravascular recanalization becomes a major issue.

Continuous wave lasers, such as the Nd:Yag, argon ion and carbon dioxide, as the most widely used medical lasers, destroy tissue by rapid conversion of solid matter to gas. Absorbed photon energy is converted to heat, causing water and other compounds within the tissue to vaporize [1].

This kind of photothermal ablation tends to leave a ragged surface and an adjacent area of thermal injury after atheroma ablation.

Experimental and clinical studies with 'hot-tip' systems could demonstrate results superior to balloon angioplasty in large diameter vessels like femoral arteries, but thermal injury in small vessels like the coronaries can cause thrombotic or spasm induced occlusion [9, 14, 15, 17]. Furthermore heavily

55

V. Hombach et al. (eds), Interventional Techniques in Cardiovascular Medicine, 55–61.

calcified plaque material is refractory to simple heating and the effects of thermaly injured neosurface may lead to restenosis [2, 7, 15, 17].

In contrary to thermal laser systems ultraviolet pulsed lasers such as excimer laser are capable of facile tissue ablation by photodecompensation without pathologic heating of boundary tissues. The higher peak power characteristics of pulsed laser irradiation are more effective for ablation of calcified lesions. The fact that ablation is accomplished with little change in tissue temperature, might translate into a more benign healing process, less thrombogenic residual surface and a diminished likelihood of thermal perforation [15, 16].

Moreover, pulsed laser light, at least in the ultraviolet and visible, causes photorelaxation rather than contraction, that means spasm, of vascular smooth muscle [2, 5, 14].

In the past, clinical application of excimer laser angioplasty was limited by difficulties in transmitting high peak powers via diminutive fused silica fibers. The development of resistant laser fibers, bounded into flexible catheter systems, novel means of laser fiber optic coupling and the longer pulse durations of so called 'streched' excimer lasers have facilitated fiber optic transmission, so that at present devices for clinical use are available [10, 11].

Based on extensive experimental studies including those of the own group [7, 22] we have started to apply excimer laser angioplasty in human coronary arteries, the first clinical experiencies of which will be reported below.

Methods

Energy source and catheter system

In our study laser energy was supplied by the XeCl excimer laser MAX 10 (TM) system (TECHNOLAS Company, Munich). The technical specifications of the system are: wavelength: 308 nm, pulse duration: 60 nsec, laser energy per pulse: 30 to 160 mJ, repetition rate: 20 to 160 Hz.

In our clinical study laser coronary angioplasty (ELCA) usually was performed with repetition rates of 20 Hz. Laser energy was applicated by multifiber ring catheters with a length of 140 cm and outer diameters of 4, 5 and 5.5 French (Table 1). 18 to 20 silica fibers with a diameter of 100 μm are concentrically arranged around a central lumen for taking up a conventional 0.014 Inch guide wire and for flushing. The fibers are welded together at the tip, the end is rounded and polished to avoid injury to the vessel. A gold mark near the catheter tip allows radiographic control of the position during the procedure. The native laser beam is focused by an optical lens (focus length 30 cm) and coupled to the fibers by a specially designed coupling system. Laser power was adjusted, so that the maximum possible energy was delivered to the plaque. Energy output was monitored by an energy meter before and after angioplasty.

Table 1. Vessel characteristics, catheter size, results and complications of ELCA and following PTCA

Case	Vessel	Catheter	Stenosis (% diameter)			Complications
no.		(French)	Prelaser	Post laser	Final result[a]	
1	CFX	4	73.5	55.3	14.4	Spasm
2	LAD	4	70.1	62.6	41.3	Spasm, dissection after PTCA
3	LAD	4				no passage of laser catheter[c]
4	LAD	5	85.3	43.4	20.0	Dissection after ELCA occlusion after 24 h
5	LAD[b]	5	68.8	43.6	33.3	Thrombotic occlusion after ELCA
6	LAD[b]	5	67.0	50.0	10.1	–
7	CFX[b]	5	84.3	43.1	42.1	–
8	RCA[b]	5	61.2	49.8	38.4	Spasm, thrombus and dissection after ELCA
9	CFX	5.5	80.8	41.8	14.3	–
10	LAD[b]	5.5	84.4	72.4	21.1	Thrombotic occlusion after ELCA

[a] After PTCA.
[b] Restenosis 2 to six months after successful PTCA.
[c] PTCA was performed without difficulties using a 3.0 mm Simson ultra low profile catheter.

Procedure

Laser angioplasty was performed by the conventional transfemoral approach in Judkins technique using a 9 French guiding catheter. After control angiography, a high torque floppy guide wire was advanced into the periphery of the obstructed vessel. After that, the multifiber catheter was positioned over the wire in front of the lesion and very slowly pushed forward performing laser energy application carefully avoiding mechanical forces. After crossing the lesion, delivery of laser pulses was stopped immediately. Under radiographic control laser application was continued during repeated pulling back and pushing forward of the catheter over the obstructed vessel segment. After each crossing of a lesion, control angiography was performed. Number of passages, application time and pulse numbers varied in dependency of the actual angiographic result. ELCA was stopped immediately in appearance of complications like spasm, thrombus formation, dissection or vessel occlusion. In these cases and in cases with unsatisfactory laser angioplasty result, the laser catheter was exchanged over a guide wire extention for a balloon catheter to perform conventional PTCA. A total number of 440 to 1742 (mean 1022) pulses per patient treatment were applied. Passage number varied from 2 to 6 (mean 3.9) and energy at the begin of the procedure ranged from 6 to 14 mJ. In most instances a considerable loss of energy per pulse was observed after angioplasty, mean values differed from 9.2 ± 2.4 mJ before to 6.6 ± 3.8 mJ after laser application.

The stenosis degree was determined by an electronically caliper by measuring the pre- and stenotic diameter in two planes. The stenoses were expressed as percent diameter stenosis. Values were presented as mean ± standard deviation. Statistical significances was calculated using the student T-test for paired variables. Statistical significance was assumed, when p values ranged < 0.05.

Medications

Premedication consisted in oral application of ASS, nitrates and diltiazem several days and the morning before angioplasty, 10,000 units of Heparine i.v. and 0.1 mg Nitrogycerine i.c. immediately before the procedure. Infusion of heparine (30,000 units/24 h and nitroglycerine (2 mg/h) was continued for 24 h after ELCA.

Patients

Our preliminary results are based on 10 patients with stable coronary heart disease, 2 females and 8 males, aged 37 to 61 (mean 52.7) years. All patients suffered from symptomatic high grade coronary stenosis, 6 in the LAD, 3 in the circumflex and 1 in the right coronary artery. Five cases presented restenosis 3 to 6 months after primary successful PTCA (Table 1).

Before the procedure, the experimental nature and the possible consequences of ELCA was extensively explained to each patient and informed written consent was obtained.

Results

In 9/10 patients the stenoses could be passed by the multifiber catheter. In one case (Table 1: case no. 3) the laser catheter failed in crossing the lesion. In this patient PTCA was performed without difficulties using a 3.0 mm Simson ultra low profile catheter with appropriate result. In 5/10 patients ELCA led to a reduction of diameter stenosis immediately after the procedure of more than 20%, in 7/9 cases stenosis was reduced to equal or more than 50% (success rate 50%/70%). Overall, ELCA was able to reduce the stenoses immediately after the procedure from a mean value of 75.2 ± 8.4 to 51.3 ± 10.4% (p = 0.005). In two of these 9 patients total vessel occlusion was observed following primary significantly stenosis reduction by laser application. In case no. 4 (Table 1) this was apparent during control angiography 24 hours later, in case no. 10 30 minutes after ELCA. Further minor or major complications were frequently observed (Table 1): spasm in 3/10 patients, dissection in 3/10 patients, intravascular thrombus formation in 4/10 patients.

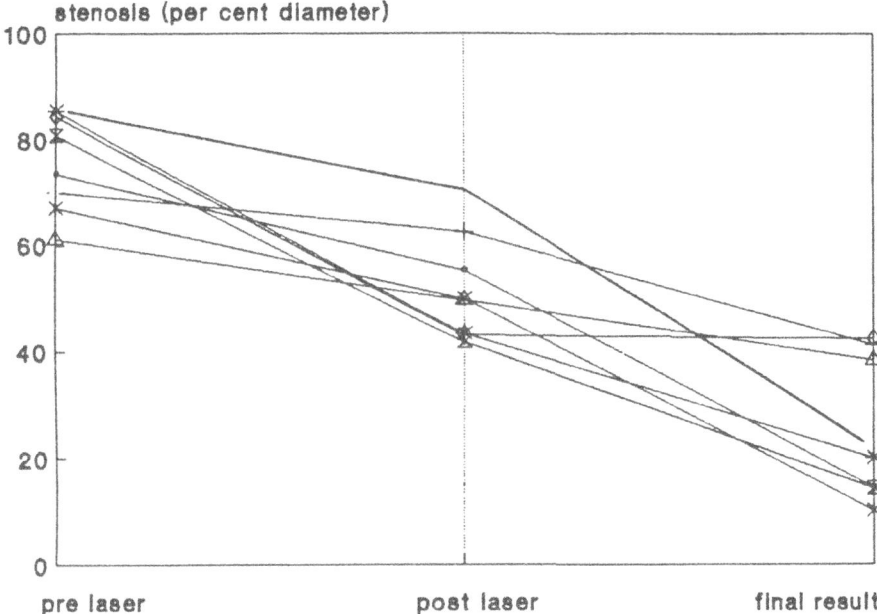

Figure 1. Percent diameter stenosis of coronary obstructions before (prelaser), after excimer laser coronary angioplasty (post laser) and following balloon angioplasty (final result) in 10 patients.

With regard to the complications described above or to the insufficient angiographic result after laser application (residual stenosis > 40%) PTCA was performed in all 10 patients with good result (stenosis after PTCA $26.4 \pm 12.0\%$, $p = 0.015$). Balloon angioplasty following laser application was not accompanied by an increased complication rate. Dissection without diminished coronary flow as the only complication in the 10 patients occured only in 1 of 10 cases. The results of stenosis reduction after laser application and after final PTCA are presented in Figure 1.

Discussion

In our experience ELCA is feasible to cross stenosis in the majority of the treated lesions and to reduce stenosis diameter significantly. But in comparison with the results of conventional PTCA the reduction of stenosis diameter was significantly minor and the acute complication rate was much higher.

The lower effect of stenosis reduction may be due to the fixed diameter of our laser catheters (4 to 5.5 French) and the minimal dispersion of laser energy into the treated plaque material. Furthermore the over the wire technique using a lumen concentrically surrounded by laser fibers causes the catheter tip to be placed in the middle part of the vessel, so that excentric plaques may not be reached by the ablating energy. Thus the plaque material may be reached only by a small portion of the energy delivered at the catheter tip.

In contrary to the theoretical considerations based on experimental studies mentioned above, in our series laser angioplasty led to a high incidence of complications like spasm and intracoronary clotting. Spasm and thrombus formation are effects typically observed using low energy thermal lasers [14, 17]. Therefore we assume, that the output energy of the presently available system is too low to perform real photoablation, but causes undesired thermal effects to the treated lesions. Furthermore mechanical effects of the catheters while crossing the stenoses should be considered. The high incidence of intracoronary thrombi in our study, which contrasts to the observation of other groups, using comparable or identical equipments, may also be due to the digital angiographic technique of our catheter laboratory, which permits the early visualisation of such complications.

Contrary to the experiences of other groups, in our experience PTCA could be performed easily and without difficulties following laser angioplasty [10] (compare also the reports of the groups from Los Angeles and Tübingen in this publication).

We presume, that higher energy and/or longer pulse duration, further improvement of the laser fibers and the catheter configuration such as excentrically guided catheters, those with larger diameter or those with dispersion of the laser energy in a predictable distance and direction would be necessary, to realize the excimer laser effect of real nonthermal photo-ablation. Thus at present PTCA seems to be superior to excimer laser angioplasty in the available configuration. Only substancial improvements of the entire system including the energy source and the catheters may realize better immediate and longterm results of these new method of great theoretical promise.

References

1. Abela GS (1989) Catheters, in: Isner J, Clarke R, (eds), *Cardiovascular Laser Therapy*, p. 173. New York: Raven Press, Ltd.
2. Deckelbaum, LI, Isner JM, Donaldson RF, Clarke RH, Laliberte S, Ahron AS and Bernstein JS (1985) Reduction of laser-induced pathologic tissue injury using pulsed energy delivery. *Am J Cardiol* 56: 662.
3. Dorros G, Cowley MJ and Simpson J (1983) Coronary angioplasty. Report of complications from the national Heart, Lung, and Blood Institute PTCA Registry. *Circulation* 67: 723.
4. Erbel R, O'Neill W, Nixdorff U, Dietz U, Rupprecht HJ, Tschollar W and Meyer J (1989) Hochfrequenz-Rotationsatherektomie bei koronarer Herzkrankheit. *Dtsch med Wschr* 114: 487.
5. Grundfest WS, Litvack IF, Goldenberg T, Sherman T, Morgenstern L, Carroll R, Fishbein M, Forrester J, Margitan J, McDermid S, Pacala TJ, Rider DM, and Laudenslager JB

(1985) Pulsed ultraviolet lasers and the potential safe laser angioplasty. *Am J Surg* 150: 220.

6. Günther RW (1989) Laserangioplastie und Gefäßendoprothesen. *Dtsch med Wschr* 114: 435.
7. Haase KK, Steiger E, Wehrmann M, Walz R and Karsch KR (1989) Einfluß von Laserstrahlen auf atherosklerotisch veränderte Gefäßabschnitte in Abhängigkeit von Wellenlänge und Pulsbreite. *Z Kardiol* 78: 701.
8. Hombach V, Höher M, Höpp HW, Kochs M, Eggeling T, Osypka P and Hilger HH (1988) High frequency current angioplasty in coronary heart disease—preliminary results. *J Am Coll Cardiol* 11: 110B.
9. Ischinger T, Coppenrath K, Weber H, Enders S, Unsöld E and Hessel S (1989) Die Nutzung der thermischen Wirkung von Laserstrahlen für kardiovaskuläre Anwendung am Beispiel des Nd: YAG-Lasers. *Z Kardiol* 78: 689.
10. Isner JM (1988) Excimer laser angioplasty: pygmalion makes it to the ball. *Lasers Surg Med* 8: 447.
11. Karsch KR, Haase KK, Mauser M, Ickrath O, Voelker W, Duda S and Seipel L (1989) Percutane transluminale koronare Excimer-Laserangioplastie. *Dtsch med Wschr* 114: 1183.
12. Kensey K, Nash J, Abrahams C, Lake K and Zarins CK (1986) Recanalization of obstructed arteries using a flexible rotating tip catheter. *Circulation* 74, Suppl II: 1821.
13. Kent KM (1988) Restenosis after percutaneous transluminal coronary angioplasty. *Am J Cardiol* 61: 67G.
14. Litvack F, Grundfest WS, Goldenberg T, Laudenslager J, Pacala T, Segalowitz J and Forrester JS (1988) Pulsed laser angioplasty. Wavelength power and energy dependencies relevant to clinical application. *Lasers Surg Med* 8: 60.
15. Litvack F, Grundfest WS, Papaioannou T, Mohr FW, Jakubowski AT and Forrester JS (1988) Role of laser and thermal ablation devices in the treatment of vascular diseases. *Am J Cardiol* 61: 81G.
16. Mohr FW, Lenz W, v Kusserow S, Greulich O, Weller, R Wolfrum J and Kirchhoff PG (1987) Excimer laser for angioplasty and cardiac valve repair. *Lasers Surg Med* 3: 93.
17. Sanborn TA (1988) Laser Angioplasty. *Circulation* 78: 769.
18. Simpson JB, Robertson GC and Selmon MR (1988) Percutaneous coronary atherectomy. *J Am Coll Cardiol* 11(2): 110B.
19. Spears JR (1986) Percutaneous laser treatment of atherosclerosis. An overview of emerging techniques. *Cardiovasc Intervent Radiol* 9: 303.
20. Strauer BE, Neubaur T, Klepzig M, Heintzen M, Zeitler E and Richter EI (1988) Perkutane periphere Laserangioplastie: erste klinische Ergebnisse. *Z Kardiol* 77: 29.
21. Werner GS, Buchwald A, von Romatowski J, Unterberg C, Sauthoff G, Wurm K, Kreuzer H and Wiegand V (1989) Excimer-Laserangioplastie bei arterieller Verschlußkrankheit. *Dtsch med Wschr* 114: 1271.
22. Wieshammer S, Hibst R, Bellekins M and Steiner R (1988) Ultraviolet laser ablation of biologic tissues. Quantification of etch rate as a function of incident fluence. *Lasers Life Sci* 2: 125.

7. Result of a pilot study on percutaneous coronary excimer laser ablation in patients with coronary artery disease

K. R. KARSCH, K. K. HAASE, M. MAUSER, W. VOELKER and
L. SEIPEL

Summary

The clinical results of conventional percutaneous transluminal coronary angioplasty are limited by a restenosis rate that approaches 40%. Laser ablation of atherosclerotic plaque using an excimer laser and a new catheter device for energy transmission has been suggest to be one alternative approach for treatment of obstructive lesions. This pilot study was designed as a first clinical trial in patients with coronary artery disease to determine the feasibility, efficacy and safety of this alternative method. In 55 of 60 patients which were included in this trial excimer laser ablation could be performed. In 23 patients the results of laser treatment was sufficient and no additional intervention necessary. In 32 patients, however, subsequent balloon angioplasty was performed. In eleven of these 32 patients additional PTCA was necessary due to early vessel closure immediately after laser ablation and in 21 patients because the qualitative result was not sufficient in reduction of the initial degree of stenosis of more than 50%. Three serious complications were encountered in this series. One patient died after early vessel closure 2 hours after intervention and in 2 patients a Q-wave infarction occurred after persistent vessel closure following laser ablation. Vessel perforation or extravasation of dye, however, did not occur.

   The results of this pilot study suggest that coronary excimer laser angioplasty is feasible. The acute success rate of this method, however, is reduced in comparison to conventional PTCA. Thus, improvement of the catheter system is mandantory before further clinical studies are performed. Furthermore, the incidence of restenosis after laser ablation has to be determined and compared to PTCA in further randomized studies.

Introduction

Balloon angioplasty is an accepted method of coronary reperfusion with a 90–95% primary success rate. Restenosis, however, is the major problem of

V. Hombach et al. (eds), Interventional Techniques in Cardiovascular Medicine, 63–71.
© 1991 Kluwer Academic Publishers.

current angioplasty practice and limits the clinical efficacy [1, 3]. The frequent occurrence of restenosis is not surprising in view of the potential for accelerating pathogenetic mechanisms following balloon angioplasty [4]. It is hypothesized that by removing atherosclerotic obstructions through ablation of plaque, pulsed laser angioplasty may be more effective than balloon angioplasty and may reduce restenosis rate [5]. To date, however, this technique has been limited by inadequate delivery systems.

Most recent studies have suggested that excimer laser ablates vascular tissue by a mechanism different from that of visible or infrared continuous wave lasers [6,8]. Excimer laser energy, operating at an ultraviolet wavelength, has been shown to cause a photothermal and chemical disruption of the molecular bonds in tissue, resulting in ablation [9]. Both in vitro and in vivo animal experiments have shown that the excimer laser may be superior than the conventionally used medical lasers for intravascular use since incision margins are sharp and adjacent normal tissue damage is minimal [7, 10, 13]. It has already been shown that coronary excimer laser ablation is feasible in patients with obstructive lesions with and without additional balloon angioplasty [14,15]. The current investigation reports on our combined clinical experience with excimer laser angioplasty in the first 60 consecutive patients with coronary artery disease undergoing elective percutaneous transluminal coronary balloon angioplasty.

Methods

Laser-technique. A commercial excimer xenon chloride laser (Technolas Inc., MAX-10, Munich, FRG) that delivered pulses at a pulsewidth of 60 nsec and at a wavelength of 308 nm was used. The laser was operated at a frequency of 20 Hz. The beam was coupled into a specially designed 1.3 mm catheter device, consisting of 20 concentric 100 μm quartz fibers around a central lumen for an 0.014 inch diameter flexible guide wire. The fibers were fixed at the proximal and distal end only to ensure maximal catheter flexibility. Energy transmission per pulse was approximately 5 mJ/mm^2. Before and after each irradiation series the actual transmitted energy at the catheter tip of each systems was measured. In prior in vitro studies the ablative threshold of this device was found to be approximately 4 mJ/mm^2 [13].

Study protocol. The patients were prepared for laser angioplasty using standard angioplasty techniques by way of the percutaneous femoral approach. After a heparin bolus (10.000 U given intraarterially) and intracoronary nitroglycerin application (100 μg left coronary artery, 50 μg right coronary artery) biplane control angiography of the ischemia related artery was performed and confirmed the severity of the lesion in all but one patient who showed a total occlusion of the right coronary artery at the site of a subtotal lesion one week before at diagnostic catheterization. After intervention all patients were monitored for 24 hours in the coronary care unit; ECGs and blood samples for enzyme levels of CK and CKMB were taken every 3 hours. The introducing sheat was left in place for 24 hours until control angiography was performed. Intravenous Heparin was administered for 24 hours after intervention at a rate of 1000 IU/hour. During all interventions a surgical team for emergency bypass operation was available.

Patients. All 60 patients had been previously selected for percutaneous transluminal coronary angioplasty on the basis of symptoms and angiographic findings. 49 patients were markedly limited by severe extertional angina pectoris despite medical therapy and 11 patients had unstable angina with reversible ST-T segment changes at rest despite vigorous therapy with nitroglycerine, β-blocking agents and calcium antagonists. Patients with angiographic evidence of intracoronary thrombi or evolving myocardial infarction were excluded. The patients baseline characteristics are provided in Table 1. The protocol of excimer laser angioplasty was approved by the Institutional Review Board Committee at the University of Tuebingen. Informed consent was obtained from each patient before the intervention.

Table 1. Patients baseline characteristics.

Total Group	N:	60
Gender	Male	49
	Female	11
Mean age (years)		59 ± 6
Extent of CAD		
	1-Vessel disease	41
	2-Vessel disease	13
	3-Vessel disease	6
Target vessel		
	Left anterior descending artery	43
	Circumflex artery	7
	Right coronary artery	10
Unstable angina		11

Laser angioplasty procedure. With a 9F lumen guiding catheter (ACS) in place in the ostium of the ischemia related artery, a 0.014 inch diameter and 180 cm long steerable guide wire (USCI) was advanced through the lesion or total occlusion into the distal vessel and the location confirmed by angiography. The tip of laser catheter was then positioned close to the lesion. In all cases, further advancement of the laser catheter across the lesion was performed with gentle pressure and during 8–10 seconds excimer laser energy delivery. The advancement was slowly performed up to the end of the lesion. After the lesion was passed additional irradiation of the lesion was performed during slow withdrawal of the catheter. This procedure was repeated at least twice for approximately 10–15 seconds per cycle. After each cycle the laser catheter was pulled back into the guiding catheter and control angiography was performed. Laser angioplasty was stopped if no visible change in comparison to the result of the pervious laser delivery was observed.

Balloon angioplasty procedure.   Following excimer laser angioplasty conventional balloon angioplasty was performed to ensure an adequate lumen. In most patients the laser catheter device including the guide wire were exchanged and conventional balloon angioplasty was performed.

Qualitative coronary analysis.   The coronary angiograms were reviewed by three experienced angiographers unaware of the clinical data. The coronary lesions were classified by a consensus of the three angiographers on the basis of qualitative analysis of the lesion in at least two projections.

Results

A total group of 60 patients were scheduled for excimer laser angioplasty. In 5 of these patients the laser catheter could not be positioned in an axial direction within the vessel. Since in these patients the laser beam was directed to wards the 'normal' vessel wall laser irradiation was not initiated to avoid vessel injury, i.e., perforation.

Figure 1.   Diagram of the results achieved by stand alone excimer laser angioplasty and after additional balloon angioplasty

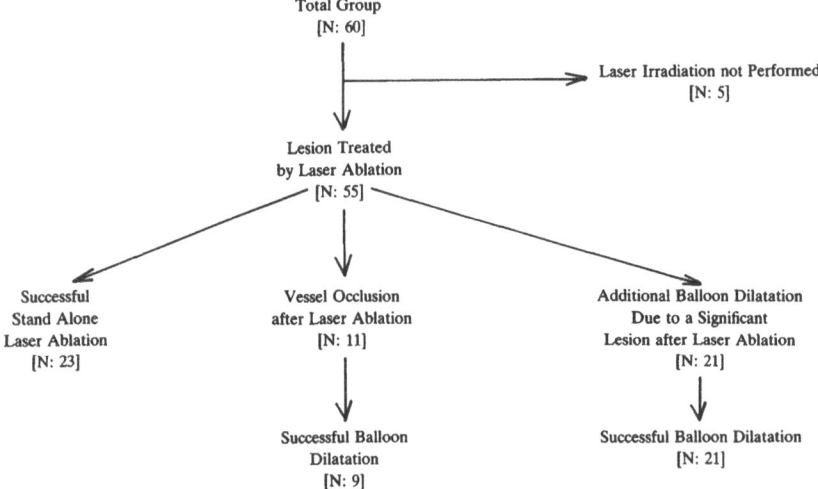

In 55 patients, in whom laser angioplasty was possible, percent stenosis decreased from ($\times \pm$SD) 81 $\pm$ 17% before to 37 $\pm$ 17% after laser treatment. The minimal lumen diameter increased from 0.45 $\pm$ 0.36 mm to 1.66 $\pm$ 0.47 mm after laser ablation. In 23 of these 55 (42%) patients no additional balloon angioplasty was performed (Figure 1). Percent stenosis decreased from 76 $\pm$ 14% before to 27 $\pm$ 17% after laser angioplasty and was 34 $\pm$ 15% at the 24 hour control angiogram. The minimal lumen diameter increased from 0.53 $\pm$ 0.34 mm to 1.78 $\pm$ 0.45 mm after laser angioplasty and was 1.77 $\pm$ 0.6 mm 24 hours later. In 32 patients percent stenosis decreased from 85 $\pm$ 14% to 44 $\pm$ 14% after coronary excimer laser treatment and conventional balloon angioplasty was performed resulting in a residual percent stenosis of 24 $\pm$ 15%. At the 24 hours control angiography percent stenosis increased not significantly to 32 $\pm$ 24% in 27 patients. Subgroup analysis between those patients undergoing laser ablation alone and those having adjunctive balloon angioplasty revealed no significant differences of the baseline angiographic parameters, i.e., percent stenosis and minimal lumen diameter. Coronary occlusion after laser angioplasty occurred within 2–10 minutes later in 11 patients and was treated with balloon dilatation. The initial result immediately after laser angioplasty was 42 $\pm$ 15% degree of stenosis and 1.45 $\pm$ 0.55 mm minimal lumen diameter in these 11 patients. No significant differences between patients in whom complications ocurred and those with an uncomplicated procedure were found in regard of the baseline angiographic characteristics. In none of these patients angiographic evidence of intracoronary thrombi or severe dissection was found. Intracoronary nitroglycerin failed to relieve vessel closure in all cases. In 9 patients balloon angioplasty was successful with persistent patency of the target vessel. In two patients the vessel could not be reopened by balloon dilatation. Both patients developed Q-wave infarctions in the perfusion area of the target vessel with a rise in CK and CKMB.

One of the 9 patients with successful balloon dilatation after vessel occlusion following laser angioplasty developed anterior ST-T segment elevation, hypotension and ventricular tachycardia suggestive of abrupt vessel closure three hours after intervention and could not be resuscitated. Thus, percutaneous transluminal coronary excimer laser angioplasty was uncomplicated and successfully accomplished in 44 of 60 patients. In all 44 patients no significant EGG changes or rise in CK and CKMB levels indicative of distal embolisation occurred within the control period. All of these patients tolerated the intervention very well without symptoms like chest pain or burning sensations. There was no evidence of vessel perforation or extravasation of contrast medium in any patient.

In the subgroup of 11 patients with unstable angina laser irradiation of the ischemia related lesion was impossible in one patient, could be performed in 10 and was successful in 2 patients only. In the remaining 8 patients additional balloon angioplasty was necessary due to acute vessel closure in four patients and due to an insufficient result in the residual four patients. In five of these 8 patients additional balloon angioplasty was successful and the following clinical course unremarkable.

However, one patient of this group died early after the intervention and two patients experienced a myocardial infarction. Thus, all three serious complications occurred in patients with unstable angina.

Energy transmission of the laser catheter was found to be 30 ± 5 mJ/mm^2. Energy transmission was above the ablative threshold in all catheteres pre-intervention. Mean irradiation time was 123 ± 65 sec. Energy fluence after treatment was found to be 16 ± 10 mJ/mm^2. The decrease of transmitted energy did not seem to be dependent on lesion length and was furthermore independent on the initial energy transmission. Additionally, the angiographic success and incidence of complications was not dependent on the energy theshold of the catheter pre-and post intervention.

Discussion

This represents the first report on the combined use of intracoronary excimer laser angioplasty and balloon dilatation in a larger series of patients with coronary heart disease. The novel 1.3 mm fiberoptic laser delivery catheter proved effective in partially reducing high degree lesions and occlusions. All patients tolerated the intervention well without symptoms like chest pain or burning sensations. It seems that with careful technique the risk of perforation with this device in comparison to the bare fiber technique or thermal laser angioplasty [16–19] is minimal. The possibility of undue thrombogenesis cannot be ruled out in this series although we saw that the incidence of occluding thrombi seems to be low at least in the acute setting.

We were unable to cross the lesion in five patients due to tortuosities of the vasculature. Although only gentle pressure was used coronary spasm occurred at the distal end of the lesion most probably as a result of mechanical manipulations. These problems might be solved using more flexible catheters with improved steerability.

In this series 55 lesions were crossed during application of excimer laser energy and a definite lumen was produced. Interestingly, the lumen diameter achieved by excimer laser irradiation was larger than the diameter of the laser catheter itself. Further work, however, is needed to develop laser energy delivery devices which can provide a more definite lumen.

In the majority of our patients repeat coronary angiography demonstrated a still relevant residual lesion after laser ablation. To ensure an optimal result subsequent balloon angioplasty was performed in 32 patients which was complicated by late occlusion and cardiogenic shock due to plaque disruption and thrombus formation in one patient and by a transmural myocardial infarction in two patients.

The histologic specimen of the patient who died in cardiogenic shock suggest the occlusion being a result of balloon angioplasty. Additional injury by laser irradation, however, cannot be ruled out, since in the proximal part of the stenosis where ablation was performed fibrin formation and platelet deposition was noted. Since we encountered this serious problem after balloon angioplasty following laser ablation we feel that laser catheters with larger diameters are necessary to avoid additional balloon dilatation.

The lumen improvement compares favourably to the result achieved by conventional angioplasty [20, 21]. Taken together with prior experimental and clinical studies in peripheral vessels [8,22], the technique of percutaneous excimer laser angioplasty does have considerable potential in expanding the morphologic subsets in which angioplasty is feasible and, conceivably, may additionally diminish the incidence of restenosis. The morphometric results of the present study demonstrate that a larger lumen diameter could be achieved than the diameter of the catheter itself due to effective ablation during multiple irradiation cycles. After the first antegrade passage of the lesion a mean increase of 0.9 mm lumen diameter was achieved. During additional irradiation cycles further lumen improvement was observed in 12 patients and proved additional effective ablation of atherosclerotic tissue.

Irradiation time differed from 40 to 220 seconds and was not primarily dependent on lesion morphology. Even in some longer and subtotal lesions lumen improvement was considerable despite short irradiation. The difference in irradiation time necessary for an optimal angiographic result is most probably due to the varying components of the atherosclerotic plaque treated with excimer laser energy. Time to ablate plaque was found to be directly dependent on tissue characteristics like extent of calcification and amount of atherosclerotic material [23,24].

A further important factor for successful percutaneous transluminal coronary ablation was exact positioning of the catheter for irradiation of plaque. Intracoronary positioning is largely dependent on catheter flexibility. Fixation of the quartz fibers, however, results in a 3–5 mm long, stiff and inflexible catheter tip. Thus, the catheter has to be used as an over the wire system to avoid vessel injury. This disadvantage was expected to restrict ablation to concentric stenosis in vessels with minimal tortuosities. However, effective ablation and successful lumen improvement of eccentric lesions was found to be comparable to the ablation of concentric stenoses.

Although the technique of laser ablation is comparable to conventional balloon angioplasty two problems must be addressed. We saw an incidence of occlusive coronary spasm in 11 patients in spite of pretreatment with intracoronary nitroglycerin. Spasm occurred at the site of the lesion as well as in the distal segments and was reversible after additional application of vasodilators in all patients. Although spontaneous active vasoconstriction is well known from balloon angioplasty [25] the incidence of this complication was higher with laser irradiation. Thus, it can be hypothezised that the mechanism of early spasm after excimer laser ablation may have a different etiology than spasm following conventional angioplasty. Secondly, in some patients intraluminal lucencies were seen after successful ablation of plaque and suggest increased platelet aggregation at the site of tissue ablation. Coronary occlusion probably due to subsequent thrombus formation and spasm, was observed in 2 patients with a circumflex lesion and could not be prevented by intravenous heparin and nitroglycerin therapy.

Conclusions: The foregoing data in this pilot study lead us to conclude that (1) excimer laser angioplasty of coronary obtructive lesions is feasible, safe and effective and (2) subsequent balloon angioplasty is, at least in a subgroup of patients, unnecessary. The clinical impact of this new interventional technique, however, has to be assessed in further clinical investigations and has to be compared to the results of conventional balloon angioplasty and bypass surgery.

References

1. Grüntzig AR, Meier B (1983) Percutaneous transluminal coronary angioplasty. The first five years and the future. *Int J Cardiol* 2: 319–323.
2. Kent KM, Bentivoglio LG, Block PC, Bourassa MG, Cowley MJ, Dorros G, Detre KM, Gosselin AJ, Grüntzig AR, Kelsey SF, Mock MB, Mullin SM, Passamani ER, Myler RK, Simpson J, Stertzer SH, Van Raden MJ, Williams DO (1984) Long-term efficacy of percutaneous transluminal coronary angioplasty (PTCA): report from the National Heart, Lung and Blood Institute PTCA Registry. *Am J Cardiol* 53: 27C–31C.
3. Holmes DR, Vlietstra RE, Smith HC, Vetrovec GW, Kent KM, Cowley MJ, Faxon DP, Grüntzig AR, Kelsey SF, Detre KM, Van Raden MJ, Mock MB (1984) Restenosis after percutaneous transluminal coronary angioplasty (PTCA): a report from the PTCA Registry of the National Heart, Lung, and Blood Institute. *Am J Cardiol* 53: 77C–81C.
4. Spears JR (1987) Percutaneous transluminal coronary angioplasty restenosis: potential prevention with laser balloon angioplasty. *Am J Cardiol* 60: 61B–64B.
5. Sanborn TA (1988) Laser angioplasty: what has been learned from experimental studies and clinical trials? *Circulation* 78: 769–774.
6. Linsker R, Srinivasan R, Wynne JJ, Alonso Dr (1984) Farultraviolet laser ablation of atherosclerotic lesions. *Lasers Surg Med* 4: 201–206.
7. Grundfest WS, Litvack F, Forrester JS, Goldenberg T, Swan HJC, Morgenstern L, Fishbein M, McDermind S, Rider DM, Pacala TJ, Laudenslager JB (1985) Laser ablation of human atherosclerotic plaque without adjacent tissue injury. *J Am Coll Cardiol* 5: 929–933.
8. Grundfest WS, Litvak IF, Goldenberg T, Sherman T, Morgenstern L, Carroll R, Fishbein M, Forrester J, Margitan J, McDermind S, Pacala TJ, Rider DM, Laudenslager JB (1985) Pulsed ultraviolet lasers and the potential for safe laser angioplasty. *Am J Surg* 50: 220–226.
9. Murphy-Chutorian D, Selzer PM, Kosek J, Quay SC, Profitt D, Ginsburg R (1986) The interaction between excimer laser energy and vascular tissue. *Am J Cardiol* 112: 739–745.
10. Abela GS, Normann S, Cohen D, Feldman RL, Geiser EA, Conti CR (1982) Effects of carbon dioxide, Nd-YAG and argon laser radiation on coronary atheromatour plaques. *Am J Cardiol* 50: 1199–1204.
11. Lee G, Ikeda R, Herman C (1983) The quantitative effects of laser irradiation on human atherosclerotic disease. *Am Heart J* 105: 885–889.

12. Abela GS, Norman SJ, Cohen DM, Franzini D, Feldman RL, Crea F, Fenech A, Pepine CH, Conti CR (1985) Laser recanalization of occluded atherosclerotic arteries in vivo and in vitro. *Circulation* 71: 403–411.
13. Haase KK, Wehrmann M, Walz R, Duda S, Karsch KR (1990) Intracoronary excimer laser angioplasty: study on postmortem hearts with angiographic control. *Z Kardiol* 79: 183–88.
14. Karsch KR, Haase KK, Mauser M, Ickrath O, Voelker W, Duda S, Seipel L (1989) Percutaneous coronary excimer laser angioplasty: initial clinical results. *Lancet*: 8664, Vol. II, 647–650.
15. Karsch KR, Haase KK, Mauser M, Voelker W (1989) Initial angiographic results in ablation of atherosclerotic plaque by percutaneous coronary excimer laser angioplasty without subsequent balloon dilatation. *Am J Cardiol* 64: 1253–1257.
16. Sanborn TA, Faxon DP, Haudenschild C, Ryan TJ (1985) Experimental angioplasty: circumferential distribution of laser thermal energy with a laser probe. *J Am Coll Cardiol* 5: 934–939.
17. Abela GS, Normann SJ, Cohen DM, Franzini D, Feldman RL, Crea F, Fenech A, Pepine CH, Conti CR (1985) Laser recanalization of occluded atherosclerotic arteries in vivo and in vitro. *Circulation* 71: 403–407.
18. Choy DSJ, Stertzer SH, Myler RK, Marco J, Fourunial G (1984) Human coronary laser recanalization. *Clin Cardiol* 7: 337–343.
19. Ginsburg R, Wexler L, Mitchell RS, Proffit D (1985) Percutaneous transluminal laser angioplasty for treatment of peripheral vascular disease: clinical experience with 16 patients. *Radiology* 156: 619–626.
20. Grüntzig AR, Senning A, Siegenthaler WE (1979) Nonoperative dilatation of coronary artery stenosis. *N Engl J Med* 301: 61–68.
21. Kent KM, Bentivoglio LG, Block PC (1982) Percutaneous transluminal coronary angioplasty: report from the Registry of the NHLBI. *Am J Cardiol* 49: 2011–2020.
22. Abela GS, Seeger JM, Barbieri E, Franzini D, Fenech A, Pepine CJ, Conti CR (1986) Laser angioplasty with angioscopic guidance in humans. *JACC* 8: 184–192.
23. Müller G, Berlien HP, Biamino B, Dörschel K, Kar H (1988) Photoablation threshold of human aorta as a function of wavelength, in: Waidelich W, Waidelich R (eds), *Laser Optoelectronics in Medicine*. pp. 38–41. Proceedings of the 7th Congress of the International Society for Laser Surgery and Medicine in connection with Laser 87 Optoelectronics. Berlin-Tokyo: Springer.
24. Murphy-Chutorian D, Selzer PM, Kosek J, Quay SC, Profitt D, Ginsburg R (1986) The interaction between excimer laser energy and vascular tissue. *Am Heart J* 112: 739–745.
25. Fischell TA, Derley G, Tse TM, Stadius ML (1988) Coronary artery vasoconstriction routinely occurs after percutaneous transluminal coronary angioplasty. *Circulation* 78: 1323–1334.

8. Excimer-laser coronary angioplasty: clinical experience with high-grade stenosis and recanalization of chronic occlusions

G. S. WERNER, A. BUCHWALD, C. UNTERBERG, E. VOTH.
H. KREUZER and V. WIEGAND

Summary

A high restenosis rate of conventional coronary angioplasty (PTCA) and an even higher reocclusion rate of recanalized vessels encourages the development of new interventional techniques. Percutaneous Excimer laser angioplasty (PTLA) provides an alternative technique to ablate the obliterating atherosclerotic plaque without thermal damage to the surrounding tissue.

Laser energy of a pulsed XeCl Excimer Laser (308 nm, pulse width 55 ns) was transmitted via multifiber-catheters (MF) or 4–6 F diameter containing 20–40 fibers á 100 μm and a central lumen for a guide-wire. In 10 patients, examined 1–6 months after coronary occlusion, and in 14 patients with high-grade ($> = 90\%$) stenosis, PTLA successfully reopened the vessel lumen to the width of the MF (1.4–2.0 mm) leaving a residual stenosis of 42 ± 13%. The pulse energy ranged from 5 mJ (4 F MF) to 16 mJ (6 F MF), the total pulse count was 6872 ± 3242 with a pulse repetition rate of 10–20 Hz. No complications such as vessel perforation were observed. To reduce the residual stenosis to less than 30%, PTLA was followed by PTCA in 17/24 cases. After PTCA 5/17 vessels showed angiographic evidence of varying degrees of dissection. Angiographic control after 24 h showed reocclusion in 2/10 recanalizations, and no deterioration of the primary result of the PTLA-treated stenosis.

PTLA promises to be a safe and feasible alternative to conventional PTCA for the treatment of high-grade stenosis and coronary occlusions. However, long term results have to be awaited to evaluate the potential benefit of PTLA over PTCA, but further advancements in catheter design towards PTLA without the need for additional PTCA are required.

Introduction

Percutaneous transluminal coronary angioplasty is the standard technique for the nonsurgical treatment of symptomatic coronary heart disease [1].

V. Hombach et al. (eds), Interventional Techniques in Cardiovascular Medicine, 73–80.

While the advances in balloon technologies have increased the immediate success rate, the long term outcome is limited by the high rate of restenosis, which is even more discouraging for recanalized coronary arteries [2].

Presently, two principle alternative methods to improve the long term results are under clinical investigation: mechanical devices (atherectomy, rotablation) and laser devices. The technological difficulties of laser transmission [3] have now been overcome by the development of multifiber catheter systems which are flexible enough to be advanced into coronary arteries, and which achieve a sufficient energy fluence to reach the ablation threshold of atherosclerotic tissue.

After having become familiar with the application of laser angioplasty in peripheral occlusive arterial disease [4]. We report on our clinical experience with coronary laser angioplasty in patients with severe coronary stenosis and symptomatic coronary occlusions.

Method

Study group

Percutaneous coronary laser angioplasty was performed in 24 patients according to a protocol approved of by the university's commission on

Table 1a. Laser angioplasty of coronary occlusions (0)

Pat	Age/ sex	CAD	Vessel	Infarct	Occl. since	pre PTLA	post PTLA	addit. PTCA	Cath Size	Power pre	power post	Pulse-count	Frequency (Hz)
01	51 m	1	RCA	HWI	1	100	80	yes	4	4.0	3.5	4091	15
02	63 f	1	CX	LI	6	100	75	yes	4	2.5	0.0	8631	15
03	60 m	2	CX	HWI	2	100	65	yes	4	6.0	6.0	12130	20
04	54 m	3	RCA	HWI	3	100	60	yes	4	5.5	5.5	4060	20
05	69 m	3	RCA	no	3	100	50	yes	4	5.8	3.5	11520	20
06	78 m	1	RIVA	VWI	2	100	60	yes	4	6.5	4.0	6280	20
07	44 m	1	RCA	HWI	4	100	65	yes	5	12.0	8.5	4520	20
08	52 m	3	RCA	HWI	na	100	60	yes	5	11.0	8.0	6940	20
09	71 f	3	RIVA	no	2	100	70	yes	5	10.0	7.5	4000	20
010	53 m	2	CX	LI	1	100	45	no	5	11.0	4.0	4810	20
x	60				2.7	100	63		4F/5F	5.1/11	3.8/7	6671	
±SD	11				1,6		11			1.5/0.8	2.1/2.0	3075	

Summary of clinical and technical data of PTLA. CAD = number of vessels with significant stenosis; Occl. since indicates the time in months since occlusion was detected or suspected because of the date of a previous myocardial infarction. The percent reduction of vessel lumen diameter is given before (pre PTLA) and after (post. PTLA); addit. PTCA indicates the succession of PTLA by conventional balloon angioplasty; the power of the employed catheters (4 and 5F) is given in mJ before (pre) and after (post) performing PTLA with the catheter; the number of pulses/frequency yields the time of lasing in seconds.

Table 1b. Laser angioplasty of coronary stenoses (S)

pat	Age/ sex	CAD	Vessel	Infarct	Pre PTLA	Post PTLA	Addit. PTCA	Cath size	Power pre	Power post	Pulse-count	Frequency (Hz)
S1	65 f	1	RIVA	no	90	55	no	4	5.0	2.5	7250	20
S2	62 m	2	RIVA	VWI	80	60	yes	4	5.0	5.0	3060	20
S3	61 m	1	RIVA	no	90	50	no	4	4.0	4.0	1060	20
S4	60 m	1	RCX	no	95	75	yes	4	5.5	1.0	9020	20
S5	36 m	1	RIVA	VWI	90	65	yes	4	6.0	2.0	12660	20
S6	62 m	1	RCA	HWI	85	60	yes	6	16.0	14.0	4440	20
S7	60 m	2	RCA	HWI	85	50	no	6	14.0	11.0	1680	20
S8	73 f	1	RCA	no	95	65	yes	5	8.0	9.5	3200	20
S9	44 m	1	RIVA	no	95	40	no	5	12.0	11.0	4400	20
S10	57 m	3	CX	no	85	50	no	5	10.0	6.5	5900	20
S11	50 m	2	RIVA	VWInQ	90	60	yes	5	12.0	0.0	3400	20
S12	66 m	2	RIVA	VWI	85	60	yes	5	11.0	2.0	8480	20
S13	61 f	1	CX	no	90	90	yes	5	11.0	6.5	4700	20
S14	76 f	1	RIVA	no	90	50	no	5	11.0	11.0	3600	20
x	60				89	57		4F/5F	5.1/10.8	2.9/6.6	5204	
±SD	11				5	9			0.7/1.4	1.6/4.3	3175	

For abbreviations see Table 1a.

ethical standards in medical research; all patients had given written consent. After the diagnostic angiography patients were selected for laser angioplasty if a high-grade stenosis ($> = 90\%$ diameter narrowing) was found, and at least one of two noninvasive tests (thallium scintigraphy and/or bicycle ergometer ECG) indicated the significance of the lesion for the occurrence of ischaemia during exercise. Similarly, in patients with complete occlusion of a vessel, the occurrence of ST segment changes or exercise induced ischemia during thallium scintigraphy were required to make them eligible for laser recanalization. Table 1 summarizes the clinical data of patients with chronic occlusion and high-grade stenosis.

Laser source

Laser angioplasty was performed by using a XeCl-Excimer Laser (MAX 10, Fa. Technolas) emitting pulsed laser energy of 50-120 mJ/pulse at a wave length of 308 nm. The pulse width was 58 ns, and the pulse repetition was selectable between 2 and 40 Hz. A 4 or 5 F multifiber catheter system was coupled with the laser source, consisting of 15 to 28 quartz fibers of 100 µm concentrically aligned around a central lumen for a 14 to 18/1000 inch guide wire. The transmitted pulse energy ranged from 4–6 mJ for the 4 F catheter to 10–12mJ for the 5 F system. The calculated energy density per fiber surface was 42–51 mJ/mm^2.

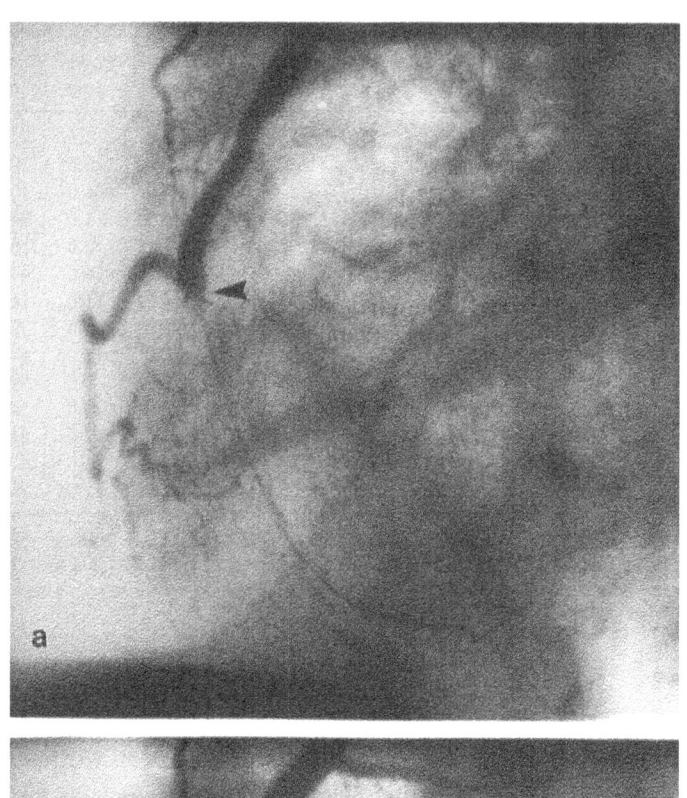

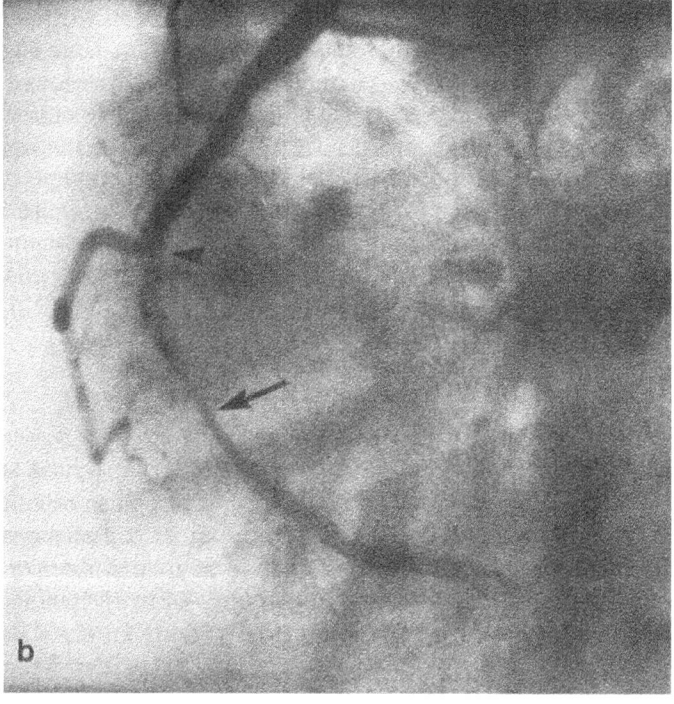

Procedure

To avoid perforation of the vessel wall a guide wire system was applied. For both recanalization of occlusions and angioplasty of stenosis it was required to pass a 14/1000 or 18/1000 inch guide wire through the lesion. If necessary, a recanalization guide wire was used. Then the laser catheter of 4–5 F outer diameter (see Table 1) was placed next to the vessel lesion or occlusion and lasing started at a constant frequency of 20 Hz. The individual data of energy transmitted and lasing time is summarized in Table 1. After the laser angioplasty a biplane control angiogram was taken, and according to the degree of the residual stenosis it was decided whether to follow laser angioplasty by additional balloon angioplasty or not. Routine control angiograms were taken after 24 hours.

Statistical analysis

Group means of numerical data are expressed as mean ± standard deviation. The vessel obstruction was described as maximum percent lumen diameter narrowing as compared with the average of pre and poststenotic segment diameters. The assessment was done with a caliper by an independent observer not involved in the laser procedure.

Results

Percutaneous laser coronary angioplasty (PTLA) was performed in 24 patients. In 10 patients with total occlusions the average residual stenosis after lasing was 63% (Table 1a). In all but one patients a balloon angioplasty succeeded PTLA in order to achieve a residual stenosis of less than 30%. In 2 patients the 24 hour control angiogram showed a reocclusion (Table 1a: 04 and 05), while in 8 patients the vessel remained open. In these latter patients the pre PTLA findings of localized ischemia in the target vessel region provided by bicycle ergometer and/or thallium scintigraphy had improved. Figure 1 shows one patient with a chronic occlusion of the right coronary artery (inferior infarction 4 months before PTLA). After PTLA the residual stenosis was still significant, and therefore a PTCA followed the laser recanalization.

In 14 patients a high grade stenosis (average 89%) was treated by PTLA. There was only one case in which the laser catheter could not be advanced

Figure 1. Chronic coronary occlusion (arrow head) in a 44 year old man with inferior infarction four months before angiography. After passage of the occlusion by 14/1000[11] guide wire (a) lasing with a 5 F catheter lead to reopening of the vessel lumen (b) with a significant residual stenosis (arrow). Lasing was therefore followed by conventional balloon angioplasty (not shown).

through the stenosis. Here, a sharp angle of the circumflex artery branch from the main stem made it impossible to advance the catheter close enough towards the obstruction to achieve contact of the fiber surface and the plaque (Table 1b: S13).

After lasing the residual stenosis was 57%. Therefore in 8 of 14 procedures an additional balloon angioplasty followed lasing, to further reduce the vessel obstruction below 30%. Vasospasm or acute occlusion during PTLA was not observed, local dissections were not observed as well. In contrast, after conventional balloon angioplasty local dissections were observed, and in one case had to be treated by a balloon expandable stent (Table 1b: S8). The primary success after PTLA was such that no balloon angioplasty was performed; an exercise test before discharge showed no sign of exercise ischemia in contrast to the pre PTLA test.

The duration of lasing depended on the passage of the laser catheter across the obstruction. If the residual stenosis was no longer completely occluded by the catheter, it was assumed, that further lasing would not induce a further enlargement of the lumen, as the laser effect depends on a slight contact with the target tissue without inhibition by hemoglobin. Thus, the effective time of lasing ranged from 53 to 630 s (mean: 298 s).

During PTLA angina pectoris was observed only during immediate occlusion of the residual lumen by the catheter itself, no matter whether lasing was performed. Peripheral occlusion of small coronary branches was not observed, and none of the patients showed increase in serum creatinine kinase after the procedure.

In the two groups of patients treated by Excimer Laser Coronary Angioplasty alone or in conjunction with conventional balloon angioplasty we observed only one major complication, which was caused by a guide wire loop leading to a local wall dissection (Table 1a: S9). During the following procedures only completely radio opaque guide wires were used, and no such problem reoccurred.

Discussion

The ablation of atherosclerotic lesions by laser energy can be achieved either by a thermal effect when using visible or infrared wave lengths of Nd-YAG or Argon laser sources, or by a so called photoablative effect of pulsed ultraviolet excimer laser sources [5]. The latter has the advantage of minor damage to adjacent tissue because of the negligible amount of heat that is produced during lasing [6]. It is also expected to avoid coronary spasm and thrombosis [7]. Furthermore, the transmitted excimer laser energy is high enough to ablate calcified plaques, in contrast to thermal laser techniques [8]. The application of this new technique had been previously shown to be feasible and safe in human peripheral artery disease [4]. Now there are miniaturized catheters of 4 to 6 F outer diameter available that can be used in the coronary artery system. Multiple, concentrically arranged fibers provide a good flexibility and still enough energy transmission for the ablation of atherosclerotic plaques.

For this initial clinical study to test the feasibility of PTLA in coronary arteries we chose two groups of patients with a relatively high risk of restenosis after conventional PTCA: patients with chronic occlusions, and patients with proximal high grade stenosis [1,2]. The complications observed during PTLA were not laser associated (one guide wire caused dissection), and most of them were due to the necessity of additional balloon angioplasty leading to localized wall dissections. The latter problem is inherent of PTCA, which emphasizes the need for the development of a stand-alone laser angioplasty. This would enable us to compare the potential benefits of lasing without adjacent tissue damage with balloon angioplasty.

Presently there were two major problems that became obvious during this study: firstly, the geometry of the laser catheter limits the achievable vessel lumen and restricts its applicability to concentric lesions; secondly, the lasing effect required the contact of the fiber surface and the target lesion, possibly leading to a loss of transmittable energy during the procedure by causing damage to the fibers. The use of a guide wire to align the catheter within the center of the vessel lumen was necessary to avoid the danger of vessel perforation. On the other hand, this lead to primary failures of recanalization as the guide wire could not pass the stenosis. These patients could be treated by laser angioplasty only if a guiding system would be applied that could detect atherosclerotic plaques. While such systems are tested in vitro [9] and in peripheral vessels [10], the applicability to the coronary system with the specific problem of moving vessels in the beating heart lies in the future.

At the present time it is felt that the advantage of ablating atherosclerotic plaques with only minor damage to the adjacent tissue and vessel wall by this new technique is still hampered by technological problems of the catheter design, which frequently requires additional balloon angioplasty. In order to assess the potential benefit of laser angioplasty, these limitations have to be overcome to enable a comparative large scale study with conventional balloon angioplasty.

References

1. Guidelines for percutaneous transluminal coronary angioplasty (1988) A report of the American College of Cardiology/American Heart Association task force on assessment of diagnostic and therapeutic cardiovascular procedures. *Circulation* 78: 486.
2. Liu MW, Roubin GS, King SB (1989) Restenosis after coronary angioplasty. *Circulation* 79: 1374.
3. Allison SW, Gillies GT, Magnuson GW, Pagano TS (1985) Pulsed laser damage to optical fibers. *Appl Opt* 24: 3140.
4. Werner GS, Buchwald A, Romatowski J v et al. (1989) Percutaneous transluminal excimer laser angioplasty in the treatment of peripheral vascular disease: preliminary results. *Dtsch med Wschr* 114: 1271.

5. Forrester JS, Litvack F. Grundfest WS (1986) Laser angioplasty and cardiovascular disease. *Am J Cardiol* 57: 990.
6. Isner JM, Donaldson RF, Deckelbaum LI et al. (1985) The excimer laser: gross, light microscopic and ultrastructural analysis of potential advantages for use in laser therapy of cardiovascular disease. *JACC* 6: 1102.
7. Steg PG, Rongione AJ, Gal D, DeJesus ST, Clarke RH, Isner JM (1989) Pulsed ultraviolet laser irradiation produces endothelium-independent relaxation of vascular smooth muscle. *Circulation* 79: 189.
8. Murphy-Chutorian D, Seltzer PM, Kosek J, Quay SC, Profitt D, Ginsburg R (1986) The interaction between excimer laser energy and vascular tissue. *Am Heart J* 112: 739.
9. Laufer G. Wollenek G, Hohla K et al. (1988) Excimer laser-induced simultaneous ablation and spectral identification of normal and atherosclerotic arterial tissue layers. *Circulation* 78: 1031.
10. Geschwind HJ. Dubois-Rande JL, Bonner FR, Boussignac G, Prevosti LG, Leon MB (1988) Percutaneous pulsed laser angioplasty with atheroma detection in humans (abstract). *JACC* 11: 107A.

9. High speed arteriosclerotic lesion ablation for treatment of coronary artery disease

R. ERBEL, M. HAUDE, U. DIETZ, P. STÄHR,
H. J. RUPPRECHT, R. ZOTZ and J. MEYER

Summary

Percutaneous high frequency coronary rotablation using the rotablator is able to remove arteriosclerotic material from the vessel wall. A diamond-coated (15–30 μm) brass burr drill fastened to a flexible drive shaft rotating and tracking along a coaxial guide wire is used. The turbine rotates the drive shaft at 150,000–180,000 rpm. High speed rotational angioplasty was successful in 27 of 28 patients. In about 40%, additional PTCA was necessary due to limited experience with the deuce and limited diameter of burr initially. Only one patient went to bypass surgery and myocardial infarction (CK < 150 u/l) occurred in only one of 28 patients. No vessel perforation was observed. All vessels were open at 24 hours post-procedure. By cineventro-culography, echocardiography and 201-Thallium-scintigraphy no signs of peripheral embolism induced myocardial ischemia were detected. Also, coronary flow reserve was not reduced, but increased, similar to the effect observed after PTCA. Side effects were coronary spasm in 7/28 patients, bradycardia in 5/28 and AV block in 1/28 patients possible related to microbubbles. An important indication for high frequency rotational angioplasty seems to be rigid sclerotic lesions, which cannot be treated by a conventional balloon catheter. Future studies will judge the restenosis rate of this method.

Introduction

One of the most important problems of PTCA [21, 22] is the high restenosis rate in patients with stable angina of 20–35% [3, 9, 20, 24, 27, 28, 31, 32, 35, 37, 38, 44, 45, 59] and with unstable angina pectoris of 30–40% [17, 37, 38, 44] reaching 55% in smokers [20]. In patients with chronic occlusions and successful recanalization, restenosis rate is about 50% [10, 23, 31, 50]. Also after myocardial infarction high restenosis rates were observed [13, 36]. In order to reduce restenosis rate acetylsalicylic acid [49], calcium

V. Hombach et al. (eds), Interventional Techniques in Cardiovascular Medicine, 81–93.
© 1991 *Kluwer Academic Publishers.*

82   R. Erbel et al.

antagonists [63] and molsidomine [5] were used, but unsuccessfully. Others suggested, that prolonged dilation time would increase success rate and decrease restenosis rate, but prolonged balloon inflation times (up to 10 min) using premedication with nitroglycerine and nifedipine was not effective in reducing restenosis rate [11]. Also the use of special designed catheters for continuous coronary perfusion and prolonged PTCA was not able to reduce restenosis rate [9, 11, 12]. Other methods are stent implantation [16, 39–41, 46, 47, 48, 51, 53].

In order to increase the success rate of recanalization of chronic occluded vessels and reduce the restenosis rate, laser [1, 29], high frequency [25, 56], and alternative mechanical methods were developed. Using these methods, intimal or medial dissections, which occur during PTCA [7, 26, 33, 34, 62] should be avoided. Nearly all systems use rotation. At the catheter tips balls, burrs or cutting devices are mounted [30, 50, 51, 54, 55, 57, 60, 61]. One of the most promising devices is high speed rotational angioplasty [2, 7, 8, 13, 14, 15, 18, 19, 43].

Methods

High frequency rotational angioplasty, developed by David Auth, Washington, has been used in experiments and peripheral arteries [2, 43].

ROTABLATOR

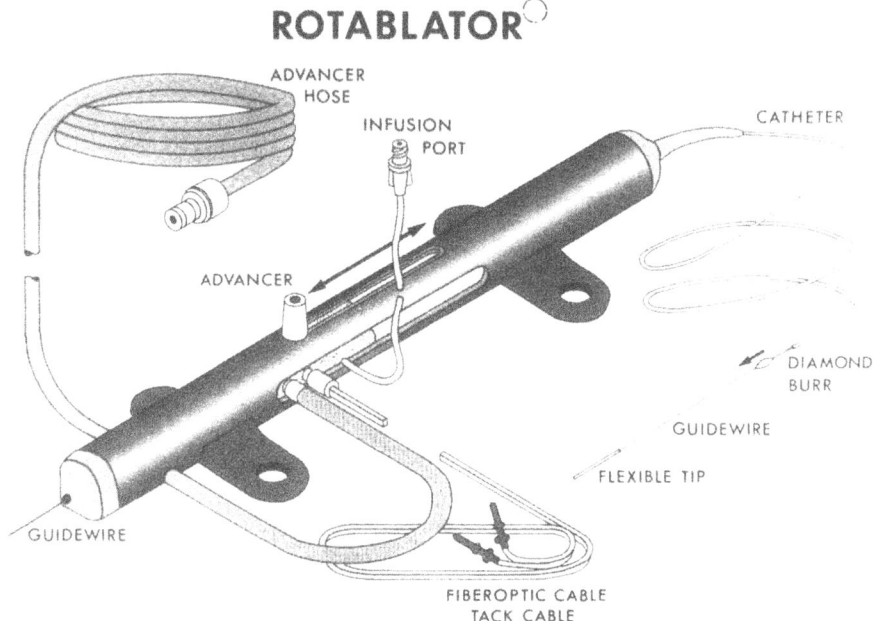

Figure 1. Schematic drawing of the Rotablator with demonstration of the pressure air line, the infusion line, the fiberoptic cable, the advancing knob and the guide wire with the diamond-coated burr.

The Rotablator^R has a diamond-coated burr fastened to a flexible drive shaft that rotates and tracks along a central coaxial guide wire (0.009 inch) (Figure 1). 15–30 μm diamond chips are inbedded in the nickel/brass burr. The drive shaft is encased within a protective plastic sheath to form a system capable of delivery as a flexible catheter. The drive shaft is connected to a turbine and driven by compressed air. The turbine rotates the drive shaft at 150–180,000 rpm. A fiberoptic light probe measures the number of revolutions per minute (rpm) which is displayed on a control panel and recorded on a stripchart recorder. The speed can be controlled by a dial on the control panel. The turbine also pumps sterile saline irrigation solution into the plastic sheath to lubricate and cool the rotating drive shaft and burr at a rate of 12 ml/s. By moving the control knob on the top of the plastic casing the operator can advance the burr along the guide wire. There is no electrical contact between the system and the patient so that a high safety level is provided [14].

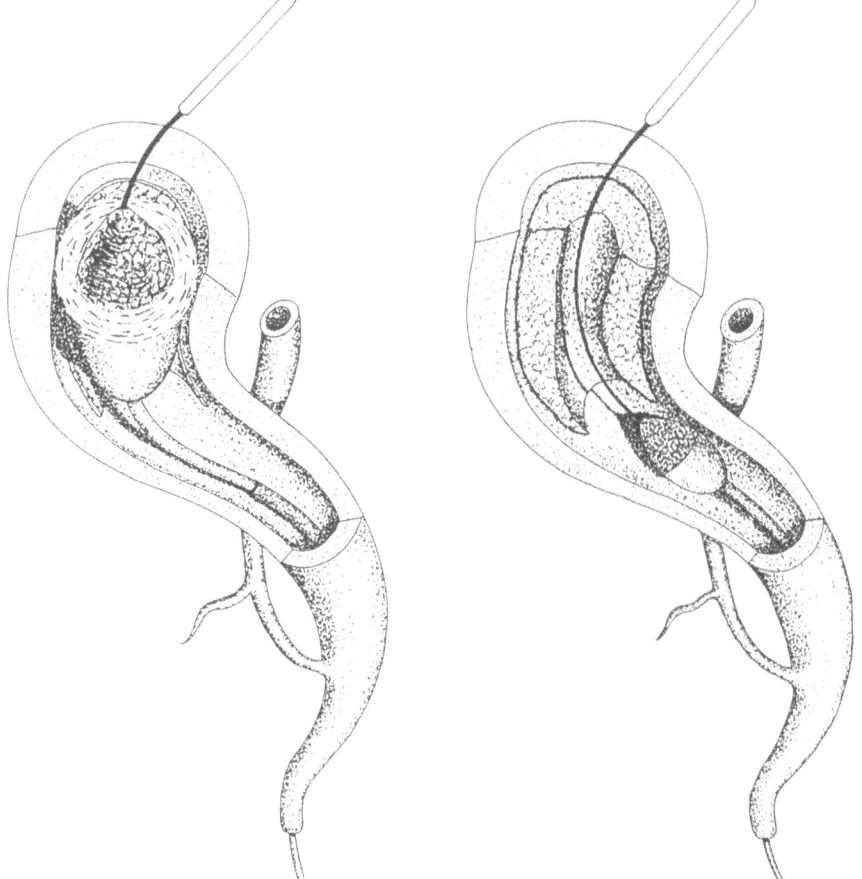

Figure 2   Schematic drawing of the effect of the Rotablator on arteriosclerotic plaques reducing arteriosclerotic plaque by micro-ablation

Mechanism

The mechanism of action of high speed rotation angioplasty is by ablation of arteriosclerotic lesions. Arteriosclerotic plaque material is converted into particles of which are > 90% smaller than erythrocytes [2] (Figure 2). In order to analyze the safety of the system the Rotablator™ was used in pig hearts with normal coronary arteries and postmortem arteriosclerotic human hearts [7, 8, 14, 42]. An important advantage is that intima and media dissections can be avoided. They are only found, when the burr is pushed too hard so that a Dotter effect or excessive rotational shear force is induced [14].

Premedication and procedure

Premedication consists of 20 ml dextran (Promit°) as hapten and 100 ml/l Rheomacrodex°, intravenous injection of 10,000 IU heparine, 1,000 IU heparine/h, 3 mg/h nitroglycerine and 0.5 mg/h nifedipine. The guide wire is placed in the coronary artery and advanced distal to the lesion, the burr is advanced over the guidewire with a minimum speed of 150,000 rpm. The speed is limited by the driving pressure of the turbine which was not allowed

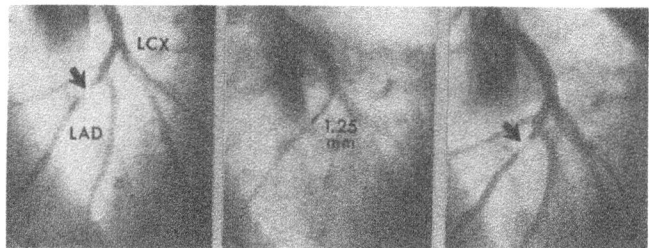

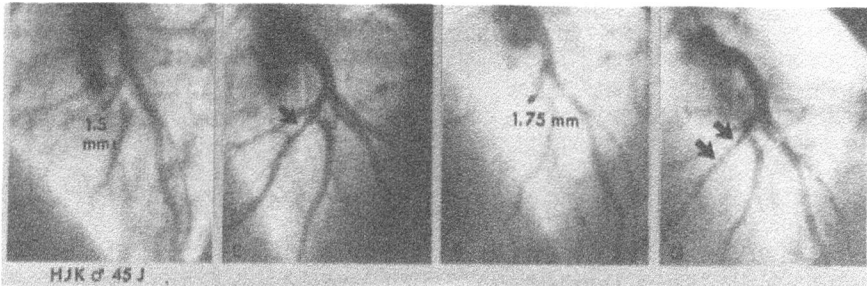

Figure 3.   Stenosis of left anterior descending (LAD) coronary artery (A) with successful use of the Rotablator, first with a 1.25 mm burr (B/C) then with a 1.5 mm burr (D/E) and 1.75 mm burr (F/G).

to exceed 60 psi. The burr size ranged between 1.25 and 2.0 mm. After early experience we now start with a 1.25 mm burr increasing the burr size to 1.5, 1.75 and 2 mm in order to avoid any Dotter effect leading to a dissection of the vessel. Large guiding catheters (9 F, Interventional Medical Systems) are used [14].

Meanwhile 28 patients have been treated with a success rate of more than 90% using the same criteria of success as described for PTCA. Typical examples are shown in Figures 3 and 4. The mean coronary luminal stenosis was reduced from 82 ± 17% to 37 ± 14%. In about 40% of our patients additional angioplasty could not be avoided (Figure 5). The final luminal stenosis measured 26 ± 15%. The main reason for using additional angioplasty was the limited experience with high speed rotablation and the limited range of burr sizes available initially. It appears, that hard, sclerotic lesions can be treated most effectively as also described by others [19].

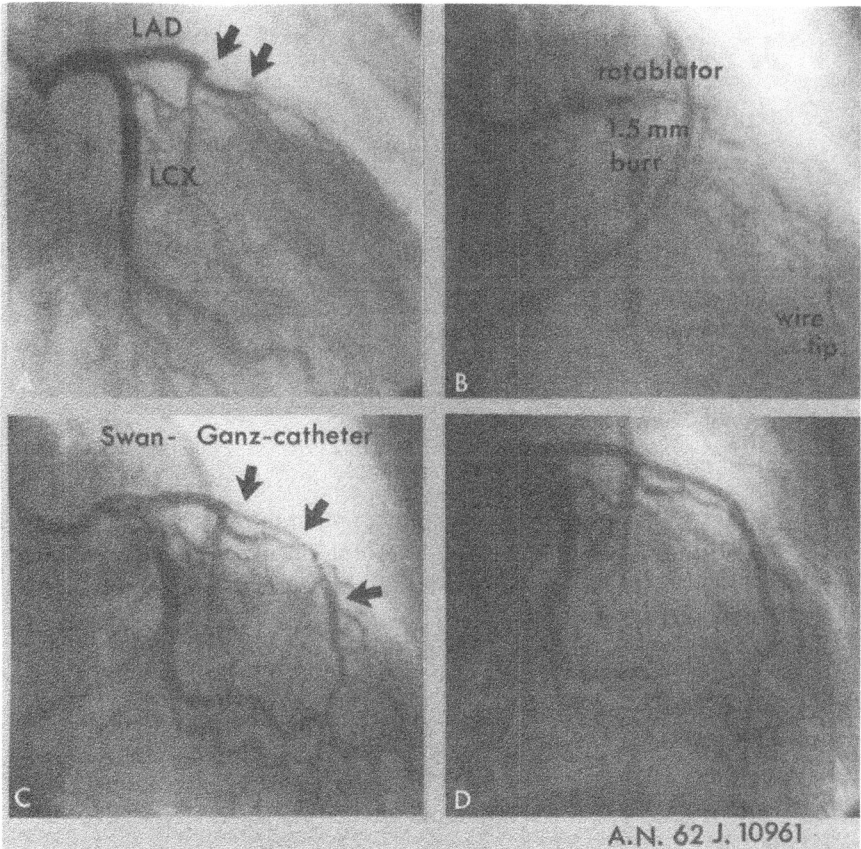

Figure 4. Occluded left anterior descending coronary artery (LAD) (A) with successful reopening with a 1.5 mm burr (B). The control angiogram is shown in C. After additional PTCA an excellent result is visible (D).

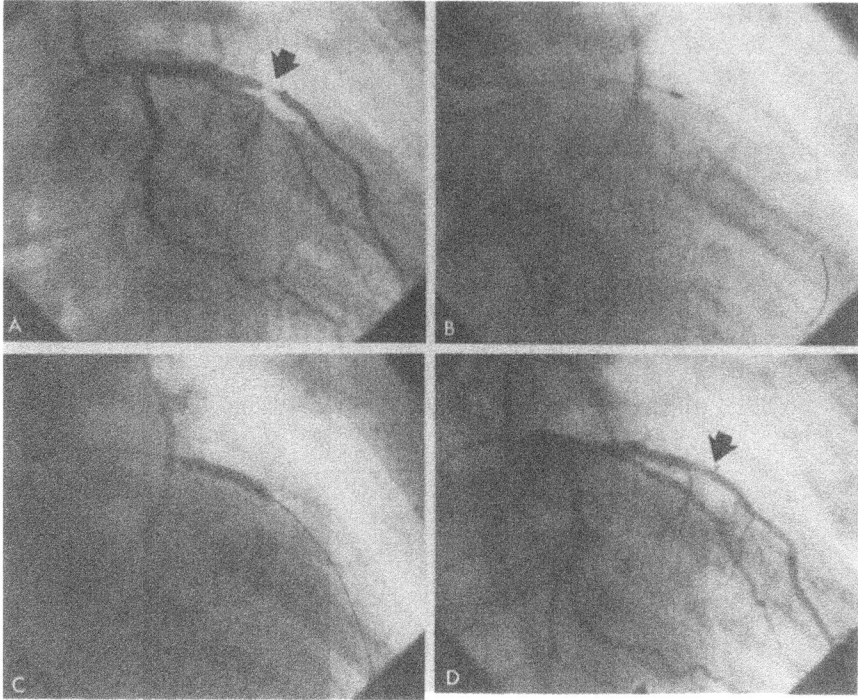

E.K.54J. 11064

Figure 5.   Proximal LAD stenosis before and with treatment with a 1.25 mm burr (A/B). After usage of a balloon (C) successful luminal increase occurs (D). Balloon dilation was used because of coronary spasm and angina pectoris.

Side effects and complications

Symptoms
During the procedure the patients did not complain of any discomfort. After numerous periods of treatment with different burrs, 5 patients reported chest pain different from usual angina lasting for up to 20 min without ECG changes or CK elevation.

ECG
ECG remained unchanged in most patients, but showed transient ST-segment depression in 8 patients similar to PTCA, disappearing during a recovery period of 30–60s. Persistent changes with CK elevation (n = 2) occurred with negative T wave development.

Embolism
The danger of peripheral embolism of arteriosclerotic or thrombotic material is principally possible with all mechanical and thermal devices

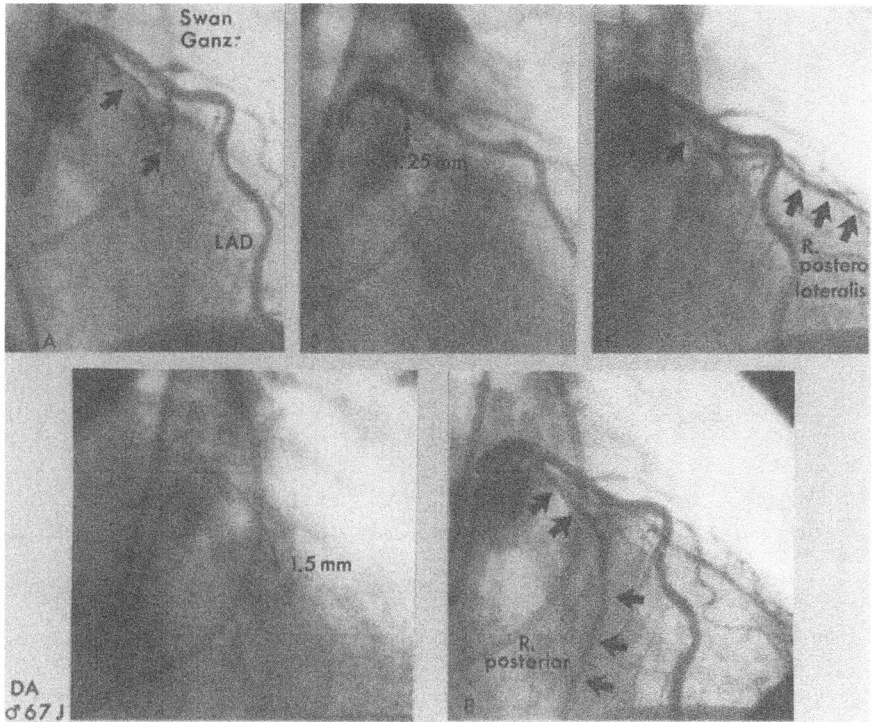

Figure 6. Occluded left circumflex coronary artery and proximal subtotal occlusion (A). Improvement of coronary lesion with 1.25 mm burr and reperfused postero-lateral branch (C), opening of the posterior branch with a 1.5 mm burr (D) and excellent first result (E).

including laser angioplasty [25, 55, 56]. In only one of our patients was an embolism of a side branch of a diagonal coronary artery observed with CK elevation up to 150 U/l.

Perforation
Perforation was not seen. According to experimental studies with high speed rotational angioplasty, perforation has to be taken considered [2]. It cannot be excluded, that one observed pericarditis was due to an adventitia touching of the device in a patient with an occluded left circumflex coronary artery (Figure 6). The danger of perforation is much higher with laser angioplasty. Perforations are rare but can also be observed after PTCA [26] and are a possible danger for medium speed rotational angioplasty [30], where a guide wire is not used. Perforation can be caused with high speed, guidewire directed angioplasty if the burr size selected is larger than the native artery.

Coronary dissection
Coronary dissection was observed in one patient, who had to be sent to surgery (Figure 7). This complication is well known for balloon angioplasty

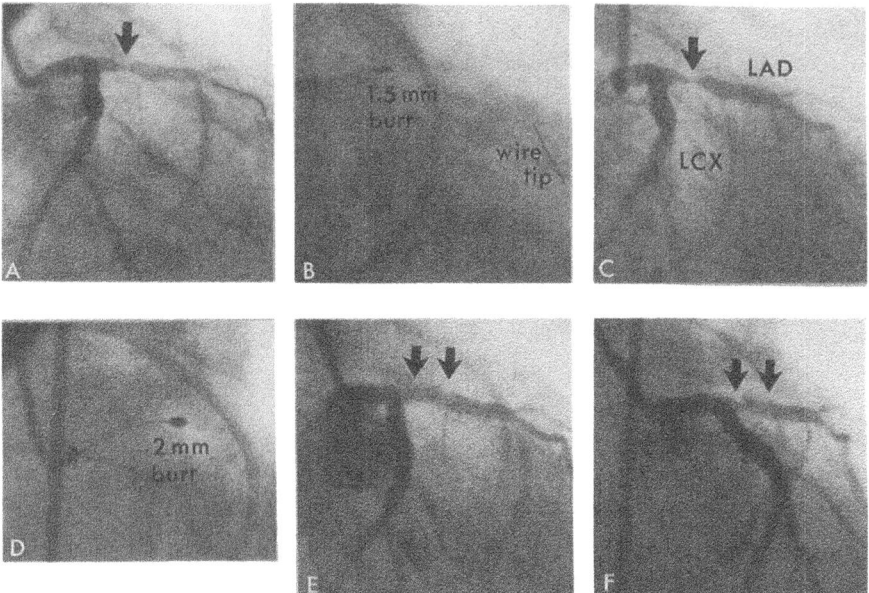

Figure 7.   Proximal lesion of the left anterior descending coronary artery (A) during and after usage of an 1.5 mm burr. After usage of 2.0 mm burr irregular surface (D/E) and flow reduction. Patient went to surgery.

[4, 33, 34, 35, 58, 62] and is observed by angiography in 10–20% of the PTCA patients and by autopsy in nearly all PTCA specimens [6, 52]. For rotational angioplasty stand-by surgery is also necessary.

Coronary spasm
Coronary spasm was observed in 2 of 28 patients. This rate is much lower than the intermittent observed occlusion rate of 20% of coronary vessels using excimer lasers [29], also related to coronary spasm.

Wall motion
The analysis of left ventricular volumes and regional wall motion before and after the procedure demonstrated that no myocardial ischemia induced by ablation of arteriosclerotic material and peripheral embolism occurred. Only in the patient with embolism and CK elevation (< 150 U/l) was a circumscript wall motion abnormality observed [14].

201-Thallium scintigrams demonstrated improved perfusion and no newly developed perfusion defects. Also coronary Doppler flow measurement showed an improvement of flow reserve and not a decline.

Microcavitations
In the first patient with a right coronary artery lesion with the start of the rotation a 2: 1 AV block occurred without moving the burr. This rhythm

disturbance was unexpected because during PTCA such an effect is rare and only occurring after occlusion of the vessel or prolonged balloon inflation.

Transthoracic and transesophageal echocardiographic studies during high speed rotational angioplasty could not detect any wall motion abnormality [64]. This may be related to the short period of rotation. It emphasizes, however, that the AV block cannot be related to ischemia. Unexpected transient enhancement of myocardial contrast during high speed rotational angioplasty occurred in the myocardial area representing the perfusion area of the treated vessel [64]. The echocardiographic images were similar to what can be seen during LV contrast and have been published for i.c. studies. Thus, it is suspected, that high speed rotational angioplasty produces microcavitations, i.c. microbubbles. In order to evaluate these effects an in vitro model was developed.

In vitro model

In a tube a catheter sheath with the burr was inserted and scanned by a 3.5 MHz conventional echo transducer in a water bath. During the rotation transient contrast appeared in the previous echo free tube. This contrast was dependent on the speed and duration of rotation. It was more intense in blood than in sparkling water, 0.9% sodium chloride (NaCl) or destilled water. In blood at 100,000 rpm echo contrast appeared, in 0.9% NACl at 150,000 rpm. The disappearance time was linearly related to rotational speed. In blood, echo contrast intensity was related to speed in a sigmoid curve reaching a maximal effect at 120,000 rpm. With the other fluids, this maximum was not reached.

The hypothesis that high speed rotational angioplasty induces micro-bubbles responsible for rhythm disturbances like AV blocks and sinus arrest could also be supported by using the Bernoulli equation for calculation of the production of gase cavitation from fluid. The critical limit of 14.6 m/s for normal blood pressure and atmospheric pressure is exceeded by high speed rotation. Using a burr size of 1.25 mm, the speed at the outer edge is > 9 m/s and for a 2.0 mm burr > 15 m/s at a speed of 150,000 rpm. Thus, high speed rotational angioplasty can produce microbubbles, perhaps the reason for transient myocardial echo contrast, explaining arrhythmia abnormalities like AV block observed with the onset of high speed rotational angioplasty.

Conclusion

High speed rotational angioplasty is able to ablate arteriosclerotic plaque material and to induce a step by step increase in the luminal diameter. In vitro studies have demonstrated, that high speed rotational angioplasty produces microbubbles by cativation of dissolved gas, because the velocity at the surface of the burr can exceed the critical value of 14.6 m/s according to the Bernoulli equation. Using short rotation period at high speed and avoiding any Dotter effect, the complication rate is low. Analysis of cine-ventriculograms before and 24 h after the procedure and two-dimensional echocardiograms have not been able to demonstrate wall motion abnormalities. 201-Thallium-scintigrams did not demonstrate new perfusion defects and Doppler coronary flow measurements showed an increase of flow reserve similar to PTCA.

References

1. Abela GS, Normann J, Cohen DM, Franzini D, Feldman RI, Crea F, Fenech A, Pepine CJ, Conti CR (1985) Laser recanalization of occluded atherosclerotic arteries in vivo and in vitro. *Circulation* 71: 403.
2. Ahn SS, Auth D, Marcus R, Moore S (1988) Removal of focal athero matous lesions by angioscopically guided high-speed rotary atherectomy. *J Vasc Surg* 7: 292.
3. Bredlau C, Roubin GS, Leimgruber PP, Douglas J Jr, King SB, Grüntzig AR (1985) In-hospital morbidity and mortality in patients undergoing elective coronary angioplasty. *Circulation* 72: 1044.
4. Cowley MJ, Dorros G, Kelsey SF, van Raden M, Detre KM (1984) Emergency coronary bypass surgery after coronary angioplasty: the National Heart, Lung, and Blood Institute's percutaneous transluminal coronary angioplasty registry experience. *Am J Cardiol* 53: 22C.
5. Darius H, Erbel R, Schmucker B, Reusch U, Meyer J (1988) Effects antiischémique du SIN-1, métabolite de la molsidomine, au cours de l'angioplastie coronarienne et effets antiplaquettaires chez l'homme. *Nouv Press méd* 17: 1033.
6. Düber C, Jungbluth A, Rumpelt HJ, Erbel R, Meyer J, Thoenes W (1986) Morphology of the coronary arteries after combined thrombolysis and percutaneous transluminal coronary angioplasty for acute myocardial infarction. *Am J Cardiol* 58: 698.
7. Dietz U, Erbel R, Iversen S, Nixdorff U, Pannen B, Haude M, Meyer J (1989) Safety-test of rotational angioplasty in post mortem human and pig coronary arteries. *Eur Heart J* 10, suppl, abstr: 199.
8. Dietz U, Erbel R, Auth D, Haude M, Nixdorff U, Pannen B, Meyer J (in preparation) Hochfrequenz-Rotationsangioplastie normaler und arteriosklerotischer Koronararterien. Experimentelle Befunde.
9. Dorros G, Stertzer SH, Cowley M, Myler RK (1984) Complex coronary angioplasty: multiple coronary dilations. *Am J Cardiol* 53: 126C.
10. Erbel R, Clas W, Busch U, von Seelen W, Brennecke R, Blömer H, Meyer J (1986) New balloon catheter for prolonged percutaneous transluminal coronary angioplasty and bypass flow in occluded vessels. *Cath Cardiovasc Diagn* 12: 116.
11. Erbel R, Diefenbach C, Schreiner G, Pop T, v. Oshausen K, Rupprecht HJ, Aydin A, Meyer J (1986) Recanalization of totally occluded coronary vessels by percutaneous transluminal coronary angioplasty, in: Höfling B (ed), *Current problems in PTCA*, p. 109, Darmstadt: Steinkopff.
12. Erbel R, Rupprecht HJ, Busch U, Darius H, Pop T, Blömer H, Meyer J (1987) Continuous coronary perfusion and prolonged balloon inflation during stenosis dilatation. *Z Kardiol* 76, Suppl 6: 49.
13. Erbel R, Pop T, Diefenbach CH, Meyer J (1989) Long-term results of thrombolytic therapy with and without percutaneous transluminal coronary angioplasty. *J Am Coll Cardiol* 14: 276.
14. Erbel R, O'Neill W, Auth D, Haude D, Nixdorff U, Dietz U, Rupprecht HJ, Tschollar W,

Meyer J (1989) Hochfrequenz-Rotationsatherektomie bei koronarer Herzkrankheit. *Dtsch med Wochenschr* 114: 487.

15. Erbel R, O'Neill W, Auth D, Haude M, Nixdorff U, Rupprecht HJ, Dietz U, Meyer J (1989) High-frequency rotablation of occluded coronary artery during heart catheterization. *Cath Cardiovasc Diagn* 17: 56.

16. Erbel R, Schatz R, Dietz U, Nixdorff U, Haude M, Aichinger S, Pop T, Meyer J (1989) Ballondilatation und koronare Gefäßstützenimplantation. *Z Kardiol* 78: 71.

17. Faxon DP, Detre KM, McCabe CH, Fisher L, Holmes DR, Cowley MJ, Bourassa MG, v. Raden M, Ryan TJ (1983) Role of percutaneous transluminal coronary angioplasty in the treatment of unstable angina. *Am J Cardiol* 3: 131C.

18. Fourrier JL, Auth D, Lablanche JM, Brunetaud JM, Gommeaux A, Bertrand ME (1988) First percutaneous coronary rotational atherectomies in man. *Eur Heart J* 9, suppl I: 336.

19. Fourrier JL, Bertrand ME, Auth DC, Lablanche JM, Gommeaux A, Brunetaud JM (1989) Percutaneous coronary rotational angioplasty in humans: preliminary report. *J Am Coll Cardiol* 14: 1278.

20. Galan KM, Deligonul U, Kern MJ, Chaitman BR, Vandormael MG (1988) Increased frequency of restenosis in patients continuing to smoke cigarettes after percutaneous transluminal coronary angioplasty. *Am J Cardiol* 61: 260.

21. Grüntzig A (1976) Perkutane Dilatation von Koronarstenosen – Beschreibung eines neuen Kathetersystems. *Klin Wochenschr* 54: 543.

22. Grüntzig A, Riedhammer HH, Turina M, Rutishauser W (1976) Eine neue Methode zur perkutanen Dilatation von Koronarstenosen – tierexperimentelle Prüfung. *Verh Dtsch Ges Kreislaufforsch* 42: 282.

23. Hartzler GO, Rutherford BD, McConahay DR, Johnson WL, McCallister BO, Gura GM, Conn RC, Crockett JE (1983) Percutaneous transluminal coronary angioplasty with and without thrombolytic therapy for treatment of acute myocardial infarction. *Am Heart J* 106: 965.

24. Holmes DR, Vliestra BE, Smith HC, Vetrover GW, Kent KM, Cowley MJ, Faxon DP, Grüntzig AR, Kelsey SF, Detre KM, van Raden MJ, Mock MB (1984) Restenosis after percutaneous transluminal coronary angioplasty (PTCA). A report from the PTCA registry of the National Heart, Lung and Blood Institute. *Am J Cardiol* 53: 77C.

25. Hombach V, Höher M, Arnold G, Osypka P, Koch M, Eggeling T, Höpp HW, Hirche H, Hilger H (1987) Die Hochfrequenzangioplastie – eine neue Methode zur Rekanalisation verschlossener arterieller Gefäße. *Cor Vas* 2: 67.

26. Jungbluth A, Düber C, Rumpelt HJ, Erbel R, Meyer (1988) Koronararterienmorphologie nach perkutaner transluminaler Koronarangioplastie (PTCA) mit Hämoperikard. *Z. Kardiol* 77: 125.

27. Kaltenbach M, Kober G, Scherer D (1980) Mechanische Dilatation von Koronararterien-stenosen (Transluminale Angioplastie). *Z Kardiol* 69: 1.

28. Kaltenbach M, Beyer J, Klepzig H, Schmidt L, Hübner K (1982) Effect of 5 kg/cm² pressure on atherosclerotic vessel wall segments, in: Kaltenbach M, Grüntzig A, Rentrop K, Bussman WD (eds), *Transluminal Coronary Angioplasty and Intracoronary Thrombolysis* p. 189. New York: Springer.

29. Karsch KR, Haase KK, Mauser M, Voelker W, Ickrath O, Seipel L (1989) Perkutane transluminale coronare Examer Laser Angioplastie. *Z Kardiol* 78: 27.

30. Kensey KR, Nash E, Abrahams C, Zarins CK (1987) Recanalization of obstructed arteries with a flexible rotating tip catheter. *Radiology* 165: 387.

31. Kober G, Hopf R, Reinemer H, Kaltenbach M (1985) Langzeitergebnisse der trans-luminalen koronaren Angioplastie von chronischen Herzkranzgefäßverschlüssen. *Z Kardiol* 74: 309.

32. Levine S, Ewels CJ, Rosing DR, Kent KM (1985) Coronary angioplasty: clinical and angiographic follow-up. *Am J Cardiol* 55: 673.

33. Leimgruber PP, Roubins GS, Anderson HV, Bredlau CE, Whitworth HB, Douglas JS,

King SB, Grüntzig AR (1985) Influence of intimal dissection on restenosis after successful coronary angioplasty. *Circulation* 72: 530.

34. Leimgruber PP, Roubin GS, Hollman J, Cotsonis GA, Meier B, Douglas JS, King SB, Grüntzig AR (1986) Restenosis after successful coronary angioplasty in patients with single-vessel disease. *Circulation* 73: 710.

35. Matthews BJ, Ewels CJ, Kent KM (1988) Coronary dissection: a predictor of restenosis? *Am Heart J* 115: 547.

36. Meyer J, Merx W, Schmitz H, Erbel R, Kiesslich T, Dörr R, Imbert CH, Bethge C, Krebs W, Bardos P, Minale C, Messmer BJ, Effert S (1982) Percutaneous transluminal coronary angioplasty immediately after intracoronary streptolysis of transmural myocardial infarction. *Circulation* 66: 905.

37. Meyer J, Schmitz RJ, Kiesslich T, Erbel R, Krebs W, Schulz W, Bardos P, Minale C, Messmer BJ, Effert S (1983) Percutaneous transluminal coronary angioplasty in patients with stable and unstable angina pectoris: analysis of early and late results. *Am Heart J* 106: 973.

38. Meyer J, Erbel R, Pop T, Rupprecht HJ (1987) Derzeitiger Stand der intrakoronaren Ballondilatation. *Internist* 28: 736.

39. Palmaz JC, Sibbitt RR, Tio FO, Reuter SR, Peters JE, Garcia F (1986) Expandable intraluminal vascular graft: a feasibility study. *Surgery* 99: 199.

40. Palmaz JC, Kopp DT, Hayashi H, Schatz RA, Hunter G, Tio FO, Garcia O, Alvarado R, Rees C, Thomas SC (1987) Normal and stenotic renal arteries: experimental balloon-expandable intraluminal stenting. *Radiology* 164: 705.

41. Palmaz JC, Windeler SA, Garcia F, Tio FO, Sibbitt RR, Reuter SR (1986) Atherosclerotic rabbit aortas. Expandable intraluminal grafting. *Radiology* 160: 723.

42. Pannen B, Dietz U, Erbel R, Iversen S, Nixdorff U, Meyer J, Auth D (1989) Ultrastructural changes in coronary arteries after rotational angioplasty. Possible relevance of Dotter effects. *Eur Heart J* 10, Suppl: 323.

43. Ritchie JL, Hansen DD, Intlekofer MJ, Hall M, Auth DC (1987) Rotational approaches to atherectomy and thrombectomy. *Z Kardiol* 76, suppl 6: 59.

44. Rupprecht HJ, Erbel R, Brennecke R, Pop T, Jung D, Kottmeyer M, Hering R, Meyer J (1988) Aktuelle Komplikationsrate der perkutanen transluminalen Koronarangioplastie bei stabiler und unstabiler Angina. *Dtsch med Wochenschr* 113: 409.

45. Rupprecht HJ, Brennecke R, Erbel R, Pop T, Jung D, Kottmeyer M, Hering R, Meyer J (1987) Early and long-term outcome after PTCA in stable versus unstable angina. *J Am Coll Cardiol* 9: 150, abstr.

46. Schatz RA, Palmaz JC, Tio FO, Garcia O, Reuter SR (1987) Balloon-expandable intra-coronary stents in the adult dog. *Circulation* 76: 450.

47. Schatz RA, Leon MB, Baim DS, Ellis SG, Erbel R, Hishfled JW, Goldberg S, Penn JM (1989) Balloon expandable intracoronary stents. Initial results of a multicenter study. *Circulation* 80, suppl II: 174.

48. Schatz RA, Leon MB, Baim DS, Ellis SG, Marco J, Erbel R, Goldberg S, (1990) Short term clinical results and complications with the Palmaz-Schatz coronary stents. *J Am Coll Cardiol* 15, suppl A: 117A.

49. Schwartz L, Bourassa MG, Lespérance J, Aldridge HE, Kazim F, Salvatori VA, Henderson M, Bonan R, David PR (1988) Aspirin and dipyridamole in the prevention of restenosis after percutaneous transluminal coronary angioplasty. *New Eng J Med* 318: 1714.

50. Serruys PW, Umans V, Heyndrickx GR, v.d.Brand M, de Feyter PJ, Wijns W, Jaski B, Hugenholtz PG (1985) Elective PTCA of totally occluded coronary arteries not associated with acute myocardial infarction. Short-term and long-term results. *Eur Heart J* 6: 2.

51. Serruys PW, Beatt KJ, Bertrand M, Meier B, Puch J, Richards T, Sigwart U (1989) Restenosis rate after coronary stent implantation. Angiographic assessment of the initial series. *Circulation* 80, suppl: II–173.

52. Shiu MF, Silverton NP, Oakley D, Cumberland D (1985) Acute coronary occlusion during percutaneous transluminal coronary angioplasty. *Br Heart J* 54: 129.
53. Sigwart U, Puel J, Mirkovitch V, Joffre F, Kappenberger L (1987) Intravascular stents to prevent occlusion and restenosis after transluminal angioplasty. *N Engl J Med* 316: 70.
54. Simpson JB, Selmon MR, Robertson GC, Cipriano PR, Hayden WG, Johnson DE, Fogarty TJ (1988) Transluminal atherectomy for occlusive peripheral vascular disease. *Am J Cardiol* 61: 96G.
55. Simpson JB, Robertson GC, Selman MR, Sipperle ME, Brader LJ, Hinohara T (1989) Restenosis following successful directional coronary atherectomy. *Circulation* 80, suppl: II–582.
56. Slager CJ, Hugenholtz PG, Bom N, Lancée CT, Schuurbiers CH, Serruys PW (1988) Spark erosion: an alternative to laser recanalization, in: *Advances in Laser Medicine*, p. 244. Landsberg: Ecomed.
57. Stack RS, Quigley PJ, Sketch MJH, Stack RK, Walter K, Hofman PU, Philips HR (1989) Treatment of coronary artery disease with the transluminal extraction-endarterectomy catheter: initial results of a multicenter study. *Circulation* 80, suppl, III: 583.
58. Steffenino G, Meier B, Finci L, Velebit V, v. Segesser B, Faidutti B, Rutishauser W (1988) Acute complications of elective coronary angioplasty. A review of 500 consecutive procedures. *Br Heart J* 59: 151.
59. Vandermael MG, Deligonul U, Kern MJ, Harper M, Presant S, Gibson P, Galan K, Chaitman BR (1987) Multilesion coronary angioplasty: clinical and angiographic follow-up. *J Am Coll Cardiol* 10: 246.
60. Vallbracht C, Schweitzer M, Kress J, Bamberg W, Kollath J, Liermann D, Paaschs C, Rauber K, Roth FJ, Prignitz J, Beinborn W, Landgraf H, Breddin K, Schoop W, Kaltenbach M (1988) Rotationsangioplastik. Erste klinische Ergebnisse bei peripheren Gefäßverschlüssen. *Z Kardiol* 77: 352.
61. Vallbracht C, Kreis J, Schweitzer W, Schneider M, Wendt Th, Ziemen M, Kollath J, Bamberg W, Kaltenbach M (1987) Rotationsangioplastik – ein neues Verfahren zur Gefäßeröffnung und –erweiterung. Experimentelle Befunde. *Z Kardiol* 76: 608.
62. Waller BF, Gorfinkel HJ, Rogers FJ, Kent KM, Roberts WC (1984) Early and late morphologic changes in major epicardial coronary arteries after percutaneous transluminal coronary angioplasty. *Am J Cardiol* 53: 42C.
63. Whitworth HB, Roubin GS, Hollman J, Meier B, Leimgruber PP, Douglas JS, King SB, Grüntzig AR (1986) Effect of nifedipine on recurrent stenosis after percutaneous transluminal coronary angioplasty. *J Am Coll Cardiol* 8: 1271.
64. Zotz R, Wittlich N, Erbel R, Stähr P, Meyer J (1989) Erkennung von myokardialem Kontrast während hochfrequenter Rotablation von atherosklerotischen Plaques mittels transösophagealer Echokardiographie. *Z Kardiol* 78, suppl 1: 131.

10. A new balloon-expandable coronary tantalum stent in atherosclerotic minipigs: angiographic and histologic findings 4 weeks after implantation

A. BUCHWALD, C. UNTERBERG, H. TILL, K. NEBENDAHL, P. GRÖNE and V. WIEGAND

Summary

Minipigs (20–30 kg bodyweight) were fed an atherogenic diet (2% cholesterol), starting 4 wks prior to endothelial balloon-denudation in one coronary artery. Another 4 weeks later, a balloon-mounted tantalum-stent (2.0–4.0 mm diameter) was implanted at the site of previous endothelial damage. Animals were given 10,000 U heparin immediately before PTCA and stent-implantation. 100 mg acetyl-salicylic acid per day were given orally afterwards. Stent-implantation could be performed at the selected site in all cases without complications due to good radiopacity of the tantalum-stent. 4 weeks later, repeat angiography for assessment of stented vessel patency and eventual stenoses was performed. Subsequently, hearts were perfusion-fixed with glutaraldehyde for histologic examination. All vessels were patent (left circumflex, n = 4) left anterior descending coronary artery, n = 1) on angiography. Stents were covered by endothelium. Results 3 months after stent-implantation are currently assessed.

Introduction

Despite continuous improvement in balloon catheter technology, percutaneous transluminal coronary angioplasty (PTCA) today still is limited by a rate of 2 to 5% of acute occlusions and a restenosis rate of 20 to 40% [1, 2].

Among the new techniques designed to reduce either rate, intracoronary stents possibly constitute a principle, that enables the interventional cardiologist to handle acute coronary occlusions after PTCA as well as reduces the rate of restenosis.

Problems of these stents include thrombosis and difficult control of positioning in the coronaries because of the poor radiopacity of thin stainless steel wires [3]. Recently, a new, balloon-expandable tantalum stent has been introduced, that is characterized by good visibility on fluoroscopy and

95

V. Hombach et al. (eds), Interventional Techniques in Cardiovascular Medicine, 95–99.

low thrombosis rates in an atherosclerotic pig model without prior balloon-denudation [4].

The present study was performed to investigate the feasability of this stent, acute and long-term patency of stented coronary arteries and the histologic reactions in stented vessels. Because of possible influences of serum-cholesterol levels on restenosis rates and thus, vessel reaction to the implanted stent, we chose an athersclerotic minipig model.

Methods

Göttingen minipigs of either sex weighing between 22 and 28 kg were fed a standard diet supplemented with 2% cholesterol and 10 g Na-cholate per day. After 4 weeks on this diet, a standard balloon angioplasty catheter was introduced via a carotid artery, inflated and moved back and forth several times in one coronary artery to set an endothelial injury. The left anterior descending coronary artery (LAD) was treated in one animal and the left circumflex coronary artery (RCx) in 4 other minipigs. Another 4 weeks later, a stent was implanted at the site to prior dilatation. 4 weeks after stent-implantation, coronary angiography was performed. Thereafter, the hearts were rapidly excised and the aorta was fixed to a canula allowing extensive flushing of the heart, followed by perfusion-fixation with gluta-raldehyde. The stented segment was then excised and embedded in a special plastic, that allowed cutting of the stent-wire by a special saw without movement against the newly formed tissue around the stent.

Blood for serum-cholesterol measurement was collected at 4 timepoints during the experimental protocol: Control values were obtained before putting the animals on the cholesterol-diet, and the rise in serum-cholesterol was measured 4 weeks later at balloon-denudation of the endothelium, at stent-implantation and at termination of the experiment.

Medication: The animals received 10000 units of heparin i.v. immediately before each arterial catheterization. Starting with the balloon-denudation, they were given acetyl-salicylic acid (100 mg/day) orally.

Results

The stents are easily seen on fluoroscopy, what allows precise control of positioning of the stent at the predetermined site within the coronary artery. All stented vessels were patent 4 weeks after stent-implantation. Figure 1 shows a stented left circumflex coronary artery. While there was no angiographic evidence for a stenosis in 4 animals, one segment showed a signification luminal narrowing by about 70%.

Histology in this segment revealed an organized thrombus, that had partially obstructed the free lumen of the vessel without completely occluding

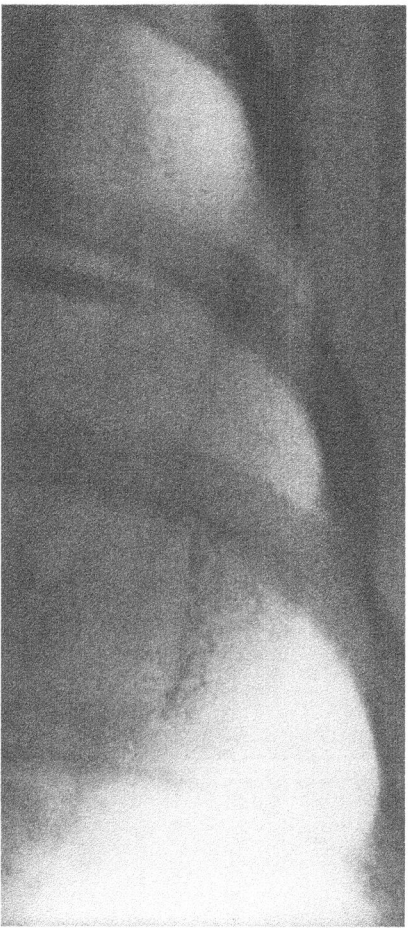

Figure 1.   An example of a stent implanted in the left circumflex coronary artery and documents the excellent radiopacity of the stent.

it. In the remaining four stented segments without angiographic evidence for stenosis (Figure 2), we found a neointima covering several regular layers of fibroblasts, while the stent-wire is found almost within the media of the arterial wall, surrounded by irregularly growing fibroblasts and few mono-nuclear cells, indicating an active tissue reaction around the stent.

Conclusions

The superior visibleness of this new tantulum stent on radioscopy allows precise control of stent positioning. In atherosclerotic minipigs, coronary

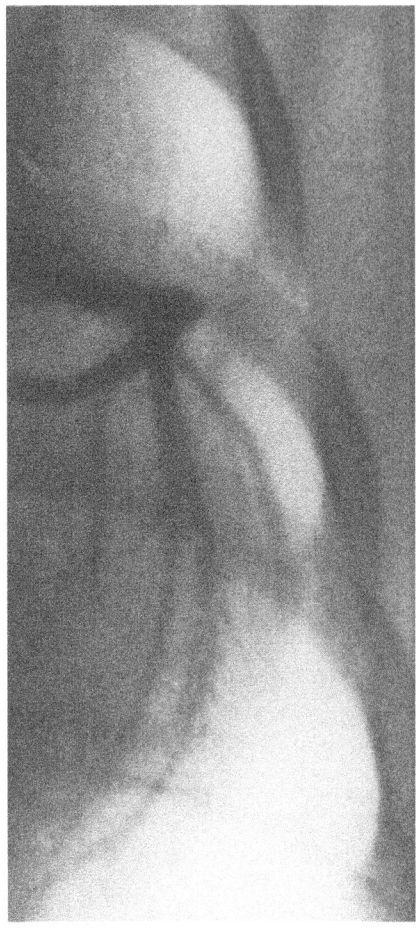

Figure 2.   The angiogram of this artery performed 4 weeks after implantation. The artery is open without luminal narrowing within the stented segment.

arteries, that had been stented 4 weeks after balloon denudation, were patent after 4 weeks.

Histologic examination 4 weeks after stent implantation showed, though there was an active tissue reaction around the stent, that a neointima had formed, and that the tissue reaction did not result in luminal narrowing.

Since this stent allows exact control of positioning and good acute patency, it might prove beneficial in the management of acute occlusions after PTCA.

References

1. Simpfendorfer C, Belardi J, Bellamy G, Galan K, Franco I, Hollman J (1987) Frequency, management and follow-up of patients with acute coronary occlusion after percutaneous transluminal angioplasty. *Am J Cardiol* 59: 267.
2. Mabin TA, Holmes DR, Smith HC, Vliestra RE, Bove AA, Reeder GS, Chesbro JH, Bresnahan JF, Orzulack TA (1985) Intracoronary thrombus: role in coronary occlusion complicating percutaneous transluminal coronary angioplasty. *J Am Coll Cardiol* 5: 198.
3. Sigwart U, Urban P, Golf S, Kaufman U, Imbert C, Fischer A, Kappenberger L (1988) Emergency stenting after coronary balloon angioplasty. *Circulation* 78: 1121.
4. White CW, Ramee SR, Ross TC, Banks AK, Wiktor D, Graeber GM Goldstein RE, Price HL, Isner JM (1988) A new percutaneous balloon expandable stent. *Circulation* 78, suppl II: 409.

11. Autoperfusion catheter for preservation of myocardium during coronary artery obstruction after failed PTCA

H. KORB, A. HOEFT, U. TEBBE, A. BOROWSKI and
E.R. DE VIVIE

Summary

The aim of this study was to examine whether myocardial function can be maintained by a catheter system designed for coronary autoperfusion in emergency cases due to coronary artery obstruction (CAO) after failed PTCA.

Experiments were performed in open-chest dogs with coronary artery ligation. Ischemic stress was quantified by the energy deficit during ischemia occurring as difference between oxygen demand and uptake and by changes of regional myocardial wall function measured with a new electromagnetic distance measuring system.

During control occlusions a reproducible energy deficit with accompanying systolic bulging was observed. These changes failed to occur after subselective positioning of the catheter beneath the occlusion side and religation of the artery.

The results—confirmed by first clinical observations—suggest that in emergency cases with CAO autoperfusion of myocardium through the catheter system is obviously sufficient to maintain myocardial energetic and functional intergrity until revascularisation is achieved by surgery.

Introduction

With increasing application of percutaneous transluminal coronary angioplasty (PTCA) cardiac surgeons are more frequently concerned with emergency coronary bypass surgery resulting from CAO by major dissection, spasm or thrombosis during catheterisation. Despite the availability of emergency surgical backup, myocardial infarction or death may occur, if coronary blood flow is not reestablished immediately and mortality of the operative intervention may be increased under these circumstances [2].

This study describes the experimental use of an autoperfusion catheter designed to reestablish and maintain myocardial blood flow after coronary artery occlusion during PTCA.

101

V. Hombach et al. (eds), Interventional Techniques in Cardiovascular Medicine, 101–106.
© 1991 *Kluwer Academic Publishers.*

Methods

Conventional open-chest dog preparation was performed in mongrel dogs under piritramide anaesthesia and artificial respiration [9].

As parameters for the occurrence of ischemia the difference (oxygen debt; dO_2, ml O_2/min) between myocardial oxyen consumption (MVO_2) and energy demand (E_t), as well as changes of regional myocardial wall function were measured.

Oxygen debt

MVO_2 was calculated from continuous recordings of coronary blood flow by electromagnetic flow-meter and coronary venous oxygen saturation by a fiberoptic system. E_t was determined indirectly from monitored hemo-dynamic data according to the Bretschneider equation giving the energy demand per 100 g left ventricular weight [1]. The continuous monitoring of these parameters has been established as very sensitive method for the

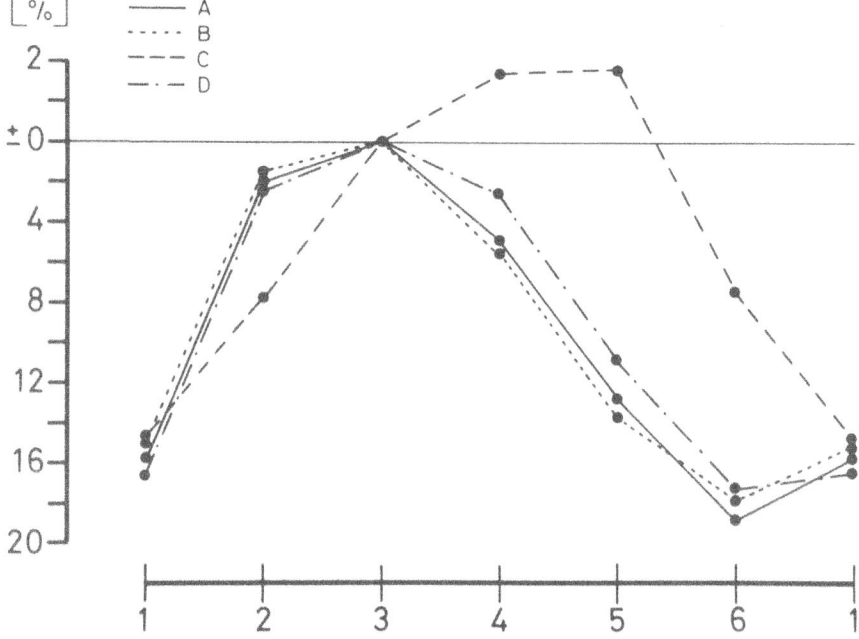

Figure 1.   Regional wall function, coronary occlusion and catheter perfusion. (A) Baseline conditions. (B) Perfusion catheter in LAD artery position. (C) Ligation of the LAD artery around the perfusion catheter with an occluding guidewire in place leads to systolic bulging with systolic enlargement of the epicardial area. (D) When the guidewire is withdrawn and coronary blood supply is solely dependent on transluminal perfusion by the catheter no impairment of regional wall function can be observed.

All values are average values of 8 measuring periods, standard variations are less than 1%.

quantification of disturbances in myocardial energy balance as occurring in ischemia [7].

Regional wall function

Changes of wall function were assessed by a newly designed electromagnetic device for continuous distance measurements, modified to quantify wall function from epicardial area changes. Electromagnetic transducers forming a triangle on the epicardial surface were positioned within the later ischemic zone. By continuous recordings of the three distances between the transducers the changes of the area of the triangle, representing the systolic and diastolic wall function, can be determined. Three diastolic and systolic measurements were made during a single heart action: in the early diastole at the end of the isovolumetric relaxation (point 1), in the late diastole at the beginning of P-wave in the ECG (point 2), at the end of diastole at the beginning of left ventricular pressure rise (point 3), during isovolumetric tension development (point 4), during the midsystolic ejection phase (point 5) and at the end of systole at closure of the aortic valve (point 6) (see Figure 1).

Experimental protocol

Measurements were performed (A) under basic conditions, (B) after subselective positioning of the autoperfusion catheter into the left anterior descending (LAD) artery, (C) after insertion of an occluding guidewire to the top of the autoperfusion catheter and simultaneous ligation of the LAD artery and (D) after removal of the occluding guidewire from the autoperfusion catheter but with ligation of the LAD artery in place.

The sequence of measurements was repeated in a single experiment 5 to 10 times with recovery periods of 30 min. All data are given as mean values.

For autoperfusion, a standard 3F coronary infusion catheter ('coronary infusion catheter with sideholes'; Advanced Cardiovascular Systems, Inc. Mountain View, CA, USA) with 36 sideholes arranged in a spiral pattern over the distal 10 cm has been used.

Results

In vitro results showed [1] that the fluid flow through the autoperfusion catheter is practically independent from the catheters position within the stenosis and [2] that a pressure gradient of about 50 mmHg is sufficient to drive a flow of 70–80 ml/min (data not shown). Based on these results, five in vivo experiments were performed in open-chest mongrel dogs.

Figure 2 shows the continuous monitoring of the difference (oxygen debt; dO_2, ml O_2/min) between myocardial oxygen consumption (MVO_2) and energy demand (E_t).

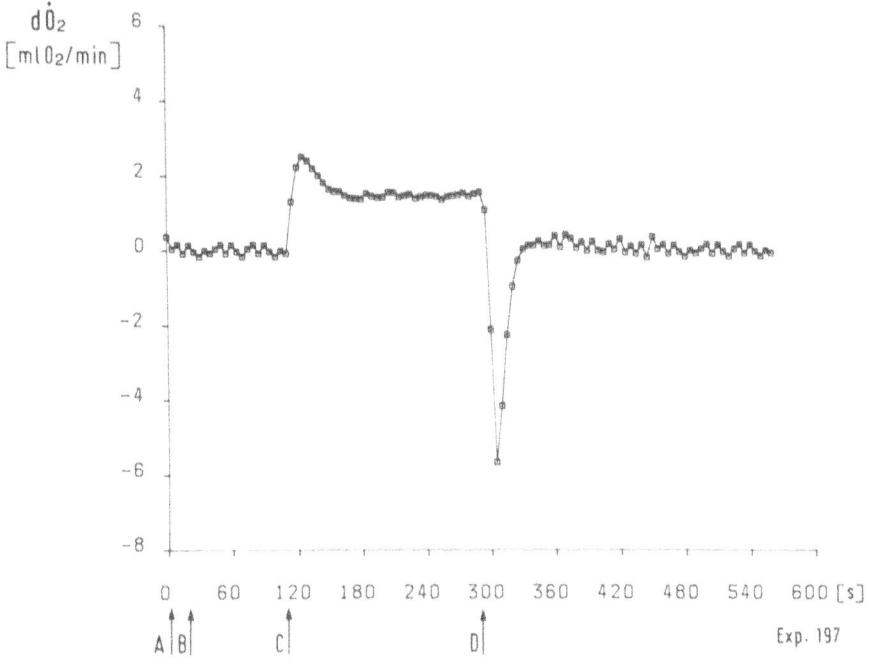

Figure 2.   Myocardial oxygen debt (dO_2), coronary occlusion and catheter perfusion. (A) Under baseline conditions the relationship between myocardial energy demand and oxygen uptake is balanced ($dO_2 = 0$). (B) The introduction of the perfusion catheter into the LAD does not disturb this balance. (C) Ligation of the artery around the catheter with an occluding guidewire in place leads to the development of an oxygen debt (dO_2 ca. 1.5 ml O_2/min). (D) A reactive hyperemia can be observed when the guidewire is withdrawn, the oxygen supply to the heart by transluminal perfusion is sufficient to match myocardial energy demands ($dO_2 = 0$).

Values are average values of 8 measuring periods performed in a single experiment.

Under baseline conditions (point A) the relationship between MVO_2 and E_t is balanced. Subselective positioning of the catheter into the LAD artery does not alter this balance (point B) demonstrating that the catheter itself does not impair blood flow or even obstruct the artery. A marked energy deficit can be observed when the artery is ligated around the catheter with an occluding guidewire in place (point C). After removal of the guidewire autoperfusion immediately takes place even allowing a reactive hyperemia (point D). After the hyperemic response no difference between MVO_2 and E_t can be observed showing that autoperfusion is sufficient to match myocardial energy demands.

These energetic data are confirmed by measuring changes of regional wall function (Figure 1). Curve A represents regional wall function under control conditions. With beginning of systole (point 3) the area of the triangle becomes smaller reaching its minimal size at the end of systole at closure of the aortic valve (point 6). The subsequent increase in size reflects the filling of the ventricle during diastole (points 1–3). Curve B shows that the introduction of the catheter into the LAD has no influence on the wall function. A systolic enlargement of the area reflecting the systolic bulging of the ischemic myocardium can be observed when the artery is ligated around the catheter with an occluding guidewire in place (curve C). This bulging completely disappears and no further impairment of regional wall function can be seen, when the occluding guidewire is removed and autoperfusion is allowed (curve D).

Discussion

Coronary artery obstruction during PTCA occurs in about 5% of all cases [3] and may result in myocardial infarction and death. This study describes our experimental results with a mechanical reperfusion device designed to reestablish coronary blood flow after an occlusive lesion.

A standard 3F catheter with sideholes on its distal end was used for autoperfusion across a total coronary artery obstruction. The perforations allow blood to enter through the side of the catheter under proximal aortic pressure (see in vitro — results). The blood flows through the obstruction and out of the sideholes and endhole of the reperfusion catheter distal to the obstructing lesion.

The effectiveness of the device was clearly supported by our results demonstrating that coronary blood flow by autoperfusion is sufficient to match the energetic demands even for the metabolic and functional recovery of ischemic myocardium. This has been verified by the prevention of any further imbalance between myocardial oxygen consumption and energy demands and by the disappearance of the systolic bulging as parameter for the impairment of regional wall function.

Compared to other attempts with continuous [5] or intermittent [8] intracoronary perfusion the described autoperfusion technique seems to be an effective and easily applicable method to reestablish coronary blood flow after coronary artery obstruction. First clinical results attest to this concept as demonstrated by dramatic relief of chest discomfort and ST-segment elevation [6], by the absence of electrocardiographic changes after corrective bypass surgery [4] and by the results of follow-up radionuclide angiograms [10] after successful placement of the reperfusion catheter.

References

1. Bretschneider HJ (1971) Die hämodynamischen Determinanten des O_2-Bedarfs des Herzmuskels. *Arzneimittel-Forschung/Drug Res* 21: 3–11.
2. Cowley MJ, Dorros G, Kelsey SF et al. (1984) Emergency coronary bypass surgery after coronary angioplasty: the National Heart, Lung, and Blood Institute's percutaneous transluminal coronary angioplasty registry experience. *Am J Cardiol* 53: 22C–26C.

 3. Detre K, Holubkov R, Kelsey S et al., and the Co-investigators of the National Heart, Lung and Blood Institute (1988) Percutaneous transluminal coronary angioplasty in 1985–1986 and 1977–1981. The National Heart, Lung, and Blood Institute Registry. *N Engl J Med* 318: 265–270.
 4. Ferguson TB, Hinohara T, Simpson JB et al. (1986) Catheter reperfusion to allow optimal coronary bypass grafting following failed transluminal coronary angioplasty. *Ann Thorac Surg* 42: 399–405.
 5. Fuchs M, McDonald FM, Kreuzer J et al. (1984) Myokardpotektion durch Perfusion während perkutaner transluminaler Koronarangioplastie (PTCA). *Herz/Kreislauf* 16: 549–555.
 6. Hirohara T, Simpson JB, Phillips HR et al. (1986) Transluminal catheter reperfusion: a new technique to reestablish blood flow after coronary occlusion during percutaneous transluminal coronary angioplasty. *Am J Cardiol* 57: 684–686.
 7. Hoeft A, Korb H, Baller D et al. (1984) Quantification of ischemic stress during repeated coronary artery occlusion in the dog. A method for validation of therapeutical effects. I. Estimation of O_2-debt and O_2-repayment. *Basic Res Cardiol* 79: 27–37.
 8. Hopf R, Kunkel B, Schneider M et al. (1985) Koronarperfusion bei akutem Gefäßverschluß im Rahmen der transluminalen Koronarangioplastik (TCA). *Z Kardiol* 74: 580–584.
 9. Korb H, Hoeft A, Baller D et al. (1984) Quantification of ischemic stress during repeated coronary artery occlusion in the dog. A method for validation of therapeutical effects. II. Reproducibility of the release and uptake of electrolytes and substrates. *Basic Res Cardiol* 79: 38–48.
10. Tebbe U, Ruschewski W, Korb H et al. (1989) Der Einsatz des Autoperfusionskatheters bei Koronarverschluß im Rahmen der perkutanen transluminalen Koronarangioplastie (PTCA). *Z Kardiol* 78: 63–67.

PART TWO

Peripheral vessel angioplasty

12. Balloon angioplasty

E.-I. RICHTER and E. ZEITLER

Summary

Since the introduction of PTA 25 years ago, a dramatic technical develop-ment has taken place which makes PTA a first choice treatment for radiologists, angiologists, and surgeons. There is no doubt about PTA being a locally controlled trauma of very low risk. Besides, medication or surgery invasive techniques offer an additional potential in several areas of vascular diseases. Six years ago, Dotter stated: 'Transluminal angioplasty is here to stay, at least until something better comes along'.

Introduction

At first, PTA was regarded with scepticism as a treatment of arteriosclerotic angiostenoses and occlusions. Nowadays, the conviction prevails that this 25 year-old local treatment technique helps patients with symptoms such as intermitting claudication, pain at rest, and gangrenous ulcers.

In the following, I want to present a brief survey of the historic develop-ment of PTA and currently implemented techniques.

Whereas the coaxial catheter system with its long metal tube developed by Dotter was able to dilate vascular lumen up to 12 Charriere [1], the development of the Grüntzig double lumen catheter started the era of the dilatation technique [2].

After considerable initial difficulties in finding manufacturers for the production of the appropriate balloon catheters, there is now an exponential increase in specialized producers. To the same extent, new catheters have been developed with different properties and different material. Additional enlargements of the arterial puncture causing lacerations and subsequent inguinal hematomas could now be decreased.

The balloon catheter system developed by Olbert [3] has the advantage that when completely collapsed, the balloon clings closely to the catheter,

V. Hombach et al. (eds), Interventional Techniques in Cardiovascular Medicine, 109–114.

thus considerably facilitating its introduction. Complications with a possibly defective balloon during removal have not been reported so far.

The Olbert catheter is the appropriate method for aortic bifurcation stenoses, stenoses of the pelvic, and peripheral vascular sections.

With further changes in catheters and material, the rate of intimal ruptures and lacerations, as well as the compression of the obstruction material could be considerably increased. Initially, it was only possible to dilate the internal diameter by up to 70–90% of its original lumen.

Angiographic follow-up controls have revealed that the improved hemo-dynamic flow led to a further reduction in the arterial obliteration. More-over, the induction of autofibrinolytic mechanisms have been discussed.

Efficient patho-physiological mechanisms are various which of them represents the main aspect, couldn't yet be defined [14, 15].

Morphologic documentation of the vascular changes and the classification by the La Fontaine stages have led to the appropriate indications which finally induced the success of the catheter technique.

Nowadays, PTA is indicated in patients suffering from intermitting claudication, stage II, and in the case of symptoms where walking distances of less than 500 m, disrupts professional and private life [8]. This can happen in the case of an isolated iliac stenosis, an isolated or multiple femoral stenoses, or in a popliteal stenosis.

The outcome of PTA is poorer in occlusions longer than 10 cm in the region of the femoral or popliteal arteries and the changes of the catheter technique being used in aortic or renal artery occlusions or in peripheral occlusions longer than 10 cm with an additional poor outflow out of the lower leg arteries are even worse. Also, patients older than 75 years with the additional complication of diabetes mellitus and who continue to smoke without the administration of aggregation inhibitors, have a poor prognosis.

Additional medication is an essential part of PTA [12]. When using this additional therapy the rethrombosis rate within the first 10 days decreased from 21 to 2%. Unfortunately, so far the question of how long aggregation inhibitors have to be administered to prevent the rapid formation of a thrombus and reobliteration has not been conclusively answered. At the Nurenberg Medical Center we normally administer ASA (3xo. 5g) 2 days prior to the PTA therapy. We also apply intraarterially 5 000 I.U. of Heparin following the puncture.

After the PTA procedure, the patient continues on ASA medication for up to 10 days (330 mg acetyl salicylic acid and 75 mg Dipyridamol) [12]. Prophylactic medication is started on the second or third day using Coumarin derivates.

Grüntzig balloon catheters made of polyethylene are specially lubricous, thus allowing their use in all types of vessels [2]. An additional safety precaution concerning the location of the catheter is provided by the implementation of a special lock system.

Besides the use of dilation techniques for large vessels, even more refined methods have been developed to allow application in nearly all peripheral vascular regions [4, 10, 11, 17, 19, 20]. First of all, the use in supraaortic branches has been proposed, although however, the risk of cerebral emboli with permanent lesions cannot be totally excluded. The results of vascular surgery in the region of the carotid artery are very good and the complication rate has been reported as being very low.

In the case of the lack of a patient's consent or of medical contra-indications to an operative procedure, the dilation of the carotid vessel by PTA is a good alternative. In such situations, stenoses of the internal carotid artery right below the base of the skull, which are not accessible to the vascular surgeon, or stenoses of the external carotid artery, can be dilated to improve the collateral function [17].

Fibromuscular changes of the carotid artery in the extracranial area are also treatable by PTA. The leading symptoms preceding the indication for PTA in the supraaortic branches are defective vision, vertigo, tendency to fall over, reduced hearing, steal's syndrome with ischemia of the arms and differences in the blood pressure in the upper extremities.

The dilatation of subclavian stenoses and the brachio-cephalic trunk nowadays presents no technical problems if a safe passage of the guide wire and the catheter is provided [18, 19]. The common femoral artery, as well as the axillary artery, may be used as access for the puncture and for dilatation.

Many good hemodynamic results have been reported which demonstrate the low complication rate achieved in the cerebro-vascular region.

It was Grüntzig who first applied the balloon dilatation technique to coronary arteries, one typical indication of which are short singular stenoses.

Nowadays, we count on a 77% of success rate when dilating the anterior interventricular artery, although dilatation of the circumflex artery is more difficult, with a lower success rate of 68%. The outcome at the right coronary arteries is even less favourable. However, even stenoses of aortic coronary bypasses are successfully dilated in 82% of reported cases and the usual relapse rate has been reported to be between 12 and 15% in an angiographic follow-up control after 3 to 6 month.

The risk of an acute myocardial infarction exists in 3%, while an imme-diate surgical intervention is required in only 1% due to intima lesions. In such instances, an aortic coronary bypass is required [13, 20, 21].

Occlusions and stenoses of the infrarenal abdominal aorta are low in unselected populations. The previous treatments for aortic-iliac stenoses and isolated stenoses of the distal adominal aorta were thrombend arterectomy and aortic iliac bypass, respectively. The indication for the introduction of catheter treatment is based on the angiogram, walking distance, Doppler blood pressure, and clinical characteristics. Appropriate premedication is applied as previously mentioned [12].

To choose the appropriate size of catheter in the angiogram, the diameter of the stenosis is measured distally and proximally.

A dilatation by the catheter technique is feasible up to a vessel diameter of 12 mm, which corresponds to a stenosis situated close to the aortic bifurcation. The application of two balloons placed side by side — the so-called kissing-balloon technique — is required if the diameter of the vessel is larger than 12 mm. The recording of the intra–arterial blood pressure prior and following PTD completes the procedure and provides information on the initial success.

Besides a single mode non-invasive method applied for infrarenal aortic stenoses, there is also the combined mode surgical radiological intervention. Such a procedure is preferred in cases where an isolated iliac stenosis is associated with a primary occlusion of the superficial femoral artery.

During the operation, the dilatation of the iliac stenosis is performed under direct vision and following the successful dilatation, the femoral popliteal bypass is put in place [9, 16]. The success of PTA is primarily measured by a decrease in the symptoms.

For peripheral vessels, the assessment of the brachiopedal pressure is indispensable. The difference between systolic arm and ankle blood pressures (delta p) usually approximates the systolic pressure gradient. Normally, the systolic pressure at the ankle is at least as high as the systolic arm pressure but not more than –20 or –15 mm Hg below.

A decrease of the pressure gradient indicates an improvement of the hemodynamic situation. In addition, the standard walking test, 90 steps a minute walked for 5 minutes followed by 110 steps in the same period, reveals the success or failure of the catheter treatment. The control of the pulse characteristics are also of importance [11].

Recently, digital subtraction angiography has become a less invasive method for characterizing the vascular situation of the pre- or post-therapeutic stage [5, 7]. This imaging technique is being used more and more in functional and morphological diagnosis. In complicated situations, it offers the advantage of acting as a road map which facilitates the guiding and selective intubation of the catheter [6].

DSA has also had a considerable impact on the diagnostic concept of hypertension. Depending on the DSA result, the treatment can be started earlier than any possible operative procedure.

Many researchers report on a normalization or essential improvement of hypertension in 78 to 85% of renal artery stenoses as fibromuscular dysplasia usually does not progress as fast as arteriosclerosis. The results mainly correlate with the age of the patients, the duration of hypertension, and the degree of renal insufficiency. Restenosis occurred in approximately 15% of the cases.

It may be concluded that stenoses of renal arteries in patients up to the age of 45 years can be more successfully treated using the catheter technique. Hypertension with a unilateral renal-artery stenosis is the easiest to treat. The evidence of an hemodynamically effective stenosis is the prerequisite for renal PTA. The pressure measurement in the aorta and distally to the stenosis is of great consequence for PTRD. If the gradient shows a value of more than 20 mm Hg, the dilatation catheter is introduced by the guide wire which is placed distally to the stenosis.

A pressure of 5 to 7 atm is transmitted from the balloon onto the vessel wall. This is repeated on the stenosis about three times with 10 to 20 sec intervals. The repeated pressure measurement reflects the treatment success, while the morphologic changes are documented in the final angiogram. Additional medication with anticoagulating drugs is absolutely necessary for about 6 months.

Patients with stenoses which continue after ineffective PTA, usually undergo an aortic-renal bypass operation. Dilatation procedures as the treatment mode do not negatively affect subsequent operations.

Clinical results

Numerous studies have been performed to assess the results of PTA in peripheral arteries. In a large cooperative study among 12 different centers involving 1184 patients, the primary success rate was 74% with an overall complication rate of 10%. Over 20% of the patients had occlusions greater than 10 cm in length.

For ideal lesions e.g. short femoro-popliteal stenoses, we had a success rate of between 91 and 94%; the patency rate after three years was 80%. Similar with occlusions of less than 10 cm, the rate of success varies from 74 to 91%, depending on the stage of ischemic disease. The patency rate was 70 to 75%. In occlusions longer than 10 cm, the complication rate was 5.9% with a success rate of 59% [8].

References

1. Dotter CT, Judkins MP (1964) Transluminal treatment of arteriosclerotic obstruction. *Circulation* 30: 654–670.
2. Grüntzig A, Hopff H (1974) Perkutane Rekanalisation chronischer arterieller Verschlüsse mit einem neuen Dilatationskatheter. *Dtsch med Wschr* 99: 2502.
3. Olbert F, Kasprzak P, Muzika N, Schlegel A (1982) Perkutane transluminale Dilatation und Rekanalisation. Langzeit-ergebnisse und Erfahrungsbericht mit einem neuen Kathetersystem. *VASA* 11 (4): 327–331.
4. Roth FJ, Cappius G (1980) Die Angioplastie in der Leiste gelegener Arterienabschnitte, in: Müller-Wiefel H, Harras J–P, Ehringel H, Krüger M (eds), *Mikrozirkulation und Blutrheologie*, pp. 430–432. Baden-Baden, Köln, New York: Verlag G. Witzstrock.
5. Seyferth W, Marhoff P, Zeitler E (1982) Transvenöse und arterielle digitale Videosubtraktionsangiographie (DVSA). *Fortschr Röntgenstr* 136: 3.
6. Seyferth W, Polster W (1985) Pfadfindertechnik: eine Ergänzung der Digitalen Subtraktionsangiographie im fluoroskopischen Betrieb. *Electromedica* 53: 39–45.
7. Crummy AB, Mistretta CA, Cline R (1974) An inexpensive storage system for selective catheterization procedures. *Radiology* 110: 369–372.
8. Schmidtke I, Zeitler E, Schoop W (1975) Langzeitergebnisse der perkutanen Katheterbehandlung (Dotter-Technik) bei femoropoplitealen Arterienverschlüssen im Stadium II. *VASA* 4: 210.

9. Vollmar J (1975) *Rekonstruktive Chirurgie der Arterien.* Stuttgart: Georg Thieme Verlag.
10. Zeitler E, Hüring HG, Schoop W, Schmidtke I (1971) Mechanische Behandlung von Beckenarterienstenosen mit der perkutanen Kathetertechnik. *Verh dtsch Kreisl–Forschg* 37: 402.
11. Zeitler E, Grüntzig A, Schoop W, (1978) *Percutaneous Vascular Recanalization.* Berlin, Heidelberg, New York: Springer–Verlag.
12. Zeitler E, Reichold J, Schoop W, Loew D (1973) Einfluß von Acetylsalicylsäure auf das Frühergebnis nach perkutaner Rekanalisation arterieller Obliterationen nach Dotter. *Dtsch med Wschr* 98, 1285–1288.
13. Sörensen R, Grassot A, Zühlke HV (1982) The fate of 'no angioplasty' in peripheral vascular disease, in: Kaltenbach et al. (ed), *Transluminal Coronary Angioplasty and Intracoronary Thrombolysis.* Berlin, Heidelberg: Springer-Verlag.
14. Leu HJ (1982) Morphologie der Arterienwand nach PTA Röntgenpraxis 8. *Bd* 35: 313.
15. Höhn P, Wagner R, Zeitler E (1975) Histologische Befunde nach der Katheterbehandlung arterieller Obliterationen nach Dotter und ihre Bedeutung. *Herz/Kreisl* 7: 13–23.
16. Giessler R, Schoop W, Zeitler E (1973) *Indikationen zur operativen Therapie bei coronaren und cerebralen Durchblutungsstörungen.* Bern: Huber-Verlag.
17. Mathias K, Mittermeyer Ch H, Essinger H (1980) Perkutane Katheterdilatation von Karotisstenosen. *Fortschr Röntgenstr* 133 (3): 258–261.
18. Mathias K, Steiger J, Thron A et al. (1980) Perkutane Katheterangioplastik der Arteria subklavia. *Dtsch med Wschr* 105, 16–28.
19. Mathias K, Schlosser M, Reinke M (1980) Katheterrekanalisation eines Subklaviaverschlusses. *Röfo* 132 (3): 346–347.
20. Sievert H, Kober G, Hopf R, Scherer D, Kaltenbach M (1984) Transluminale Koronarangioplastik bei Ärzten. *Herz und Gefäße* 4: 523–529.
21. Kaltenbach M, Kober G, Scherer D (1990) Transluminal coronary angioplasty: transbrachial approach and prevention of thromboembolic complications, in: Kaltenbach M, Grüntzig A, Rentrop K, Bussmann W–D (eds), *Transluminal Coronary Angioplasty and Intracoronary Thrombolysis.* Berlin, Heidelberg, New York: Springer Verlag.

13. Symptomatic occlusion of the subclavian artery: treatment by balloon angioplasty

C. DÜBER, K.-J. KLOSE, H. KOPP and W. SCHMIEDT

Introduction

Percutaneous transluminal angioplasty (PTA) has become an accepted method of treatment in patients with symptomatic stenosis of the subclavian artery (for review of literature see [1, 2, 7]. However there are only few reports on PTA in subclavian artery occlusion [11]. In this study our experience with recanalization procedures of the subclavian artery is reported.

Patients and methods

Patients

August 1987—February 1989;
8 patients: 5 men, 3 women;
age: 44–57; mean: 50;
left sided proximal occlusion: 8.

Symptoms

Arm symptoms: 8;
brachial blood pressure gradient (L/R): 30–60 mmHg; mean: 40;
cerebral symptoms: 5;
subclavian steal syndrome: 6;
occlusion of vertebral artery: 1;
aortic origin of vertebral artery: 1.

Methods

Clinical and noninvasive diagnosis: 8;
angiography (Digitron 2, Siemens, FRG);

V. Hombach et al. (eds), Interventional Techniques in Cardiovascular Medicine, 115–119.
© 1991 *Kluwer Academic Publishers.*

two step procedure:
iv. DSA (diagnostic) and ia. DSA (therapeutic): 2;
single step procedure:
combined diagnostic and therapeutic ia. DSA: 6;
femoral approach: 6;
combined femoral/brachial approach 2;
recanalization catheter:
multipurpose. sidewinder, headhunter;
balloon catheter (Medi-tech, Watertown, USA):
balloon size: 5 mm: 1; 6 mm: 1;
          7 mm: 2; 8 mm: 4;
nonionic contrast medium (Solutrast, Byk-Gulden, FRG).

Medical treatment

– Heparin 5000 units ia. during PTA;
– hydroxyethylstarch 500ml/24 hours iv. post PTA;
– aspirin 500 mg per day after PTA.

Results

Early results

Successful recanalization: 7/8;
none or moderate residual stenosis: 4/7;
severe residual stenosis: 3/7;
systolic brachial blood pressure;
gradient (L/R): 0–65; mean: 14;
clinical improvement: 7/8;
early reocclusion: 1/8;
persistent arm and cerebral symptoms: 1/8.

Complications

Asymptomatic embolization to distal subclavian artery: 1/8 (in a patient with recent thrombosis);
stenosis of brachial artery: 1/8 (combined femoral/brachial approach).

Figure 1. Occlusion of left subclavian artery with steal syndrome (b) Intravenous DSA 3 months after PTA: recanalized subclavian artery with normal vertebral blood flow.

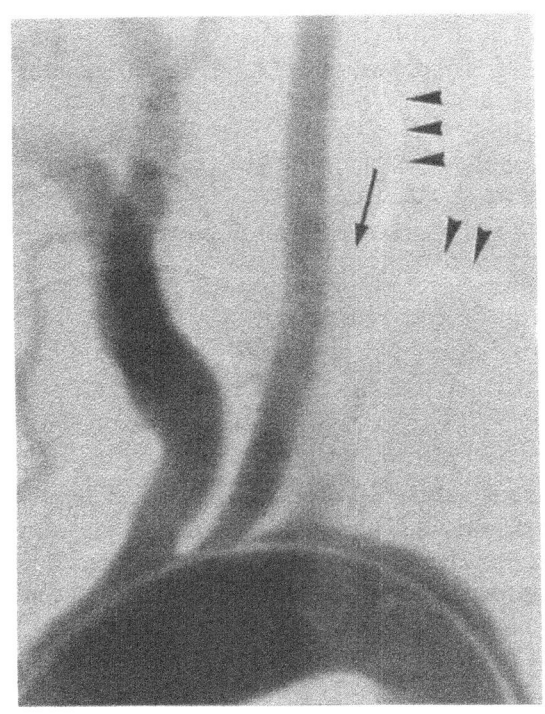

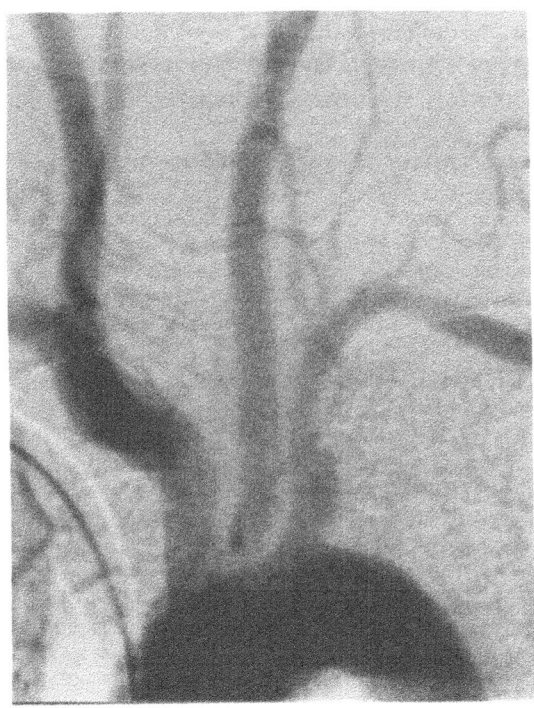

118   C. Düber et al.

Late results

Complete relief of symptoms: 4/7 (3, 4, 7, 20 months after PTA);
symptomatic reobstruction: 3/7;
restenosis: 1/7;
reocclusion: 2/7 (8, 12, 16 months after PTA);
successful second PTA: 3/7;
complete relief of symptoms or clinical improvement: 3/7 (4, 4, 4 months after second PTA).

Example: see Figure 1.

Conclusions

PTA of symptomatic subclavian artery occlusion can be performed with a high initial success rate.

The femoral approach to the arterial system is recommended. A combined brachial/femoral procedure is possible using the brachial route for recanalization and the femoral route for dilatation.

There is a risk of thrombus embolization in patients with recent onset of symptoms.

The cerebral circulation is protected against embolization in patients with preserved flow in the vertebral artery.

Late results after PTA of subclavian artery occlusion are worse than after PTA of subclavian artery stenosis with reobstruction occuring in about 50% of patients.

Restenosis or reocclusion can successfully be treated by a second PTA.

References

1. Becker GJ, Katzen BT, Dake MD (1989) Noncoronary angioplasty. *Radiology* 170: 921–940.
2. Düber C, Klose KJ, Kopp H, Schild H, Hake U (1989) Angioplastie der Arteria subclavia. Technik, Früh-und Spätergebnisse. *Dtsch Med Wschr* 114: 496–502.
3. Erbstein RA, Wholey MH, Smoot S (1988) Subclavian steal syndrom: treatment by percutaneous transluminal angioplasty. *AJR* 151: 291–294.
4. Lederer W, Dingler WH (1989) Subclaviaverschluß und Anomalie der Arteria vertebralis mit Subclavian-Steal-Syndrom. Fibrinolyse und PTA-Therapie. *Fortschr Röntgenstr* 150: 447–479.
5. Mathias K, Staiger J, Thron A, Spillner G, Heiss HW, Konrad-Graf S (1980) Perkutane Katheterangioplastik der Arteria subclavia. *Dtsch Med Wschr* 105: 16–18.
6. Mathias K, Schlosser V, Reinke M (1980) Katheterrekanalisation eines Subclaviaverschlusses. *Fortschr Röntgenstr* 132: 346–347.
7. Mathias K (1987) Katheterbehandlung der arteriellen Verschluß krankheit supraaortaler Gefäße. *Radiologe* 27: 547–554.

8. Motarjeme A, Keifer JW, Zuska AJ, Nabawi P (1985) Percutaneous transluminal angio-plasty for treatment of subclavian steal. *Radiology* 155: 611–613.
9. Ringelstein EB, Zeumer H, Brückmann H, Stübben G, Strum KW (1986) Atraumatische Diagnostik und semi-invasive Therapie des Subclaviaanzapfsyndroms mit Hilfe der perku-tanen transluminalen Angioplaste (PTA). Ein zeitgemäßes Konzept. *Fortschr Neurol Psychiat* 54: 216–231.
10. Staller BJ, Maleki M (1989) Percutaneous transluminal angioplasty for innominate artery stenosis and total occlusion of subclavian artery in Takayasu's type arteritis. *Cath and Cardiovasc Diagn* 16: 91–94.
11. Zietler E, Berger G, Schmitt-Rüth R (1983) Percutaneous transluminal angioplasty of the supra-aortic arteries, in: Dotter CT, Grüntzig A, Schoop W, Zeitler E (eds), *Percutaneous Transluminal Angioplasty*, pp. 245–261. Berlin, Heidelberg: Springer-Verlag.

14. Rotational atherectomy: current use in vascular disease with specific focus on the Simpson device

B. HÖFLING and A. von PÖLNITZ

Introduction

The percutaneous treatment of vascular disease with balloon angioplasty may be limited by inability to cross a lesion, acute re-occlusion and the relatively high long-term restenosis rate after a primarily successful inter-vantion [1, 2]. For these reasons, new techniques using either mechanical or other energy forms such as laser [3, 4], high-frequency [5] or ultrasound [6], which attempt to remove material are being developed. In this report we will focus on rotational atherectomy and devices developed with the goal of removing obstructing plaque material. In particular, we will focus on our results with the Simpson directional atherectomy catheter and its use in peripheral vascular disease.

There are rotational devices underway which were designed for crossing total occlusions. A prototype is the Rotacs wire [7, 8] which operates at a low-speed (200 rpm) and has been used successfully in peripheral and coronary vessels. In crossing an occlusion with this wire, plaque is not removed, but a channel is created that then allows passage of other devices to complete the revascularization. The Kensey catheter [9] is a flexible polyurethane catheter with a rotating cam tip at speeds up to 100,000 rpm. A fluid channel allows a fine circular jet spray for cooling and centering of the device and for contrast injection during angioplasty. Early clinical results showed success in crossing 4/10 total occlusions and in treating 10/13 stenoses [10], however perforation was noted in 8/9 unsuccessful cases, suggesting that further technical improvements are necessary.

There are currently several designs of rotational atherectomy devices in clinical use, both in peripheral and coronary vessels, which are capable of extracting or pulverizing plaque material. The rotating burr device developed by Auth [11] uses a diamond-studded abrasive tip on a flexible catheter, rotating at approximately 120,000 revolutions/min. The pulverized athero-matous particles thus generated are up to 250 microns in size, although 90% of ablated particles were measured at less than 8 microns [11]. After initial promising results in the periphery without significant embolization [12],

V. Hombach et al. (eds), Interventional Techniques in Cardiovascular Medicine, 121–131.

122   *B. Höfling and A. von Pölnitz*

coronary stenoses have also been successfully treated using shafts of 1.25 to
3.5 mm in an over-the-wire technique [13, 14]. Although Fourrier et al.
reported no procedure related complications in 12 patients [14], others [15,
16] have reported transient regional myocardial dysfunction or coronary
spasm after successful rotablation which could represent showers of emboli

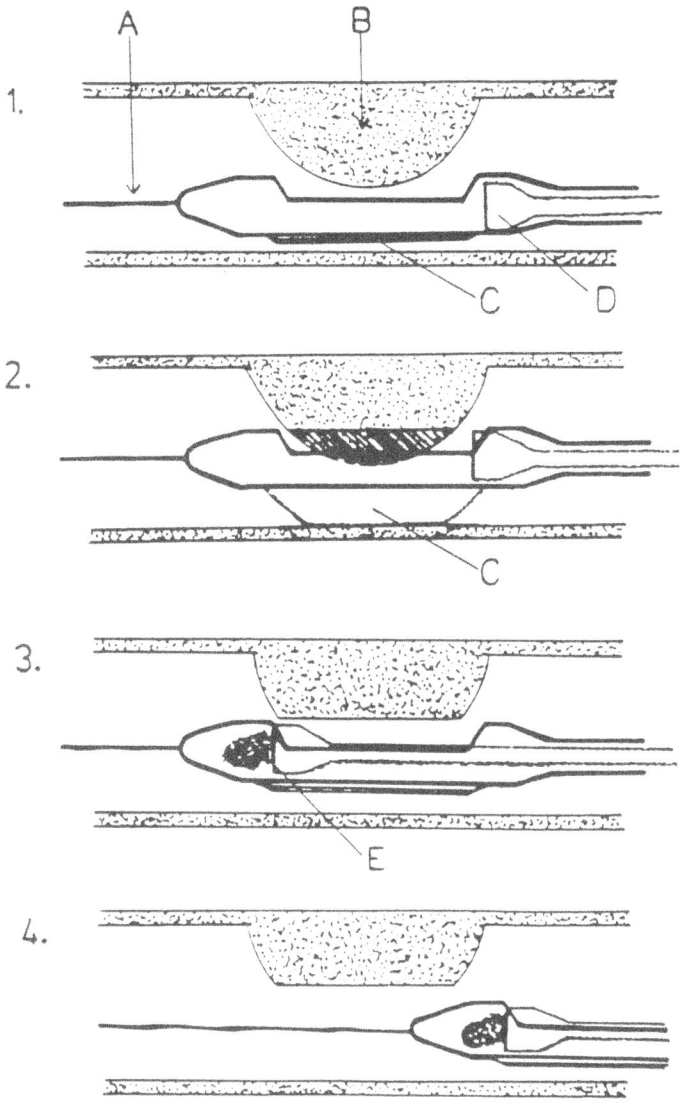

Figure 1.   Schematic illustration of the principle of directional atherectomy. The window in
the housing of the catheter is positioned against a stenosis (B). A low-pressure (2–3 atm)
balloon (C) is used to fix the position and the rotating cutting edge (D) is advanced shaving off
slices of protruding plaque material (E). These are deposited within the collecting chamber and
later removed (see Figure 2).

in the coronary microcirculation. The restenosis rate in the coronaries with this device appears to be approximately 50% [17].

The transluminal extraction catheter (TEC) uses a vacuum system to aspirate excised plaque material [18]. The advantage of this device is its flexibility as well a suction mechanism to avoid distal embolization. Stack et al. have now reported on the multicenter registry on 66 coronary patients treated with this device (42% LAD, 42% RCA, 9% Cx, 5% graft, and protected main stem 2%). There was a high procedure success rate of 92% and no cases of distal embolization. Long-term results are presently unavailable.

The Simpson directional atherectomy catheter [19, 20] utilizes a rotary cutting edge (600–2000 rpm) incorporated within a metal housing at its tip. A window in the housing is positioned against a stenosis by a low-pressure balloon opposite to the window, thus the cutting edge can be 'directed' towards the surface to be excised (Figure 1). In this report we will present long term clinical and angiographic results in 60 patients with symptomatic peripheral vascular disease treated with this catheter [21, 22]. Initial results of 260 patients undergoing coronary directional atherectomy [23, 24] show a low incidence of complications (CABG 3.5%, perforation without hemopericardium 1.2%, deaths 0%) with abrupt vessel closure occurring in only 2 patients. The overall restenosis rate has been approximately 40% [24], with the lowest rates found after treatment of the proximal LAD (26%) or larger caliber vessels (23% in vessels > 3.25 mm).

A distinct advantage of the Simpson catheter lies in its 'biopsy' mechanism, enabling retrieval of full thickness slices of excised material which may be investigated with light or electron microscopy [25–27], immunohistochemistry [28] or cell culture study [29, 30]. This access to human primary advanced plaque material and restenotic lesions may prove valuable in studying atherosclerosis and the process of restenosis and their pharmacological prophylaxis.

Methods

Patients. A total of 60 patients (48 male, 12 female) with a mean age of 64.1 ± 10.6 years and all with symptomatic disease were accepted for atherectomy. Fifteen patients had rest pain and 6 (10%) had gangrene. The majority of patients were referred because of complexity of the lesion or because they were considered poor surgical candidates because of poor distal vessels, with limb salvage as the main goal in 3 patients.

Clinical evaluation and follow-up. All patients underwent baseline doppler with calculation of the leg/arm index and standardized claudication limited walking distance evaluation (3 km/h, 12.5% incline, maximal 250 m). All parameters were repeated on the 2nd day after the procedure, as well as after 1, 3 and 6 months, at which time a control angiogram was also performed (or sooner if dictated by symptoms), and bi-annually thereafter. All patients were treated with 500 mg of aspirin prior to the procedure and continued on aspirin for 6 months post-procedure. Most patients were discharged with 48 hours of the procedure.

Atherectomy procedure.   The intervention was performed as previously described [21]. The Simpson catheter has a 4.5 cm guide wire at its distal end and its metal housing incorporates a rotary knife (2000 rpm) which is battery powered and under operator control. A window in the housing is directed towards the aspect of the lesion to be excised (thus the technique is termed 'directional' atherectomy) and a low pressure (2–3 atm) balloon is used to maintain the selected orientation. As the cutting edge is advanced slices of material protruding into the opening in the housing are shaved off and trapped in a collecting chamber (Figure 2). Passes of the cutter are continued with adjustment of position as necessary until no or minimal residual stenosis and good contrast density is achieved.

In cases of total occlusion (Figure 3), the procedure was modified in the following stepwise fashion: after creation of a channel by a mechanical dotter technique, an attempt was made to introduce the atherectomy catheter. If this was not feasible, balloon angioplasty was performed with the goal of creating a lumen large enough to allow passage of the atherec-

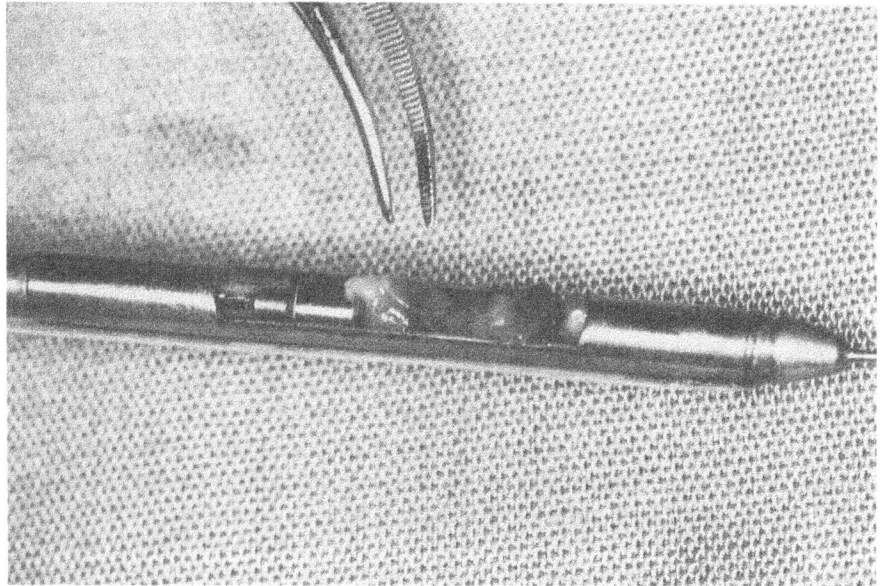

Figure 2.   Close-up of the housing of the atherectomy catheter. The rotary cutting edge has been retracted and excised plaque can be removed from the collecting chamber and submitted for investigation.

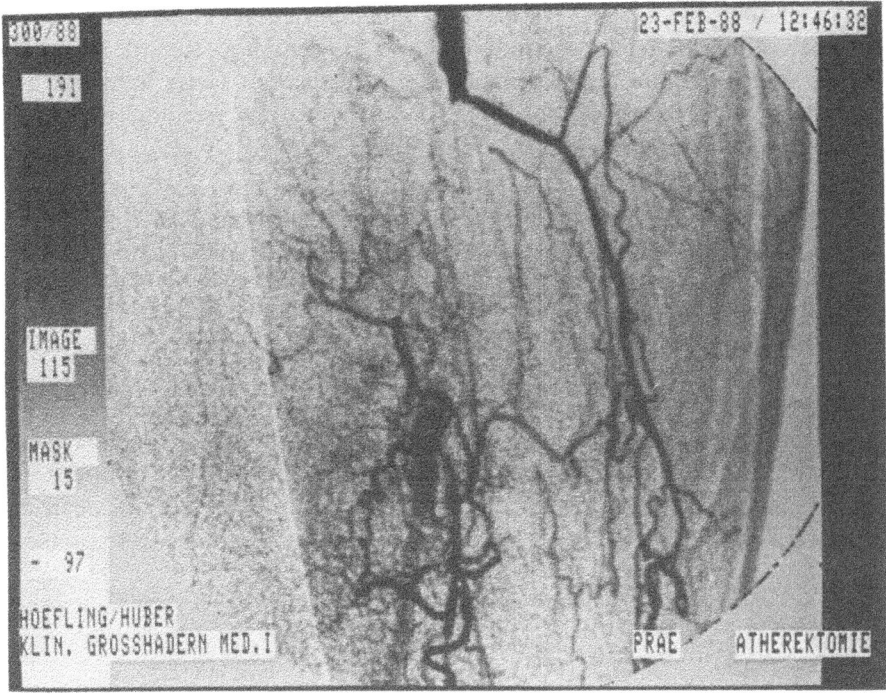

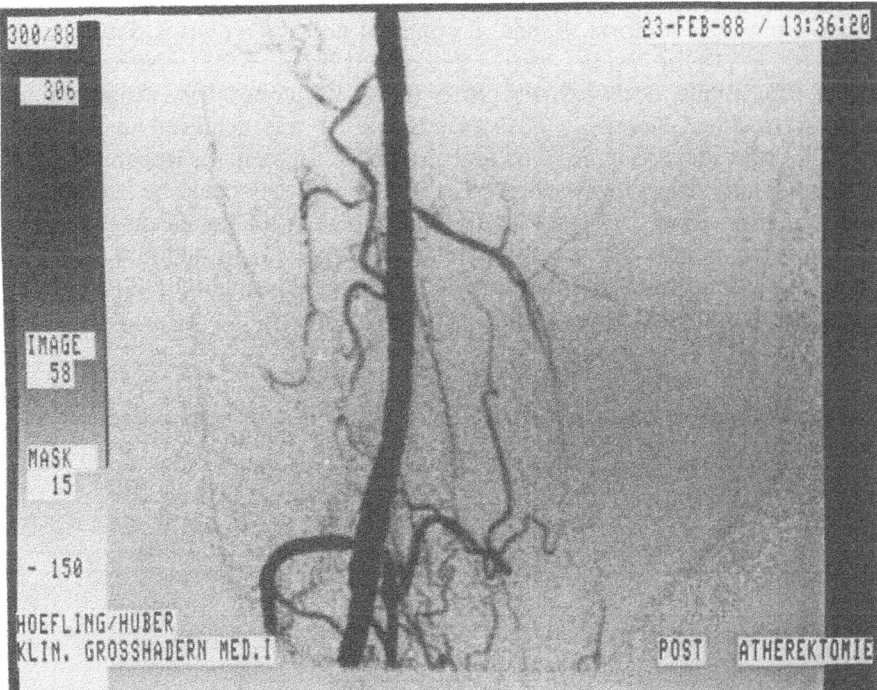

Figure 3.   Total occlusion of the right superficial femoral artery which was first crossed with a recanalization catheter. The atherectomy catheter could then be positioned within the recanalized lumen and obstructive material excised. Final results (3b) show a relatively smooth lumen without dissection.

tomy catheter, *but not achieve maximal dilatation effect.* Once introduced, the atherectomy catheter was used to remove the disrupted, stenotic material or 'cut' back into the lumen from within a dissection. Cases in which an angioplasty was considered necessary *after* atherectomy (residual diameter stenoses >50%) were considered atherectomy failures.

Angioscopy.   In addition, in 60% of treated lesions an American Edwards (USA) angioscope was introduced, and as previously described [31] used to inspect the treated site. Although angiographic results may be satisfactory, angioscopy can sometimes detect residual obstructive material or large flaps, which can be removed with additional passes of the atherectomy catheter.

Statistics.   The paired student's t-test and Mann-Whitney tests were used to calculate quantitative differences before and after the procedure and between groups while the chi-square test was used to calculate qualitative differences. Significance was based on values >0.05. Results are expressed as mean ± standard deviation.

Results

Angiographic.   60 patients with a total of 94 lesions in 65 limbs underwent atherectomy (77 femoral, 8 iliac, 8 popliteal and one anterior tibial). Over 63% (n = 60) of lesions were calcified, 51% (n = 48) eccentric, 33% (n = 31) totally occluded and 16% (n = 15) concentric. Angiographic success (residual stenosis <50%; see Table 1) was achieved in 85 of 94 (90.4%) of lesions or in 56 of 65 limbs (84.6%). In stenoses (mean length of 1.1 ± 0.5 cm) success was achieved in 90.4% and they could be successfully reduced from 83 ± 13% to 17 ± 18%. There was no significant difference between concentric and eccentric stenoses (Table 2). In addition, the presence of calcification did not preclude the achievement of a low post-procedure residual stenosis (Table 2).

Table 1. Angiographic success, defined as a residual stenosis of <50%, after atherectomy in 94 lesions

Vessel	Stenoses n = 63 Mean length 1.1 ± 0.5 cm	Occlusions n = 31 Mean length 4.2 ± 2.9 cm
Iliac	4/8 (50%)	—
Femoral	51/53 (96%)	21/24 (88%)
Popliteal	1/1 (100%)	7/7 (100%)
Tibial	1/1 (100%)	—
Total	57/63 (90%)	28/31 (90%)

Table 2. Angiographic results in 61 stenoses and 28 total occlusions in which the atherectomy procedure was completed (mean ± SD)

	No	% pre-	No	% post-	No	% 6 Mo
All stenoses	61	83 ± 13	61	17 ± 18	40	31 ± 26
concentric	15	85 ± 12	15	17 ± 12	13	44 ± 28
eccentric	46	82 ± 13	46	17 ± 17	27	27 ± 25
calcified	33	85 ± 13	33	19 ± 21	18	35 ± 20
Occlusions	28	100	28	9 ± 9	15	60 ± 34[a]

[a] p < 0.05 as compared to stenoses.

Occlusions.   Thirty-one occlusions (mean length 4.2 ± 2.9 cm) judged to be occluded for 19.2 ± 21.6 months (range 1 week to 6 yrs) were attempted, with success in 21 of 24 femoral and 7 of 7 popliteal lesions, for a total initial success rate of 90.3% (Table 1). The mean post-procedure residual stenosis was 9 ± 9%. In 17 of 28 (61%) occlusions, an initial 'Dotter' technique was followed directly by atherectomy, while in 11 of 28 (39%), a balloon angioplasty was first required to allow passage of the more stiff atherectomy catheter.

Control angiographic study at 6 months has been performed of 55 primary lesions, representing an 87.3% follow-up of the 63 lesions due for 6 month study; the mean 6 month stenosis for all lesions was 39%. Although there is a trend for a higher residual stenosis for concentric as compared with eccentric stenosis, this difference has not reached significance (44 ± 28% vs. 27 ± 26%, Table 2). Total occlusions showed a significantly higher 6 month mean stenosis of 60 ± 34%. Angiographic restenosis, defined as >50% reduction in luminal diameter, were found in 13 of 55 lesions (23.6%). When analyzing for primary morphology, restenoses were found in 3 of 13 concentric lesions (23.1%), 3 of 27 eccentric lesions (11.1%) and 7 of 15 (46.7%) total occlusions studied.

Complications.   There have been no instances of vessel perforation, acute occlusion or need for emergency surgical intervention. One patient undergoing an iliac atherectomy suffered a distal embolus to the bifurcation of the anterior and posterior tibial artery but had no long-term sequelae. In addition, two patients undergoing second atherectomies suffered groin hematomas requiring surgical evacuation on the 3rd and 6th day post-procedure. Local dissections are often seen angiographically after crossing total occlusions, but appear to be of no acute consequence.

Clinical.   In patients with a completed procedure, the mean Doppler-index improved significantly from 0.59 ± 0.18 to 0.83 ± 0.17 in 59 limbs which could be evaluated. A parallel improvement was found in walking distance, which increased from 81.4 ± 63.7 to 161.6 ± 82.8 m. Twenty-five patients who had initial successful interventions have now reached 1 year follow-up and 18 (72%) remain clinically patent, 4 (16%) have undergone repeat atherectomy and 2 (8%) surgical intervention. Of the 4 patients who have undergone repeat atherectomy, 3 have had second restenoses: 2 have since undergone surgery and 1 patient a third atherectomy (and remains clinically patent at 2 years). To date, only one patient has developed a restenosis beyond 6 months and the mean Doppler index and walking distance has been maintained up to 2 years (1 year: 0.78 index (n = 15) and 160.5 meters (n = 11) respectively; 2 years: 0.91 index (n = 8) and 188.7 meters (n = 7)).

Histological   Macroscopically, excised material ranged from shiny white to pale yellow in appearance, with a mean length of 4.9 ± 2.4 mm. Microscopic evaluation of 305 specimens from 52 lesions showed a thickened fibrotic intima in 100% of stenoses with varying degrees of 'myointimal proliferation' found in 35%. Sections of media were reached in 55% of stenoses and adventitia never. Fresh or organized thrombus material was found in 75% of stenoses and the classical atheromatous bed with cholesterol crystals could be detected in only 5.8% of cases. All 7 restenoses evaluated showed a thickened, fibrotic intima; marked cellular proliferation and organized thrombus were found in 6 of 7 and media reached in 6 of 7 [25] (Figure 4).

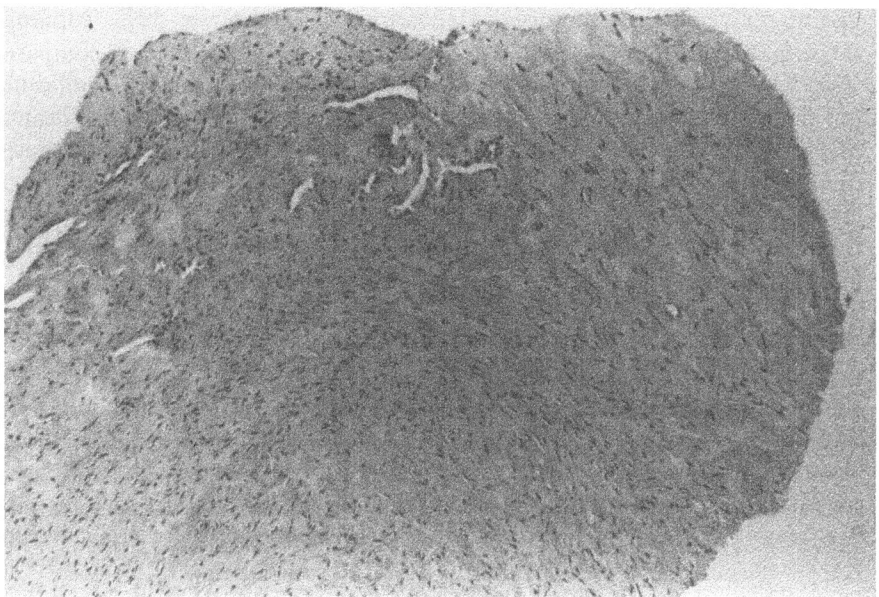

Figure 4.   Plaque material removed from a restenosis after previous atherectomy of a superficial femoral artery. An area of neo-capillarization is seen with a bed of marked cellular proliferation ('myointimal hyperplasia'). These spindle shaped smooth muscle cells with variable orientation are typical for restenosis lesions.

Electron microscopy Ultrastructurally, plaque material consisted of abundant extracellular matrix with collagen fibrils and elastic fibers or lamellae. Elongated and pancake-shaped smooth muscle cells surrounded by an amorphous basal lamina of variable width were irregularly embedded in this matrix. Variable cell phenotypes of smooth muscle cells were found, but cells particularly rich in filaments were not seen. The majority contained numerous cytoplasmic organelles, including perinuclear rough endoplasmic reticulum, golgi complex and mitochondria as well as lysosomes, suggesting increased synthetic activity. In addition, rare macrophages with intracellular lipid (foam cells) could be identified [27, 28].

Discussion

Percutaneous atherectomy with the Simpson atherectomy catheter in patients with peripheral vascular disease allows a high initial success rate and a low complication rate. This applies to eccentric and concentric stenoses as well as to total occlusions. Markedly irregular, eccentric lesions or longer occlusions may be more difficult to treat with angioplasty alone, and the removal of plaque material with this atherectomy catheter enables a favorable immediate angiographic result. Significantly, there were no incidence of procedure related acute occlusion or vessel perforation. The treatment of iliac vessels is somewhat limited by the size of the vessel and inferior to results with conventional angioplasty.

The angiographic restenosis rate of 15% for stenoses is comparable to that reported for balloon angioplasty. High-grade eccentric lesions, with a 12% angiographic restenosis rate, appear to be particularly amenable to treatment with directional atherectomy. Although good immediate results were achieved in short- and moderate length total occlusions by the combination of recanalization followed by plaque removal with atherectomy, restenosis rates remain high (47%).

The key to better long term results after percutaneous intervention, whether balloon, laser or atherectomy, will probably be in better medical prophylaxis. In this regard, the actual removal of plaque material allowed by this system, in effect a vessel wall biopsy, may prove helpful in the study of the process of restenosis.

References

1. Zeitler E, Richter EI, Roth FJ, Schoop W (1983) Results of percutaneous transluminal angioplasty. *Radiology* 146: 57–60.
2. Krepel VM, van Andel GJ, van Erp WFM, Breslau PJ (1985) Percutaneous transluminal angioplasty of the femoropopliteal artery: initial and long-term results. *Radiology* 156: 325–328.

3. Cumberland DC, Sanborn TA, Tayler DI, et al. (1986) Percutaneous laser thermal angioplasty: initial clinical results with a laser probe in total peripheral artery occlusions. *Lancet* 1: 1457–1459.
4. Sanborn TA, Cumberland DC, Greenfield AJ, et al. (1988) Percutaneous laser thermal angioplasty: initial results and 1-year follow-up in 129 femoropopliteal lesions. *Radiology* 168: 121–125.
5. Hombach V, Höher M, Arbikd O, et al. (1987) Die Hochfrequenzangioplastie — eine neue Methode zur Rekanalisation verschlossener arterieller Gefäße. *CorVas* 2: 67.
6. Siegel RJ, Cumberland DC, Myler RK and DonMichanel TA (1989) Percutaneous ultrasound angioplasty: initial clinical experience *Lancet* II: 772–774.
7. Kaltenbach M, Vallbracht C (1987) Rotationsangioplastik — ein neues Katheterverfahren. *Fortschr Med* 105: 412–414.
8. Vallbracht C, Liermann D, Prignitz I et al. (1988) Results of low speed rotational angioplasty for chronic peripheral occlusions. *Am J Cardiol* 62: 935–940.
9. Kensey KR (1987) Recanalization of obstructed arteries with a flexible, rotating tip catheter. *Radiology* 165: 387–389.
10. Snyder SO, Wheeler JR, Gregory RT et al. (1988) The Kensey catheter: preliminary results with a transluminal atherectomy tool. *J. Vasc Surg* 8(4): 541–543.
11. Ritchie JL, Hansen DD, Vracho R, Auth DC (1986) Mechanical thrombolysis: a new rotational catheter approach for acute thrombi. *Circulation* 73: 1006–1012.
12. Ahn SS, Auth D, Marcus DR, Moore WS (1988) Removal of focal atheromatous lesions by angioscopically guided high-speed rotary atherectomy. *J Vasc Surg* 7: 292.
13. Erbel R, O'Neil W, Auth D et al. (1989) Hochfrequenz-Rotations-Atherektomie bei koronarer Herzkrankheit. *Dtsch Med Wschr* 114: 487–495.
14. Fourrier JL, Bertrand ME, Auth D et al. (1989) Percutaneous coronary rotational angioplasty in humans: preliminary report. *JACC* 14: 1278–1282.
15. Tierstein PS, Ginsburg R, Warth D et al. (1990) Complications of human coronary rotablation. *JACC* 2: 57A, abstract.
16. Zacca N, Heibig J, Harris S, Kleiman N et al. (1990) Percutaneous coronary high speed rotational atherectomy: new, but how safe? *JACC* 15: 58A, abstr.
17. Niazi KA, Brodsky M, Friedman HZ et al. (1990) Restenosis after successful mechanical rotary atherectomy with the Auth rotablator. *JACC* 15: 57A, abstr.
18. Stack RS, Quigley PJ, Sketch MH et al. (1989) Treatment of coronary artery disease with the transluminal extraction-endarterectomy catheter: initial results of a multicenter study. *Circulation* II: 583.
19. Simpson JB, Selmon MR, Robertson GC et al. (1988) Transluminal atherectomy for occlusive peripheral vascular disease. *Am J Cardiol* 61 (14): 96G–101G.
20. Simpson JB, Zimmerman JJ, Selmon MR et al. (1986) Transluminal atherectomy: a new approach to the treatment of atheroscletoric vascular disease. *Angiology* 37: 409–410.
21. Höfling B, von Pölnitz A, Backa D et al. (1988) A new technique for non-operative removal of obstructive plaques in peripheral vascular disease. *Lancet* 1: 384–386.
22. von Pölnitz A, Nerlich A, Berger H, Höfling B (1990) Percutaneous peripheral atherectomy: angiographic and clinical follow-up of 60 patients. *JACC* 15: 682–688.
23. Simpson JB, Rowe M, Robertson G et al. (1990) Directional coronary atherectomy: success and complication rates and outcome predictors. *JACC* 15(2): 196A.
24. Hinohara T, Rowe M, Sipperly E et al. (1990) Restenosis following directional coronary atherectomy of native coronary arteries. *JACC* 15(2): 196A.
25. von Pölnitz A, Backa D, Remberger K et al. (1989) Restenosis after atherectomy shows increased intimal hyperplasia as compared to primary lesions. *J of Vas Med and Biol* 1: 283–287.
26. Johnson DE, Hinohara T, Selmon M et al. (1990) Primary peripheral arterial stenoses and restenoses excised by transluminal atherectomy: a histopathologic study. *JACC* 15(2): 419–425.

27. Schinko I, Höfling B, von Pölnitz A, Bauriedel G, Welsch U (1990) Electronmicroscopic evaluation of primary and restenostic lesions after percutaneous atherectomy. *JACC* 15(2): 254A.
28. Dartsch PC, Bauriedel G, Schinko I et al. (1989) Cell constitution and characteristics of human atherosclerotic plaques selectively removed by percutaneous atherectomy. *Atherosclerosis* 80: 149–157.
29. Bauriedel G, Dartsch PC, Voisard R et al. (1989) Selective percutaneous biopsy of atheromatous plaque tissue for cell culture. *Basic Res Cardiol* 84: 326–331.
30. Dartsch PC, Voisard P, Bauriedel G et al. (1990) Growth characteristics and cytoskeletal organization of cultured smooth muscle cells from human primary stenosing and restenosing lesions. *Arteriosclerosis* 10: 62–75.
31. Höfling B, von Pölnitz A, Bauriedel G et al. (1989) Angioscopically guided percutaneous atherectomy. *Am J of Cardiac Imaging* 3: 20–26.

15. Increased growth rates of percutaneously and surgically extracted plaque cells from human restenosing tissue in vitro

R. VOISARD, P. C. DARTSCH, G. BAURIEDEL,
L. LAUTERJUNG, B. HÖFLING and E. BETZ

Introduction

Migration and proliferation of smooth muscle cells (SMC) from the media into the subendothelial space are key events in the early stages of atherogenesis [1]. Thus SMC are, besides macrophages, the main cell type of atherosclerotic plaques [1, 2]. The percutaneous Simpson atherectomy catheter (p-SAC) is a clinically used device for the extraction of plaque material [3]. The excised tissue has already been used for histological, immunohistochemical and cell biological examinations [4, 5]. In this study growth rates and cell size distributions of SMC isolated from percutaneously extracted plaque material (p-SAC-SMC) and from surgically extracted plaque material (OP-SMC) were compared.

Patients and methods

Primary stenosing and restenosing plaque material of 24 patients (age: 64 ± 11 years) was extracted by a p-SAC from the femoral artery. Furthermore, primary stenosing and restenosing tissue from the femoral artery (5 patients, age: 65 ± 8 years) carotid artery (3 patients, age: 70.6 ± 6 years) and primary stenosing tissue from the abdominal aorta (2 patients, age: 56 ± 1 years) was removed during surgical intervention.

The obtained tissue was cut into small pieces and cells were isolated by an explant technique or by enzymatic disaggregation as previously described [5, 6]. Cells were cultivated in a mixture of Waymouth's MB 752/1 and Ham F-12 (1:1), supplemented with 15% fetal calf serum and standard amounts of antibiotics. For the characterisation of plaque cells by indirect immunofluoresence microscopy [5, 6], antibodies against factor VII-associated antigen (von Willebrand factor, Calbiochem, Frankfurt, FRG) and smooth muscle alpha-actin (Progen Biotechnik, Heidelberg, FRG) were used.

For the examination of growth rates and cell size distributions cells were seeded into 6 well-plates (COSTAR 3406, Tecnomara, Fernwald, FRG) at a

133

V. Hombach et al. (eds), Interventional Techniques in Cardiovascular Medicine, 133–138.
© 1991 *Kluwer Academic Publishers.*

density of 2000 to 3000 cells/cm^2. Growth properties were analysed on every third day in the following manner: Culture medium was removed, cells were washed twice with phosphate-buffered saline without calcium and magnesium and trypsinized for 10 min at 37°C to yield a suspension of single cells. Cell numbers and cell diameters were measured by a cell counter (CASY 1, Schärfe Systems, Kirchentellinsfurt, FRG). Proliferative activity and cell size distributions were monitored for 16 days after cell seeding.

Results

Cell isolation and characterisation

Both the explant technique and the enzymatic disaggregation were used successfully for the isolation and cultivation of SMC from primary stenosing and restenosing tissue (primary-SMC and re-SMC). Within 4–8 days, primary-SMC started to grow out radially from approximately 70% of all adherent explants (Figure 1a). Re-SMC migrated and proliferated from the explanted tissue already after 2–3 days.

Enzymatic disaggregation proved to be superior to the explant technique both in respect to isolated cell number and cell vitality. The first cells attached and spread within 48 hours after isolation and some cells could be isolated nearly from all extracted specimens. The vast majority of plaque cells was identified as SMC [5] by their positive reaction with antibodies against smooth muscle alpha-actin (Figure 1b). The reaction with antibodies against factor VIII-related antigen for the identification of endothelial cells [6] was negative.

Identification of two subpopulations

In all plaque cell populations, two subpopulations (SP-1 and SP-2) could be distinguished according to cell diameters (Figure 1c): SP-1 = 18.6 ± 5 μm (x ± SD) and SP–2 = 27.1 ± 3 μm (x ± SD, p < 0.01). 70% of all primary-SMC and 85% of all re-SMC were appointed to SP–1. The amount of cell debris was extremely high for primary-SMC (45% of total counts) in comparison to re-SMC (15% of total counts). With increasing in vitro age of re-SMC the amount of cell debris and the number of cells of SP–2 increased.

Figure 1.   (a) Smooth muscle cells growing out radially from plaque tissue (explant-technique) after 21 days in culture. (b) Identification of a plaque cell as SMC by positive reaction with antibodies against smooth muscle a-actin. (c) Identification of two subpopulations (SP-1 and SP-2) in all plaque cells according to cell diameters.

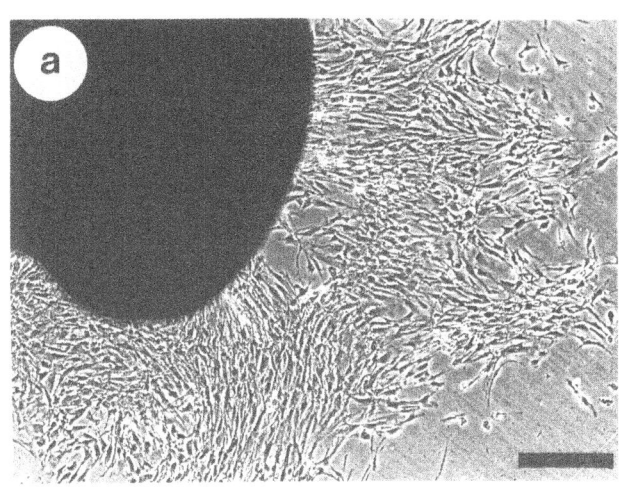

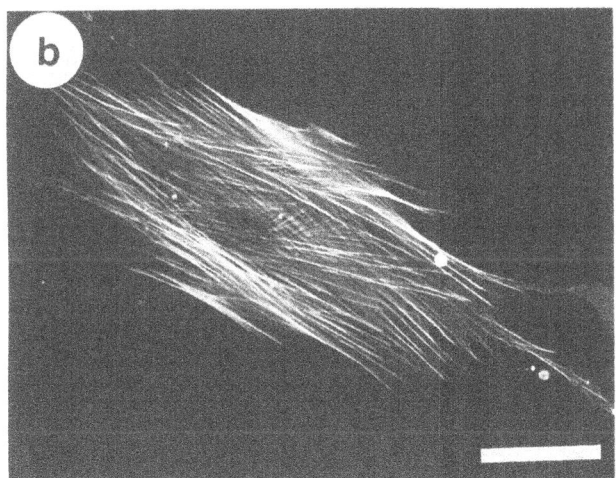

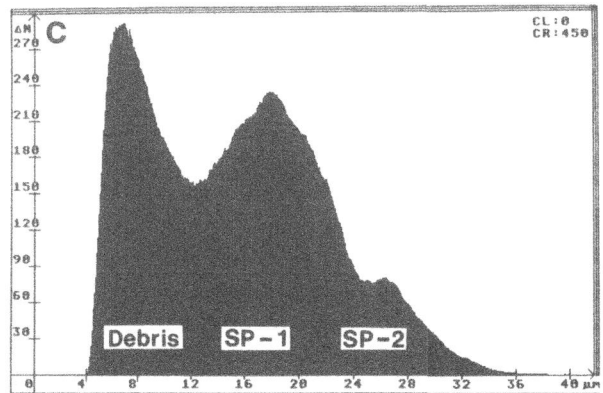

Determination of growth rates

Only SMC which had been isolated by enzymatic disaggregation were used for the determination of growth rates. A sufficient cell number was obtained in approximately 25% of total specimens. After being subcultivated twice primary-SMC did not undergo further mitoses and remained quiescent. In contrast re-SMC could be subcultivated up to 10 times. Signs of senescence such as a decreased capacity for further cell doublings or abundant amounts of cell debris were observed after 5 passages. The following survey summarizes growth rates of p-SAC-SMC and OP–SMC in first subcultures in population doublings/day (PD/day):

		primary stenosing	/	*restenosing tissue*
femoral artery	(p−SAC)	0.16 ± 0.04 (x±SD)		0.64 ± 0.15 (x±SD)
femoral artery	(OP)	0.21 PD/day		0.31 PD/day
carotid artery	(OP)	0.22 PD/day		0.27 PD/day
abdominal aorta	(OP)	0.18 PD/day		n.d.
x ± SD	(OP)	0.20 ± 0.02		0.29 ± 0.02

In both percutaneously and surgically extracted plaque material re-SMC exhibited increased growth rates in comparison to primary-SMC. The difference was highly significant for p–SAC–SMC ($p < 0.05$ for OP–SMC). There was no significant difference in growth rates of SMC from different arterial sites or between SMC from SP−1 and SP−2.

Discussion

Since both percutaneously and surgically extracted tissue have been used successfully for the cultivation of SMC, cell culture studies can be performed with tissue that was obtained by both methods. An advantage of the percutaneous technique (p-SAC) is certainly the selective capture and the early approach to the stenosing tissue.

In all plaque cell populations two subpopulations (SP-1 and SP-2) were identified according to cell diameters. Based on morphologic criteria, Björkerud et al. [7, 8] have already described small, low adhesive and enlarged, high adhesive cells. Dartsch et al. [5] demonstrated in an adhesion assay that the cells of SP-1 seem to be identical with the I-cells of Björkerud, whereas the cells of SP-2 seem to correspond to the A-cells.

In both percutaneously and surgically extracted tissue growth rates of primary-SMC were relatively low. This might be explained by a senescence of these cells, which have undergone a high number of cell doublings during atherogenesis in vivo. This interpretation was confirmed by the fact that the amount of cellular debris of primary-SMC was relatively high in comparison to fast growing re-SMC. However, with decreasing growth rates of re-SMC in higher passages, the amount of cellular debris increased as well, indicating the onset of senescene.

In comparison to primary-SMC growth rates of re-SMC were significantly increased. These results are in agreement with Hanke et al. [9], who examined the time course of SMC proliferation in restenosing lesions of rabbit carotid arteries after angioplasty. However while the difference of growth rates of primary-SMC and re-SMC from surgically removed plaque

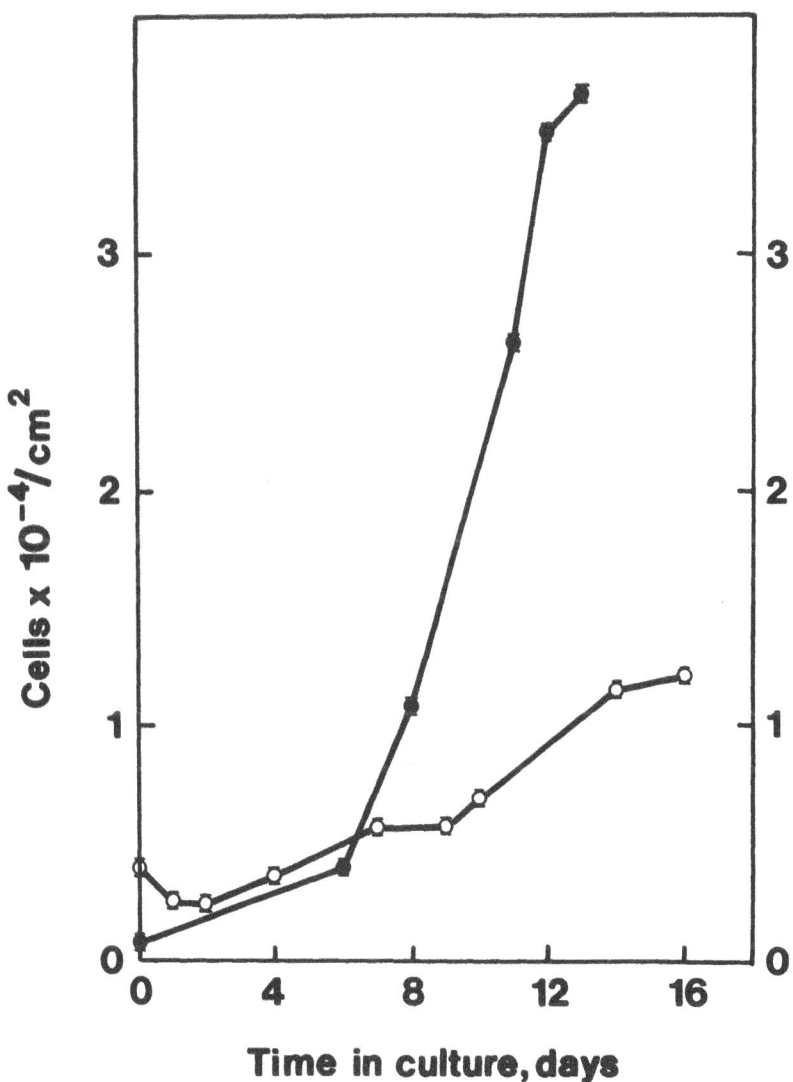

Figure 2. Comparison of growth rates of primary-SMC (□—□) and re-SMC (■—■). The calculation of population doublings/day (PD/day) gave the following results (p < 0.001, p-SAC extracted material): 0.16 ± 0.04 PD/day (x ± SD) for primary-SMC 0.64 60 0.15 PD/day (x ± SD) for re-SMC.

tissue was just significant, the difference of growth rates between primary-SMC and re-SMC from atherectomized plaque material was highly significant. The reason for this phenomenon might be a higher stimulus in vivo by the fast rotating catheter system.

With regard to the problem of restenoses after angioplasty, the search for antiproliferative drugs is of clinical interest. Drug-testing in cell cultures could be used as a prescreening system to select drugs for a scheduled test in an animal model. Cell culture techniques could possibly supply worthful additional information in the attempt to reduce restenosing events after percutaneous or surgical recanalization.

Acknowledgements

This work was supported by a grant from the MWK Baden-Württemberg, FRG (FSP 26) and Braun Melsungen AG, Melsungen, FRG.

References

1. Ross R (1986) The pathogenesis of atherosclerosis—an update. *N Engl J Med* 314: 488–500.
2. Ross R, Wight TN, Strandness E, Thiele B (1984) Human atherosclerosis: I. Cell constitution and characteristics of advanced lesions of the superficial femoral artery. *Am J Pathol* 114: 79–93.
3. Höfling B, v. Pölnitz A, Backa D, v. Arnim T, Lauterjung L, Jauch KW, Simpson JB (1988) Percutaneous removal of atheromatous plaques in peripheral arteries. *Lancet* 1: 384–386.
4. Dartsch PC, Bauriedel G, Schinko I, Weiss HD, Höfling B, Betz E (1989) Cell constitution and characteristics of human atherosclerotic plaques selectively removed by percutaneous *atherectomy*. *Atherosclerosis* 80: 149–157.
5. Dartsch PC, Voisard R, Bauriedel G, Höfling B, Betz E (1989) Growth characteristics and cytoskeletal organisation of cultured smooth muscle cells from human primary and restenosing lesions. *Arteriosclerosis*, in press.
6. Bauriedel G, Dartsch PC, Voisard R, Roth D, Simpson JB, Höfling B, Betz E (1989) Selective percutaneous 'biopsy' of atheromatous plaque tissue for cell culture. *Basic Res Cardiol* 84: 326–331.
7. Björkerud S, Ekroth R (1980) The growth of human atherosclerotic and non-atherosclerotic aortic intima and media in vitro. *Artery* 8: 329–335.
8. Bjökerud S (1985) Cultivated human arterial smooth muscle displays heterogenous pattern of growth and phenotypic variation. *Lab Invest* 53: 303–310.
9. Hanke H, Strohschneider T, Oberhoff M, Betz E, Karsch KR (1989) Time course of smooth muscle cell proliferation after angioplasty of atherosclerotic lesions of rabbit carotid arteries. *Eur Heart J* 10, suppl: 86, abstr.

16. Effect of propranolol on growth of cultured human smooth muscle cells derived from non-atherosclerotic and atherosclerotic vascular tissue

D. ROTH, P. C. DARTSCH and E. BETZ

Introduction

Intimal proliferation of smooth muscle cells (SMC) is involved in athero-genesis [8]. Several studies report that the β-adrenoreceptor antagonist propranolol has an antiatherosclerotic effect on diet- and stress-induced atherosclerosis in animal experiments [1, 5, 6, 9]. For further evaluation of this drug the influence of propranolol on growth of cultured human smooth muscle cells was tested.

Methods

Plaque material from carotid arteries was obtained from 5 patients of both sex (54-63 years of age) during thrombendarterectomy. Small pieces from human aortas were excised during autopsy 12 h postmortem (with permission of the ethical committee of the University of Tübingen). SMC were isolated by a fractionating enzymatic disaggregation with a collagenase/elastase enzyme mixture and then cultivated as described [2].

For testing the effect of propranolol cells with an in vitro age of 5–6 cumulative population doublings were seeded at densities of 2000 cells/cm^2 in 6-well plates. On days 1 and 3 after seeding, medium was exchanged and propranolol was added in concentrations ranging from 1×10^{-9} to 1×10^{-4} mol/l to the replicate sparse cultures. On day 4, cells were harvested by trypsin/EDTA treatment and cell numbers and cell size distributions were determined with a cell analyzer system (Casy I, Schärfe System, Reutlingen FRG).

Cell identification

Isolated cells were characterized as SMC by their 'hill and valley' and nodular growth patterns and their positive staining with antibodies against smooth muscle specific α-actin as described [2].

V. Hombach et al. (eds), Interventional Techniques in Cardiovascular Medicine, 139–143.

Results

Growth characteristics

SMC from primary stenosing tissue exhibited significantly lower growth rates in culture ($0,18 \pm 0,06$ population doublings per day; $\bar{x} \pm$ SD) when compared with SMC from non-atherosclerotic tissue ($0,34 \pm 0,07$).

Cell populations of plaque derived SMC consisted of two distinct subpopulations (see Figure 1a), which could be discriminated by cell size measurements: Subpopulation SP-1* contained cells with a mean cell diameter of $18,0 \pm 4$ μm ($\bar{x} \pm$ SD) and subpopulation SP-2* cells with a mean diameter of $26,0 \pm 3$ μm. In all plaque cell populations examined the smaller cells of SP−1* were predominating. In comparison, SMC derived from non-atherosclerotic tissues consisted of one population with a mean cell diameter of $14,5 \pm 3$ μm ($\bar{x} \pm$ SD) (see Figure 1b).

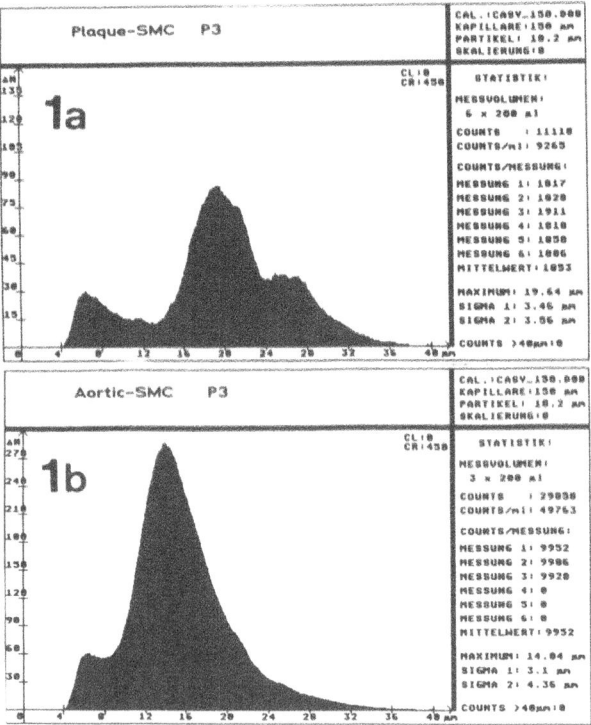

Figure 1. Original plot of cell sizes of plaque-SMC (a) and aortic-SMC (b) with an in vitro age of 6 cumulative population doublings. Note the two distinct subpopulations with different cell diameters which could be quantified by cursor settings: subpopulation SP-1* contained cells with a mean cell diameter of 18.0 ± 4 μm and SP-2* cells with a mean diameter of 26.0 ± 3 μm.

Test assay

The effect of the drug was measured by calculating cell proliferation in reference to growth in the corresponding controls (= relative cell proliferation). As shown in Figure 2, propranolol concentrations ranging from 1 $\times$ 10^{-9} to 1 $\times$ 10^{-5} mol/l had no significant influence on cell proliferation on SMC derived from non-atheroscletoric and atherosclerotic vascular tissues.

The highest concentration of 1 $\times$ 10^{-4} mol/l caused a decrease in proliferative activity of plaque derived SMC to 65% and of aortic-SMC to 60%.

Cytotoxic effects like detachment and lysis of cells were not observed during the tests. Changes in cell size distribution and cell shape after propranolol treatment were not detected.

Propranolol

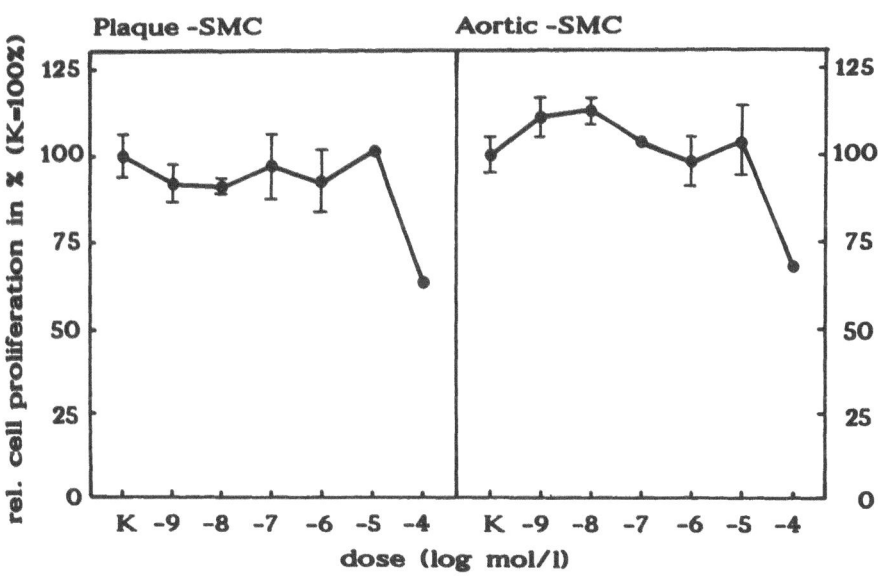

Figure 2.   Influence of propranolol concentrations ranging from 1 $\times$ 10^{-4} to 1 $\times$ 10^{-9} mol/l on growth of cultured SMC derived from non-atherosclerotic and atherosclerotic vascular tissues. Concentrations ranging from 1 $\times$ 10^{-9} to 1 $\times$ 10^{-5} mol/l show no significant effect on cell proliferation in comparison to controls (therapeutically used dosages range from 1 $\times$ 10^{-6} to 1 $\times$ 10^{-7} mol/l).

Discussion

Growth characteristics

Stenosing plaque tissues from carotid arteries obviously consisted of two SMC subpopulations SP-1* and SP-2*. Isolated SMC derived from advanced primary stenosing lesions in carotid arteries showed a lower growth rate, than SMC from normal arterial wall. This is in agreement with previous results on cultivated plaque-SMC isolated either by percutaneous trans-luminal atherectomy with a Simpson catheter or by thrombendarterectomy in coronary arteries [3, 4].

Test assay

Propranolol significantly inhibited the proliferation of cultured SMC from non-atherosclerotic and atherosclerotic tissues only at a very high concentration of 1×10^{-4} mol/l. Therapeutically used dosages which range from 1×10^{-6} to 1×10^{-7} mol/l had no significant influence on cell growth. Our results are in contrast to the findings of Orekhov et al. [7], who described a growth-stimulating effect of beta-blocking agents on cultured human smooth muscle cells isolated from non-atherosclerotic and atherosclerotic vascular tissues. However, cell culture tests of Orekhov et al. [7] were not identical to the conditions described here (e.g., Orekhov et al. used a 7-day primary culture of smooth muscle cells). This might cause the contradictory results of the effect of beta-blocking agents on SMC proliferation.

References

1. Chobanian AV, Brecher P, Chan C (1985) Effects of propranolol on atherogenesis in the cholesterol-fed rabbit. *Circ Res* 56: 755–762.
2. Dartsch PC, Roth D, Betz E (1988) Gefäßwandzellen des Menschen in Kultur. *VASA* suppl 23: 18–22.
3. Dartsch PC, Voisard R, Betz E In vitro growth characteristics of human atherosclerotic plaque cells from primary stenosing and restenosing lesions of peripheral and coronary arteries. *Res Exp Med* (submitted).
4. Dartsch PC, Voisard R, Bauriedel G, Höfling B, Betz E (1990) Growth characteristics and cytoskeletal organization of cultured smooth muscle cells from primary stenosing and restenosing lesions. *Arteriosclerosis* 10: 62–75.
5. Hirsch EZ, Maksem JA, Gagen D (1984) Effects of stress and propranolol on the aortic intima of rats. *Arteriosclerosis* 4: 526a.
6. Kaplan JR, Manuck SB, Clarkson TB, Adams MR, Weingand KW (1986) Effects of propranolol HCI on behaviorally induced atherosclerosis in hyperlipoproteinemic monkeys. *Arteriosclerosis* 6: 545A.
7. Orekhov AN, Ruda M, Baldenkov GN, Tertov W, Khashimov KA, Ryong LH, Lyakishev AA, Kozlov SG, Tkachuk VA, Smirnov VN (1988) Atherogenic effects of beta blockers on cells cultured from normal and atherosclerotic aorta. *Am J Cardiol* 61: 1116–1117.

8. Ross R (1986) The pathogenesis of atherosclerosis- an update. *N Engl J Med* Feb 20: 488–500.
9. Whittington-Coleman PJ, Carrier O, Douglas BH (1973) The effects of propranolol on cholesterol-induced atheromatous lesions. *Atherosclerosis* 18: 337–345.

17. Excimer laser angioplasty: efficiency and damage

R. HIBST, T. KOLBE, S. WEINBRENNER and V.
HOMBACH

Summary

Pulsed excimer laser light has been shown to be effective for the removal of
fibrous or calcified stenoses of vessels. In order to be able to optimize laser
parameters and irradiation mode for different clinical applications, we
investigated in vitro how radiant energy, pulse repetition rate and irradiation
geometry effect both the efficiency of the procedure and the damage of the
remaining tissue. Results are different for close contact between light
transmitting fiber and specimens and for non contact. There are no universal
optimal parameters, but the measured data allow to find the best conditions
according to the particular circumstances.

Introduction

Beginning with initial reports in 1984 [1], a lot of in vitro and in vivo
investigations have been done in order to describe and analyze the effect of
pulsed excimer laser radiation on vessel wall and different plaques. Studies
of the influence of radiant energy and wavelength on ablation [2, 3] revealed
the 308 nm emission of the excimer laser to be the most efficient radiation
for angioplasty which can be transmitted through silica fibers. Because pulse
duration does not affect tissue ablation significantly in the range from 15 ns
to 180 ns [3], relative long pulses are advantageous to overcome the
problem of fiber breakage.

In order to evaluate other parameters too, we investigated the effect of
radiant energy, repetition rate and irradiation conditions on ablation efficiency and tissue damage. Although now first experimental clinical applications are reported for peripheral vessels and even coronaries [4–6], there is
still a need for such in vitro data to optimize the clinical use of available
lasers and for the development of new laser/catheter systems. We studied
tissue ablation both for fiber/tissue contact and non contact. The contact
mode is actually the usual method. However, channel diameters are nearly as

V. Hombach et al. (eds), Interventional Techniques in Cardiovascular Medicine, 145–149.
© 1991 *Kluwer Academic Publishers*.

small as the fiber or fiber bundle. By keeping a distance between fiber end and tissue, it should be possible to enlarge the channel diameter. Conditions and limitations of this approach were evaluated.

Material and methods

Studies were performed with a short pulse excimer laser ($\tau = 17$ ns) at a wavelength of 308 nm. Light was transmitted through a PCS fiber of 600 μm core diameter. Segments of normal and atherosclerotic human cadaver aorta were irradiated under saline solution with various numbers of pulses. Radiant energies were varied from 1 to 25 mJ per pulse and repetition rates from 1 to 170 Hz.

For non contact measurements the fiber was fixed at a definite distance and angle to the aorta. The fiber end was flushed with saline solution. Contact measurements were performed for different mechanical forces which were determined by a scale. Crater depths and diameters were measured under the microscope by focusing the crater top and bottom. Damage zones were evaluated after standard histological procedures.

Results

Non contact mode

Figure 1 shows, how the ablation effiency—measured as crater depth per pulse—depends on the radiant exposure per pulse. In the energy range shown, there is a nearly parabolic relationship between the crater depth in normal aorta and the radiant exposure. Efficiency is slightly reduced for fibrous-fatty or sclerotic aorta, but it drops rapidly when plaques become calcified.

When varying the distance between fiber end and specimen from 0.5 to 1.5 mm or the angle from 90° to 45°, crater depths are also related to the radiant exposure as shown in Figure 1, when considering the irradiated area for each geometry. However, the diameters of the craters do not increase according to this area, but are roughly constant.

The data shown in Figure 1 are valid for a pulse repetition rate of 5 Hz, but ablation depth depends on the repetition rate, too. In the energy range shown in Figure 1 the ablation per pulse was maximal for a repetition rate of about 15 Hz. Maxima become more pronounced for higher radiant exposure.

Histology of the samples shows that the craters are surrounded by a small coagulation zone and a larger area with vacuols and disruptions. A systematic study of the maximum damage zone reveals, that the damage is related to the radiant exposure in nearly the same manner as the crater depth (Figure

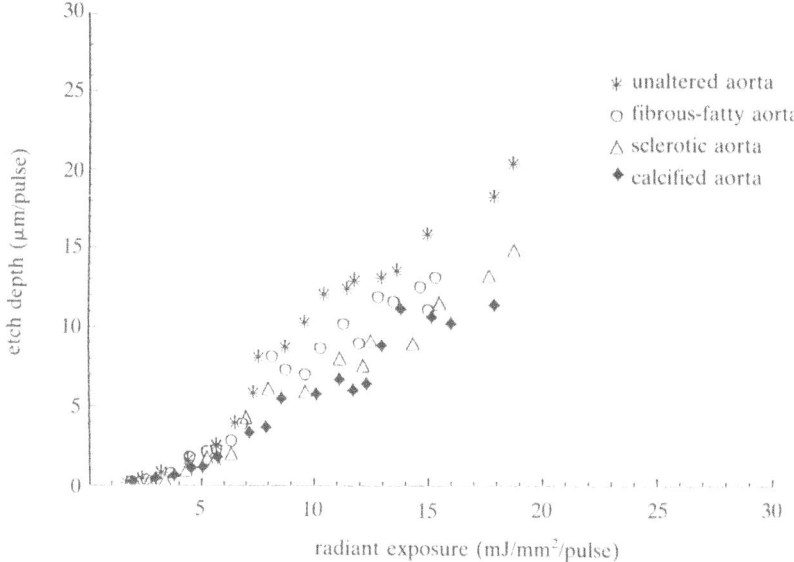

Figure 1. Crater depth per pulse vs radiant exposure ($\nu = 5$ Hz, $\alpha = 90°$).

1). For 14 mJ/mm^2 damage by disruption is up to 300μm surrounding the crater. This damage zone is only little affected by the repetition rate.

Contact mode

The relation between crater depth per pulse and radiant exposure measured for fiber/tissue contact is comparable to that measured in the non contact mode. Also the influence of plaque type is the same. The dependence of the ablation on the repetition rate, however, reveals significant differences: In the contact mode there is a linear relation between crater depth per pulse and the repetition rate in a range from 1 to 170 Hz. The slope of the lines increases with the radiant energy. This effect becomes very marked, when 5 mJ per pulse are exceeded. For 7 mJ per pulse the efficiency can be enhanced by a factor 5 when increasing the repetition rate.

Damage is of the same type as for the contact mode. Both radiant energy and repetition rate affect coagulation and disruption zone. Figure 2 shows, as an example of a systematic study which includes energies from 3 to 10 mJ and repetition rates from 1 to 170 Hz, how the repetition rate influences the damage for a definite energy of 5 mJ per pulse. When a repetition rate of 50 Hz is exceeded, the coagulation zone remains nearly constant, while disruptions increase nearby linearly in the high frequency range. Similar effects are observed when varying the radiant energy per pulse.

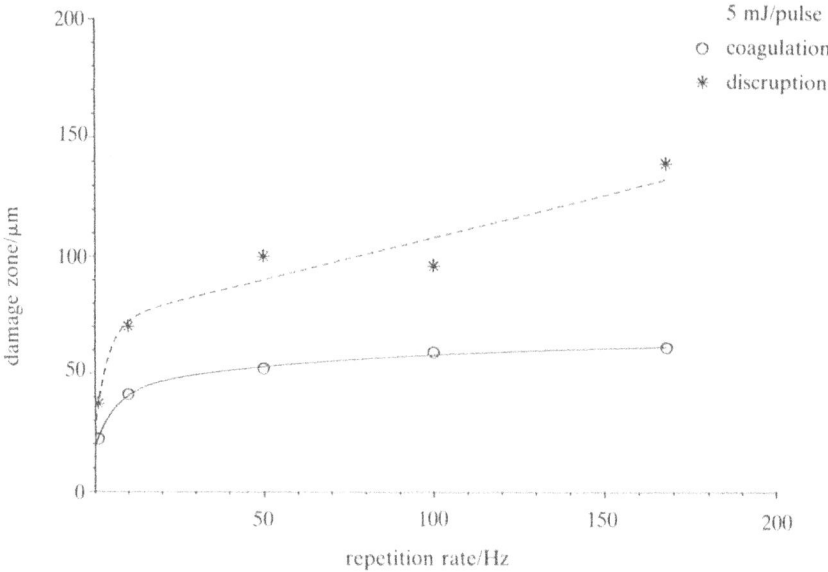

Figure 2.   Damage zone vs repetition rate (5 mJ/pulse).

Discussion

The energy dependence of ablation measured under saline solution in contact and non contact mode is in good agreement with earlier results obtained for irradiation in air [7]. Also the influence of plaque type is the same. Although crater depths measured for various distances and angles in the non contact mode fit well into the diagram of Figure 1, the diameters do not increase according to the irradiated area. This might be due to the intensity profile of the light behind the fiber. Intensity in the outer parts of a large area drops rapidly, so that the radiant exposure becomes small. Because of the parabolic dependence between crater depth and radiant exposure (Figure 1), in this case ablation is very low and negligble compared to the center.

While the energy dependence of ablation is the same in contact and non contact mode there are important differences with respect to the repetition rate. As observed for skin removal too [8], for non contact aortic ablation there is a maximum crater depth per pulse when varying the repetition rate. The decrease of ablation efficiency for high repetition rates might be due to energy absorption by ablated material, which may shield the aorta. This effect reduces the potential of the repetition rate to influence the drilling speed. The main factor in the non contact mode is the radiant exposure. Because both crater depth per pulse and damage are related to the radiant exposure in the same manner, there is no optimum. If the radiant exposure is increased to get deeper craters per pulse, damage is increased in the same way. The tolerable damage limits the radiant exposure to be used.

In contrast, for fiber/tissue contact the crater depth per pulse increases linearly with the repetition rate. Because the number of pulses per second increases linearly, too, the forward speed is related to the frequency in the second power. This makes the repetition rate for the drilling speed as important as the radiant energy per pulse. Analysis of our data shows that for high forward speed a combination of moderate energy, e.g., 5 mJ per pulse, and high repetition rate results in less damage compared to a combination with a high energy. If minimum damage is desired, both repetition rate and radiant energy have to be decreased drastically.

Conclusions

The non contact method seems actually not to be convenient for clinical use to increase lumen diameter. The intensity profile of the outcoming light has to be changed to a more homogeneous one, in order to achieve the same ablation in the flanks and the center of the irradiated area.

When applying UV excimer laser light in close contact between fiber and tissue, the repetition rate of the pulses is a very important parameter, which is often neglected. An increase of it might be sometimes more useful than an attempt to maximize the radiant energy.

References

1. Linsker R, Srinivasan R, Wynne JJ, Alonso DR (1984) Far ultraviolet laser ablation of atherosclerotic lesions. *Lasers Surg Med* 4: 201–206.
2. Bowker TJ, Cross FW, Rumsby PT, Gower MC, Rickards AF, Bown SG (1986) Excimer laser angioplasty: quantitative comparison in vitro of three ultraviolet wavelengths on tissue ablation and haemolysis. *Lasers Med Sci* 1: 91–99.
3. Litvack F, Grundfest WS, Goldenberg T, Laudenslager J, Pacala T, Segalowitz J, Forrester JS (1988) Pulsed laser angioplasty: wavelength power and energy dependencies relevant to clinical application. *Lasers Surg Med* 8: 60–65.
4. Wolleneck G, Laufer G, Grabenwöger F (1988) Percutaneous transluminal excimer laser angioplasty in total peripheral artery occlusion in man. *Lasers Surg Med* 8: 464–468.
5. Litvack F et al. (1989) Percutaneous excimer-laser and excimer-laser-assisted angioplasty of the lower extremities: results of initial clinical trial. *Radiology* 172: 331–335.
6. Karsch KR et al. (1989) Percutaneous coronary excimer laser angioplasty: initial clinical results. *Lancet* 2(8664): 647–650.
7. Wieshammer S, Hibst R, Bellekens M, Steiner R (1988) Ultraviolet laser ablation of biologic tissue. Quantitation of etch rate as a function of incident fluence. *Lasers Life Sci* 2, 125–135.
8. Kaufmann R, Hibst R (1989) Pulsed Er: YAG and 308 nm UV-excimer laser: an in vitro and in vivo study of skin-ablative effects. *Lasers Surg Med* 9: 132–140.

18. Current problems of excimer laser angioplasty

S. WIESHAMMER, M. VOGELPOHL, M. KOCHS, W. HAERER,
M. HÖHER, T. EGGELING, A. SCHMIDT, H.-H. OSTERHUES,
P. WEISMÜLLER and V. HOMBACH

Summary

Pulsed submicrosecond excimer laser irradiation provides the potential for
debulking atherosclerotic material without significant thermal injury to the
adjacent vessel wall. Considerable progress has been made during the last
few years as to the quality of the optical fibers, the design of laser-fiber
coupling devices and catheter systems, and, in particular, the development
of long-pulse excimer lasers. With these improvements in technology,
excimer laser angioplasty has become technically feasible, but most patients
require subsequent balloon angioplasty to obtain an adequate final result.
There are a number of major impediments to the clinical use of the excimer
laser for angioplasty. Among those are problems relating to (1) the heterogenous ablative characteristics of plaque, (2) the potential mismatch between
the open lumen of the vessel and the amount of atherosclerotic material that
can be removed by the laser, and (3) the failure of the cutting tip of the
catheter to engage in excentric lesions. These issues need resolution before
excimer laser angioplasty can become an alternative to balloon angioplasty.
Minor points include the distal embolization of the particulate debris and
the thrombogenicity of the lased vascular surfaces.

Introduction

The removal of atherosclerotic plaques by laser energy has been of interest
to cardiovascular interventionalists for more than 25 years [1]. Early com-
munications had generated hope that angioplasty by means of visible continuous-mode lasers would soon become a routine procedure for cleaning
out occluded vessels while recent publications raised some doubts [2, 3]. The
basic limitation to the use of visible continuous-mode lasers for angioplasty
is their potential for thermal damage to the normal vessel wall.

The introduction of submicrosecond pulsed ultraviolet lasers into angioplasty by Grundfest et al. [4] was a major advance. In contrast to the

V. Hombach et al. (eds), Interventional Techniques in Cardiovascular Medicine, 151–160.
© 1991 *Kluwer Academic Publishers*.

situation with visible continuous-mode lasers, pulsed ultraviolet laser irradiation allows for a geometrically precise removal of material without significant thermal injury to the adjacent tissue. The depth of the incision increases linearly with the number of pulses delivered while its width conforms exactly to the beam configuration irrespective of the pulse energy and the number of pulses. The underlying mechanism by which pulsed ultraviolet laser irradiation produces this distinct type of tissue ablation is incompletely understood. Potential mechanisms include photoablative decomposition involving the disruption of molecular bonds and tissue ablation due to an extremely localized thermal effect [5–8]. Laser irradiation at a wavelength of 308 nm was shown to ablate plaques containing calcified deposits which cannot be achieved with far-ultraviolet lasers [9].

Methods and results

Our initial attempts to perform excimer laser angioplasty were a rather frustrating experience. Damage to the input tip of the fiber was a frequent complication. In these early studies, we used a pulsed xenon-chloride excimer laser with a wavelength of 308 nm and a pulse width of only 15 ns. It became quickly apparent that this pulse duration was too short to allow for the fiberoptic transmission of a sufficient amount of energy per pulse. The pulse energy at the distal tip of the fiber was not high enough to ablate atherosclerotic material within a reasonably short period of time.

Considerable progress has been made during the last few years as to the quality of the optical fibers, the design of laser-fiber coupling systems and, in particular, the development of long-pulse excimer lasers. A long pulse duration reduces the enormous peak power density imposed on the silica fibers and thereby greatly facilitates the fiberoptic transmission of a given amount of energy per pulse [10]. With these improvements in equipment and technology, we were able to transfer the excimer laser from the experimental to the catheterization laboratory and have used it for peripheral vascular applications and also for coronary angioplasty since March 1989.

We currently use a xenon-chloride excimer laser system with a wavelength of 308 nm and a pulse width of 60 ns [Technolas MAX-10, Technolas Inc., Munich, FRG]. The repetition rate can be adjusted between 2 and 200 per second. The amount of energy delivered per pulse is adjustable by changing the bank voltage of the laser so that the pulse energy at the cutting tip of the catheter amouts to 6 to 25 mJ depending on the catheter design and the clinical requirements.

Angioplasty is performed by direct contact cutting in a blood environment [11]. The catheters used for angioplasty have an outer diameter of 5 to 7 F. They contain a bundle of 200–μm silica fibers which are arranged in a circular fashion around a central lumen for use with a guide wire. This

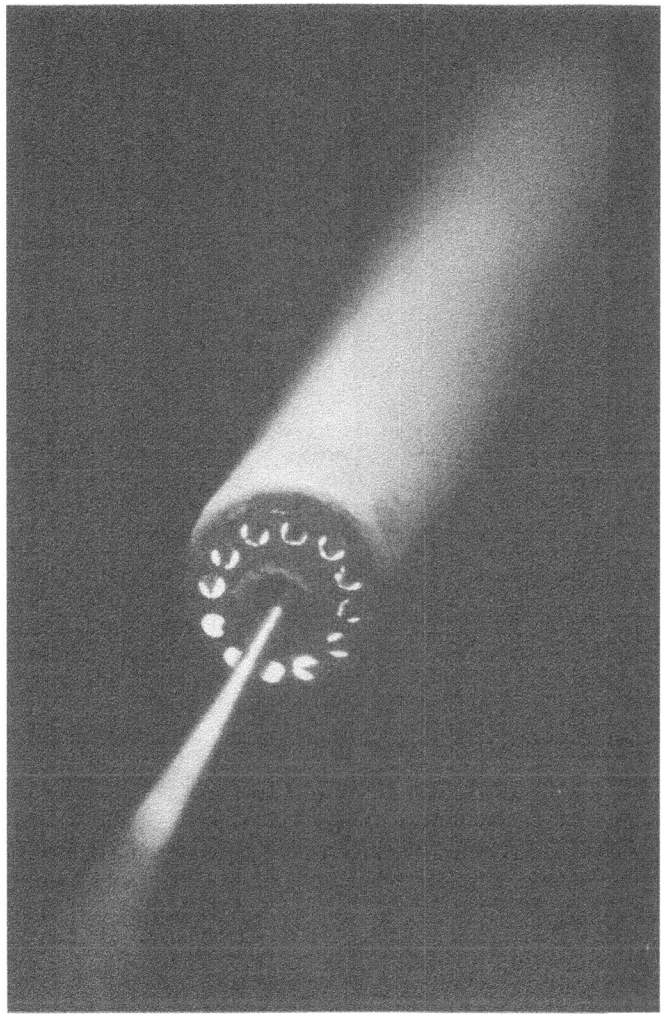

Figure 1.   Catheter design. A bundle of 200-μm silica fibers is arranged in a circular fashion around a central lumen for use with a guide wire over which the catheter is advanced to the site of stenosis. The fibers terminate in the cutting tip of the catheter. Angioplasty is performed by direct contact cutting in a blood field.

facilitates the alignment of the catheter tip with the long axis of the vessel. The fibers terminate in the non-tapered cutting tip of the catheter (see Figure 1). The catheter has a radio-opaque marker at its tip to facilitate fluoroscopic guidance. The catheters designed for angioplasty of large peripheral vessels such as the femoral artery are deliberately made rather stiff to assure an adequate axial support during advancement of the catheter across the targeted stenosis. The version designed for use in small arteries seems to

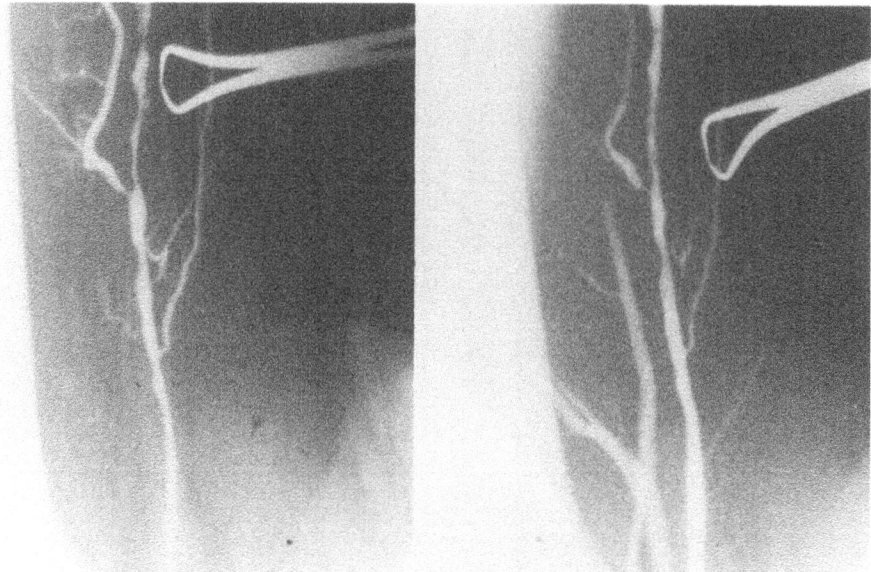

Figure 2.   Excimer laser angioplasty of a femoral artery. The pre-laser angiogram (left side) revealed several high-grade stenoses. After a total of 9000 pulses had been delivered, the post-laser angiogram (right side) was obtained demonstrating a significant reduction of the degree of stenoses. The repetition rate was 20 Hz the pulse energy was 20 mJ.

be flexible enough to maintain maneuverability in tortuous vasculatures. With these flexible catheters which are all used with a central guide wire, mechanical perforation of the vessel wall is no longer the major complication of laser angioplasty.

Figure 2 demonstrates the results of an excimer laser angioplasty of a femoral artery. The pre-laser control angiogram showed diffuse vascular disease with several high-grade stenoses. The post-laser angiogram indicated a significant reduction of the degree of stenoses. This case demonstrates that excimer laser angioplasty has become technically feasible. From a clinical point of view, technical feasibility is of only minor significance. A new interventional technique has to be evaluated against balloon angioplasty which is the gold standard. The question is not whether excimer laser angioplasty is technically feasible but whether this technique will be able to replace the balloon in certain vascular applications. In our initial clinical experience, the results of excimer laser angioplasty were less than fully satisfactory. While the degree of stenosis could be reduced by more than 30% in 10 out of 16 patients with high-grade ($\geq$ 75%) stenoses, all but 2 patients required subsequent balloon angioplasty to obtain an adequate final result. We had not included patients with total vascular occlusions in this initial series. No vascular perforations were observed but 2 patients developed acute vascular occlusions following laser angioplasty which were successfully treated by balloon angioplasty. It is noteworthy that the proportion for our patients requiring subsequent balloon angioplasty is similar to that reported by Litvack et al. [12, 13]. There should be no doubt that balloon angioplasty was the principal therapeutic intervention in the majority of cases. In these patients, the term 'excimer laser angioplasty' would be a misnomer. Conclusions from our data are limited of course by the very small number of patients. A more detailed statistical analysis were invalid and inferences concerning the prospective role of excimer laser angioplasty in different vascular indications cannot be made. Even with these limitations, it is safe to say on the basis of our experience that there are several major impediments that need resolution before the excimer laser can become an alternative to the balloon. Operator inexperience with excimer laser angioplasty is unlikely to account for our results. It is our belief that the strikingly high proportion of patients requiring subsequent balloon angioplasty and the occurrence of acute vascular occlusions following laser angioplasty relate to the currently available technology and equipment. We would like to discuss some of these issues.

Problems of excimer laser angioplasty

Among those are problems relating to (1) the heterogeneity of plaques, (2) the mismatch between the open lumen of the vessel and the volume of material that can be removed by the laser, and (3) the failure of the cutting tip of the catheter to engage in excentric lesions. Minor problems include the distal embolization of the particulate debris produced during laser irradiation [14] and the thrombogenicity of the vascular surface following laser irradiation. Recent data do not support the hypothesis that the smooth vascular surfaces produced by pulsed excimer laser irradiation are less thrombogenic than the carbonized and ragged surfaces produced by irradiation with continuous-mode visible lasers [15]. The carcinogenicity of ultraviolet light is unlikely to be a limiting factor to the use of the excimer laser for angioplasty [16].

1. Heterogeneity of plaques. Atherosclerotic plaque consists of numerous organic and inorganic compounds and there are probably no 2 plaques which are identical as to their composition and ablative characteristics. Figure 3 displays the results of an in vitro study which examined the relation between excimer laser fluence and the penetration depth per pulse in plaques [17]. It is evident from this plot of etch depth versus fluence that the penetration depth was highly variably ranging from less than 1 μm at a radiation exposure of 6 J per area unit in a calcified lesion to about 18 μm at 6 J/cm^2 in a fibrous plaque. In other words, there is a greater than twentyfold variability in ablation rate at a given radiation exposure. These in

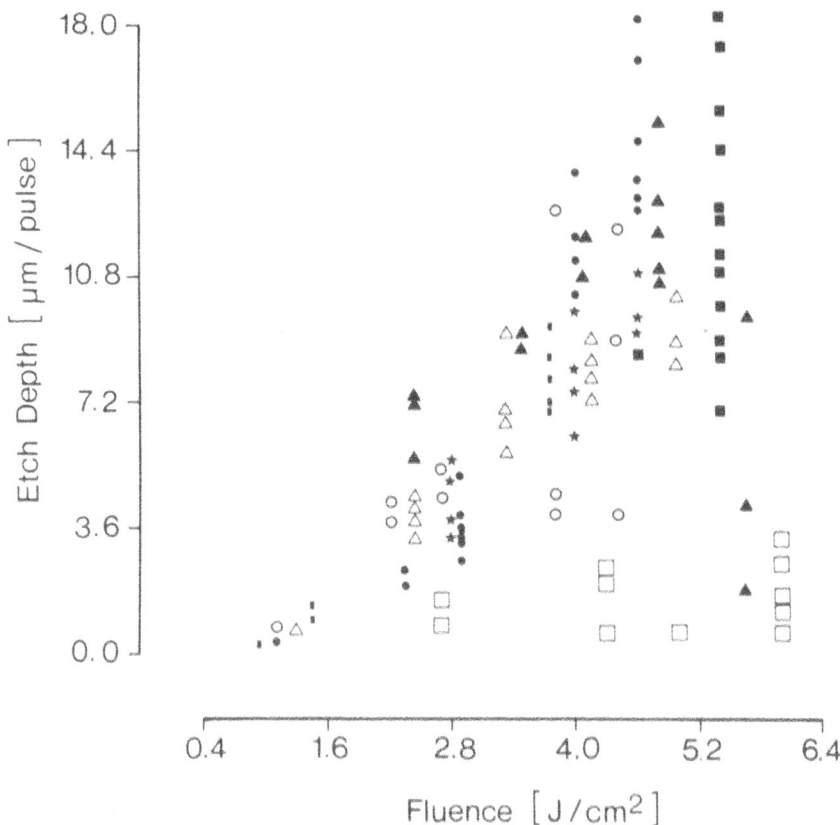

Figure 3.   Relation between excimer laser fluence and penetration depth per pulse in atherosclerotic plaque. Eight plaques were studied. The data points obtained in individual plaques are characterized by the same symbol.

vitro data are of relevance to the clinical setting because the ablation rate corresponds to the rate at which the catheter should be advanced across the targeted stenosis during lasing. The problem is that it is not yet possible to determine the ablation rate during angioplasty. The resistance encountered in advancing the catheter across a stenosis may be seriously misleading in assessing its ablative behaviour particularly if the catheter has to be advanced in a tortuous vessel. If the rate at which the catheter is advanced were greater than the ablation rate, the stenosis would be passed by the application of mechanical force and significant shear forces would be applied to the lesion. This may give rise to acute vascular occlusion. At worst, the system worked mosty like a rigid mechanical dilator as introduced by Dotter and Judkins in 1964 [18]. In this case, the expensive excimer laser system would add little beyond the appeal of the name 'laser therapy'.

2. Mismatch between lased neolumen and open lumen of the vessel. The second item we would like to address is the potential mismatch between the open lumen of the vessel and the cutting diameter of the catheter tip. The width of the lased channel corresponds to the diameter of the cutting area and so the amount of atherosclerotic material removed may be inadequate to the open lumen of the vessel as illustrated in Figure 4. A complete normalization of the vessel lumen is not achieved and the residual stenosis is still significant. We presume that this is the principal reason why most of our patients required subsequent balloon dilatation. We are not yet convinced whether laser treatment of a stenosis with subsequent balloon angioplasty is superior to balloon dilatation alone. Larger lumina can be obtained by increasing the cutting diameter of the catheter. In consideration of the cost of an excimer laser catheter, the subsequent use of catheters with serially larger cutting areas would be a rather expensive approach. Furthermore, the use of large-diameter catheters reduces the flexibility and maneuverability of the system.

3. Failure of the cutting tip to engage in excentric plaques. The laser catheter is usually maneuvered over a guide wire to the site of obstruction. When the flexible catheter is approaching an excentric stenosis, the cutting tip is taking the path of least resistance so that the wire does not guide the cutting tip into but, rather, away from the plaque and towards the normal contralateral vessel wall. So the cutting area does not effectively engage in the target lesion as shown in Figure 5. This mechanism readily accounts for our observation that the outcome of excimer laser angioplasty was less favourable in the presence of excentric stenoses. The use of very stiff catheters or bare fibers offers no solution to this problem because they do

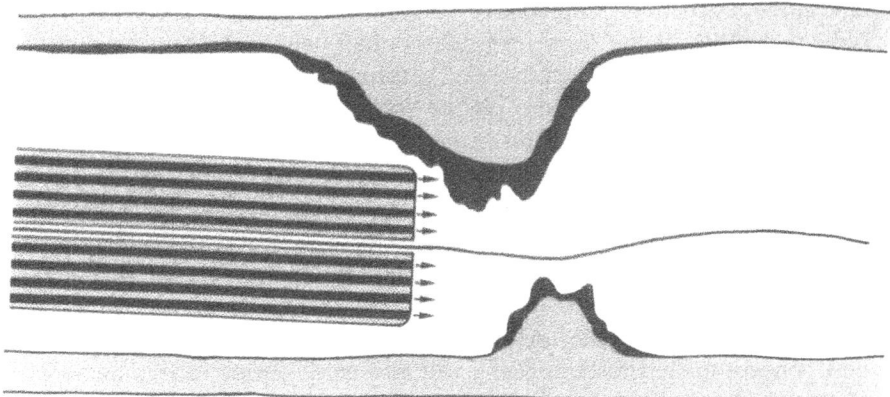

Figure 4. Mismatch between lased neolumen and open lumen of the vessel. The lased channel is of inadequate caliber so that subsequent balloon angioplasty is required.

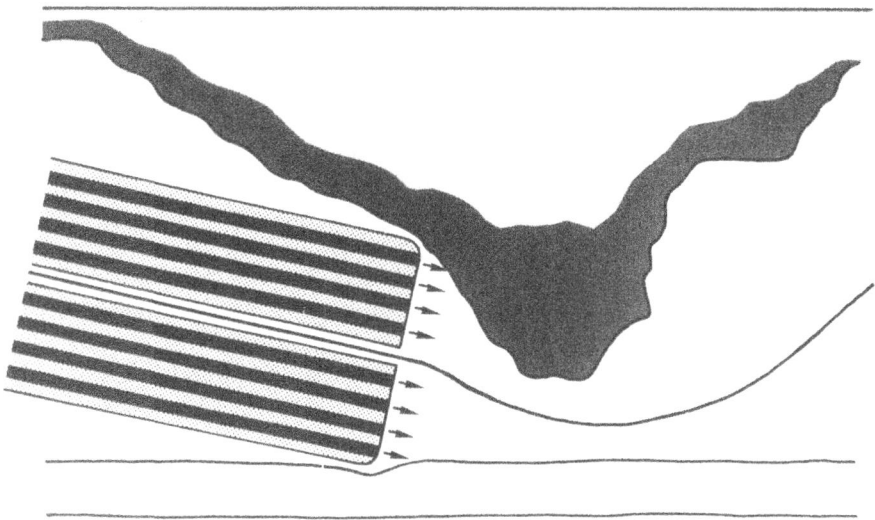

Figure 5.   Failure of the cutting tip to engage in excentric stenoses. When the flexible catheter is approaching an excentric stenosis, the cutting tip is taking the path of least resistance.

not only poke their ways into the plaque but also through the vessel wall as many early studies have shown. In an attempt to improve the efficacy of the cutting tip, we are currently testing excentric tip designs.

In conclusion, the pulsed excimer laser provides an exciting potential for debulking atherosclerotic material without significant thermal damage to the surrounding vessel wall and it seems to be more suited for angioplasty than continuous-mode visible lasers [19–21]. Although excimer laser angioplasty is technically feasible now, it will probably remain far from being an alternative to balloon angioplasty for years to come. It seems to us that quite a number of the early investigators had been too optimistic as to the laser's future role in interventional cardiovascular medicine. In 1983, an article entitled 'Poof goes the plaque with experimental laser angioplasty' appeared in the *Journal of the American Medical Association* [22]. Laser angioplasty is obviously a great deal more complicated than suggested by the title of this paper. Our future work will be directed towards the development of a novel excentric catheter tip which is able to differentiate plaque from normal artery wall by means of a real-time, pulse-by-pulse spectral analysis of the fluorescence signals. Plaque identification by spectroscopic imaging was shown to be feasible under in vitro conditions [23–25]. Whether this new concept of diagnostic imaging will also work during in vivo angioplasty remains to be seen.

References

1. McGuff PE, Bushnell D, Soroff HS, Deterling RA (1963) Studies of the surgical applications of laser (light amplification by stimulated emission of radiation). *Surg For* 14: 143–145.
2. Anonymous (1980) Surgeon develops a laser catheter to treat blockages of blood vessels. *Laser Focus* 16: 40–42.
3. Lee G, Ikeda RM, Chan MC, Lee MH, Rink JL, Reis RL, Theis JH, Low R, Bommer WJ, Kung AH, Hanna ES, Mason DT (1985) Limitations, risks and complications of laser recanalization: a cautious approach warranted. *Am J Cardiol* 56: 181–185.
4. Grundfest WS, Litvack IF, Goldenberg T, Sherman T, Morgenstern L, Carroll R, Fishbein M, Forrester J, Margitan J, McDermid S, Pacala TJ, Rider DM, Laudenslager JB (1985) Pulsed ultraviolet lasers and the potential for safe laser angioplasty. *Am J Surg* 150: 220–226.
5. Srinivasan R (1986) Ablation of polymers and biological tissue by ultraviolet lasers. *Science* 234: 559–565.
6. Sutcliffe E, Srinivasan R (1986) Dynamics of UV laser ablation of organic polymer surfaces. *J Appl Phys* 60: 3315–3322.
7. Brannon JH, Lankard JR, Baise AI, Burns F, Kaufman J (1985) Excimer laser etching of polyimide. *J Appl Phys* 58: 2036–2043.
8. Clarke RH, Isner JM, Donaldson RF, Jones G (1987) Gas chromatographic light microscopic correlative analysis of excimer laser photoablation of cardiovascular tissues: evidence for a thermal mechanism. *Circ Res* 60: 429–439.
9. Linsker R, Srinivasan R, Wynne JJ, Alonso DR (1984) Far-ultraviolet laser ablation of atherosclerotic lesions. *Lasers Surg Med* 4: 201–206.
10. Litvack F, Grundfest WS, Goldenberg T, Laudenslager J, Pacala T, Segalowitz J, Forrester JS (1988) Pulsed laser angioplasty: wavelength power and energy dependencies relevant to clinical application. *Lasers Surg Med* 8: 60–65.
11. Isner JM, Gal D, Steg G, DeJesus ST, Rongione AJ, Halaburka KR, Slovenkai GA, Clarke RH (1988) Percutaneous, in vivo excimer laser angioplasty: results in two experimental animal models. *Lasers Surg Med* 8: 223–232.
12. Litvack F, Grundfest WS, Adler L, Hickey AE, Segalowitz J, Hestrin LB, Mohr FW, Goldenberg T, Laudenslager JS, Forrester JS (1989) Percutaneous excimer-laser and excimer-laser-assisted angioplasty of the lower extremities: results of initial clinical trial. *Radiology* 172: 331–335.
13. Litvack F, Grundfest W, Eigler N, Tsoi D, Goldenberg T, Laudenslager J, Forrester J (1989) Percutaneous excimer laser coronary angioplasty (Letter). *Lancet* 102–103.
14. Haller JD, Wholey MH, Fisher ER, Krokosky EM, Srinivasan R (1987) Physical and chemical effects of ultraviolet excimer laser radiation on human atherosclerotic plaque: therapeutic implications. *Laser Med Surg* 3: 98–104.
15. Ragimov SE, Belyaev AA, Vertepa IA, Dolgov VV, Furzikov NP, Akchurin RS, Repin VS, Trubetskoy AV (1988) Comparison of different lasers in terms of thromogenicity of the laser-treated vascular wall. *Lasers Surg Med* 8: 77–82.
16. Parrish JA (1985) Ultraviolet laser ablation. *Arch Dermatol* 121: 599–600.
17. Wieshammer S, Hibst R, Bellekens M, Steiner R (1988) Ultraviolet laser ablation of biologic tissue. Quantitation of etch rate as a function of incident fluence. *Lasers Life Sci* 2: 125–135.
18. Dotter CT, Judkins MP (1964) Transluminal treatment of arterioslerotic obstruction. Description of a new technic and a preliminary report of its application. *Circulation* 30: 654–670.

19. Isner JM (1988) Excimer laser angioplasty: pygmalion makes it to the ball. *Lasers Surg Med* 8: 447–449.
20. Eldar M (1989) Laser angioplasty: a review. *Isr J Med Sci* 25: 222–228.
21. Litvack F, Grundfest WS, Papaioannou T, Mohr FW, Jakubowski AT, Forrester JS (1988) Role of laser and thermal ablation devices in the treatment of vascular diseases. *Am J Cardiol* 61: 81G–86G.
22. Gunby P (1983) 'Poof' goes the plaque with experimental laser angioplasty. *J Am Med Ass* 250: 3135–3141.
23. Laufer G, Wollenek G, Hohla K, Horvat R, Henke KH, Buchelt M, Wutzl G, Wolner E (1988) Excimer laser-induced simultaneous ablation and spectral identification of normal and atherosclerotic arterial tissue layers. *Circulation* 78: 1031–1039.
24. Leon MB, Lu DY, Prevosti LG, Macy WW, Smith PD, Granovsky M, Bonner RF, Balaban RS (1988) Human arterial surface fluorescence: atherosclerotic plaque identification and effects of laser atheroma ablation. *J Am Coll Cardiol* 12: 94–102.
25. Hoyt CC, Richards-Kortum RR, Costello B, Sacks BA, Kittrell C, Ratliff NB, Kramer JR, Feld MS (1988) Remote biomedical spectroscopic imaging of human artery wall. *Lasers Surg Med* 8: 1–9.

19. Laser angioplasty

B. E. STRAUER, M. P. HEINTZEN and T. NEUBAUR

Introduction

Clinical laser angioplasty is performed since 1983, when Ginsburg and co-workers successfully recanalized a high grade deep femoral artery stenosis [6]. The initial clinical studies using bare fiber laser systems were complicated by a significant rate of vessel wall perforation, additionally the lumen improvement by laser energy was in most of the cases insufficient [2, 7, 16, 18]. Therefore, other laser catheter systems were developed, e.g., hot tips or sapphire tips to overcome these limitations of the bare fiber technique [1, 3, 5, 15, 17, 22]. Nevertheless, bare fiber laser angioplasty offers some advantages over the other systems and subsequently in our department a novel laser catheter system was developed for clinical laser angioplasty [14, 19]. This new system allows controlled application of laser energy and thereby minimizes the risk of vessel wall damage and perforation. By rotating the oval formed laser catheter around the guide wire a larger new lumen compared to previous bare fiber systems can be recanalized.

After successful in vitro examinations 35 patients suffering from peripheral arterial occlusive disease were treated by Nd:YAG laser angioplasty with this new laser catheter system.

Methods

Patients

Thirty-five patients (mean age 61 ± 11) with stenoses (n = 26) and occlusions (n = 9) of the iliac (n = 14), superficial femoral (n = 14) and popliteal (n = 7) arteries were treated by laser angioplasty. With regard to the Fontaine classification there were 4 patients in the clinical stage IV, 3 patients in stage III, 19 patients in stage IIb and 9 patients in stage IIa.

The laser angioplasty procedure and all possible complications were explained to the patients prior to the treatment and written consent was

V. Hombach et al. (eds), Interventional Techniques in Cardiovascular Medicine, 161–168.

obtained. The study was approved by our local ethical committee to be in correspondence with the declaration of Helsinki.

Before and after treatment all patients were examined by noninvasive doppler measurements, the systolic ankle-arm index was calculated. The degree of stenosis was measured by means of the angiographies taken before and after laser angioplasty and in patients treated for iliac artery disease the directly measured transtenotic pressure gradient was recorded.

Laser equipment

The laser catheter was developed in our laboratory and was previously tested in over 100 stenosed or occluded postmortem human femoral arteries. In this study the mean degree of stenosis was improved by laser angioplasty from 89 ± 9% to 53 ± 12%, the rate of perforation was found to be only 0.9% [14, 19].

The laser catheter system has already been described in detail elsewhere [19], in brief the catheter consists of a modified 6.3 F polyethylene catheter with an oval formed X-ray dense marked tip into which an also marked 0.6 mm core silica fiber is inserted and fixed in an excentric position. The catheter is advanced over an 0.014 inch guide wire to prevent perforation. During laser energy application the catheter is manually rotated around the guide wire and is slowly advanced forward in order to recanalize an adequate new lumen while the fiber tip is constantly flushed by saline solution. The laser source is a continuous-wave Nd:YAG laser (Medilas 40, MBB, Munich) with a wavelength of 1064 nm. The laser is used in a chopped mode, pulses with an energy of 6 joule were applied with a frequency of 2 pulses per second.

Procedure

In our initial clinical study only patients with lesions below the groin were treated [9, 20, 25]. The common femoral artery was punctured by an antegrade stick, and an 8 F introducer sheath was placed intra-arterially. The stenosis/occlusion was passed by the guidewire and subsequently the laser catheter was advanced under fluoroscopy over the wire to the stenosis. Laser angioplasty was performed and the result of the recanalization was proven by intermittend injection of diluted contrast material. Finally the procedure is completed by a conventional balloon dilatation.

In the second group of patients with iliac artery disease a retrograde puncture of the contralateral common femoral artery was performed for diagnostic angiography, the ipsilateral iliac artery was punctured for laser treatment [11]. Due to complications of balloon dilatation observed in the first group of patients with lesions below the groin we decided to perform laser angioplasty of iliac arteries as a sole laser therapy. Therefore, the laser angioplasty is continued until a sufficient new lumen is recanalized. The result of laser recanalization is proven by intermittend injection of contrast material and continuous monitoring of the transtenotic pressure gradient.

All patients received platelet aggregation inhibitors prior to the procedure (acetylsalicylic acid 500 mg or acetylsalicylic acid 330 mg plus dipyridamole 75 mg). During laser angioplasty 5000–10000 IU heparine were injected intravenously. Within the following 1–2 days 25000 IU of heparine were given intravenously. The follow up medication consists of acetylsalicylic acid or a combination of acetylsalicylic acid and dipyridamole.

Table 1. Laser angioplasty procedure in femoropopliteal and iliac arteries

Femoropopliteal	Iliac
Antegrade puncture	Retrograde puncture
Angiography	Angiography
Laser angioplasty	Laser angioplasty
Angiography	Angiography
Balloon dilatation	(if necessary additional laser angioplasty)
Angiography	

Results

In 32 of the 35 patients (= 91%) laser angioplasty was angiographically successful, resulting in recanalization of an occlusion and leaving a residual stenosis of 50% or less.

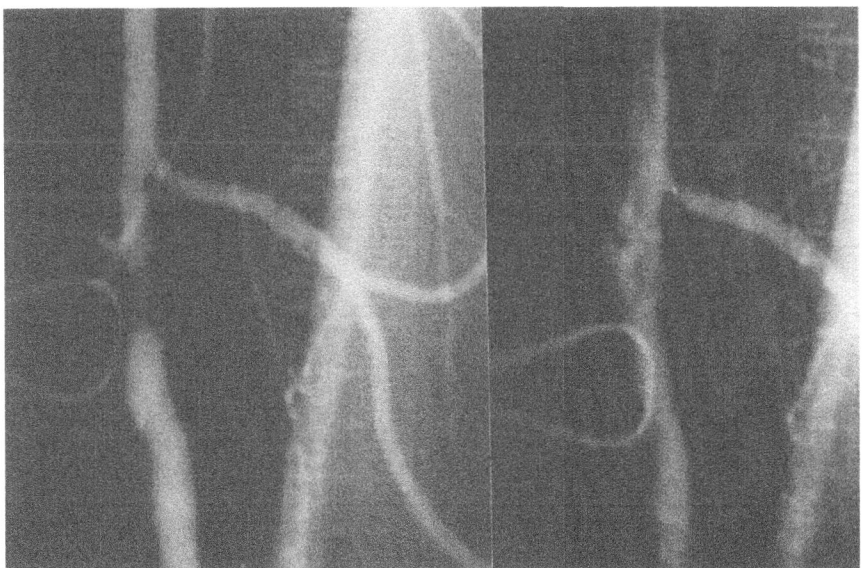

Figure 1. Angiographic result of combined laser and balloon angioplasty in a 65 year old male. Femoral artery stenosis before treatment on the left, the result after laser and balloon angioplasty on the right.

Clinically, the Fontaine stage recognized within the first week after treatment improved in 30/35 patients, in no case did it deteriorate. Therefore, the clinical success rate is 86%.

In all, the mean degree of stenosis decreased from 91 ± 10% before laser angioplasty to 20 ± 19% after laser angioplasty, the mean Doppler ankle-arm index improved from 0.63 ± 0.21 before laser angioplasty to 0.88 ± 0.18 after treatment. In patients treated for iliac artery stenoses the directly measured mean transtenotic pressure gradient decreased from 58 ± 22 mmHg before laser angioplasty to 19 ± 14 mmHg after sole laser therapy.

Related to laser angioplasty there were no acute severe complications (perforation, acute occlusion, significant embolization) requiring urgent surgical intervention. In two patients extensive hematoma at the puncture site required blood transfusion but could be treated conservatively.

In the initial group of patients with lesions in the femoropopliteal artery treated by combined laser and balloon angioplasty microembolisms were detected on the finial control angiogram taken after balloon dilatation in 7 patients. In none of these patients did any clinical symptom occur, in two cases spontaneous lysis of these emboli was proven by additional contrast

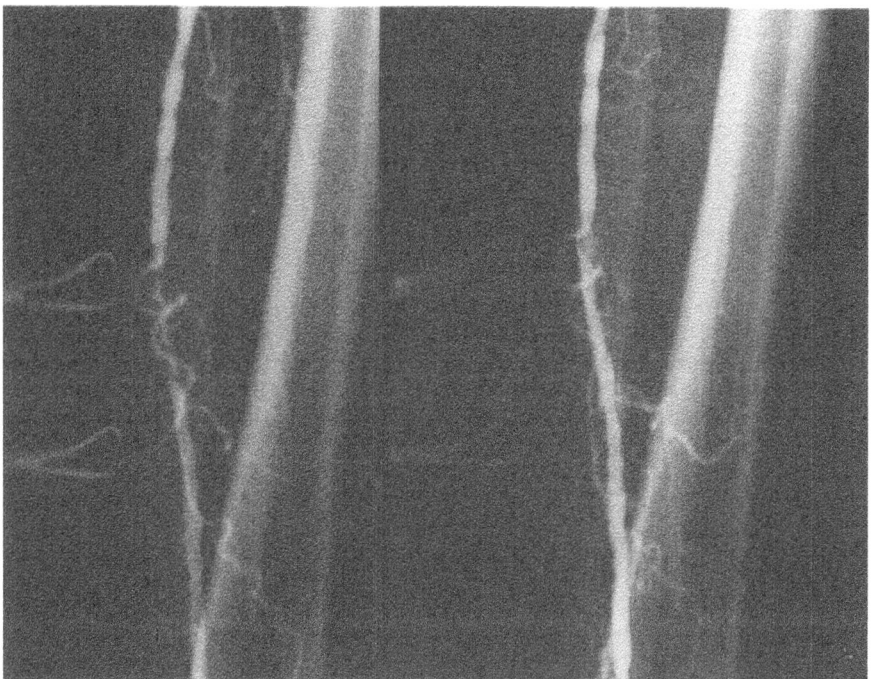

Figure 2.   Superficial femoral occlusion in a 77 year old male before (left) and after combined laser and balloon angioplasty (right).

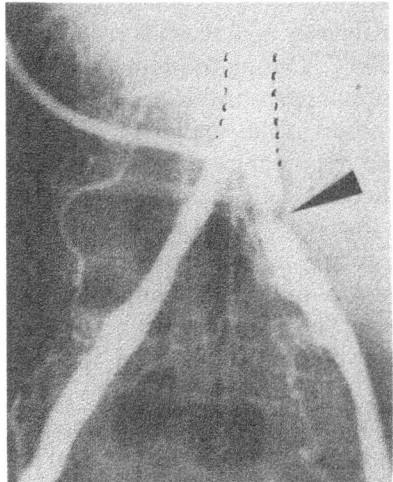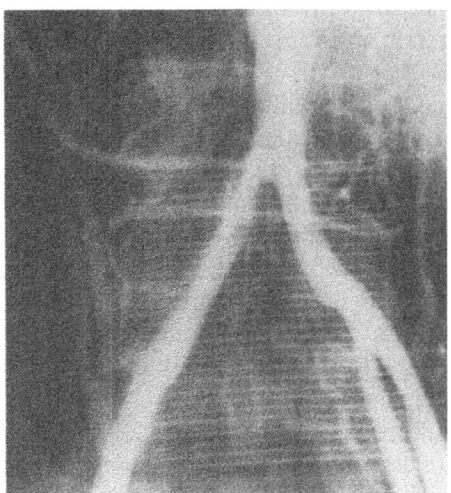

Figure 3. On the left side a high grade excentric common iliac artery in a 43 year old male, on the right side the result after laser angioplasty *without* additional balloon dilatation.

injection. In 8 patients treated by laser angioplasty and additional PTA dissections of the vessel wall were observed after balloon dilatation (= 38%). In comparison, only 2 dissections occurred in 14 patients treated by laser angioplasty alone (= 14%).

During a follow-up period of 3–24 months (mean 17 ± 5 months) 28 patients were examined, there were 4 recurrences resulting in an overall patency rate of 85%. The mean Doppler ankle-arm index after a 12 months follow-up in 23 patients was 0.76 ± 0.21.

Discussion

Laser angioplasty has become an accepted method for the treatment of peripheral arterial occlusive disease. There are several different lasers and different laser catheter systems in use for clinical laser angioplasty. Initial studies were performed with bare fibers inserted into single lumen or balloon dilatation catheters. One main problem of this technique was frequent perforation of the arterial wall due to either the cutting edges of the bare fiber or laser-induced thermal damage, another problem was the remaining significant stenosis after laser angioplasty leading to an increased rate of acute reocclusions [2, 7, 16, 18].

To overcome the risk of perforation and to attain a larger lumen compared to these bare fiber methods the socalled 'hot-tips' and 'sapphire-tips' were developed [1, 3, 5, 15, 21, 22]. The risk of perforation was deminished, but other difficulties occurred. One significant problem with 'hot-tip' laser systems is the time consuming process of heating-up and cooling-down the metal cap inside the artery. It takes approximately 3–5 seconds to heat-up the 'hot-tip' to a 'working-temperature' of 500°C. During this time the probe may cause significant thermal damage to normal parts of the vessel with the risk of subsequent formation of 'new' stenoses in the region of a former normal vessel [4]. With respect to the probe temperature and the temperature related efficacy for vaporization of atherosclerotic material the overall predictability of hot-tip laser angioplasty is low.

Compared to the hot-tip system bare fibers only need a very short time to reach high temperatures at the fiber tip (up to 1500°C within 0.1–0.2 seconds). If a chopped mode is used, a very controlled application of laser energy is possible, resulting in diminished thermal damage to the surrounding vessel wall.

In several studies [3, 15, 22] the risk of peripheral embolization using hot-tip laser angioplasty was considered to be low, nevertheless, Katzen and co-workers reported in their study on a rate of embolization of 33%, requiring surgical correction in 80% of these patients [13].

The major disadvantages of bare fiber technique (perforation, inadequate lumen improvement) were solved by the development of the new bare fiber laser catheter system in our laboratory [14, 19]. In our experimental and clinical studies the safety and efficacy of this system was shown, there were no serious complications related to laser angioplasty in 35 patients, the procedure was angiographically successful in 91% of the treated lesions [11, 20, 25].

As a part of our initial standard protocol all patients in our first study suffering from femoropopliteal artery disease were treated by combined laser and balloon angioplasty [9, 20, 25]. The balloon dilatation was performed to reduce the remaining stenosis and to smooth irregularities of the treated vessel wall. The angiographic data of these patients demonstrated, that the major part of vessel recanalization was performed by laser angioplasty, the balloon dilatation only slightly improved the final result. In addition, after balloon dilatation we observed a dissection of the treated artery in 8/21 patients (38%) and a microembolization into peripheral sidebranches of the arteries of the calf in 7/21 cases (33%). These complications are known for balloon dilatation [24]. To avoid this problem of combined laser and balloon angioplasty and to evaluate the importance of a sole laser angioplasty we treated further patients with laser angioplasty without subsequent balloon dilatation [11]. In a group of 14 patients with iliac artery stenoses we were able to achieve an angiographic success in 12/14 lesions (86%), there were only 2/14 dissections (14%) and one clinically insignificant peripheral microembolisation (7%).

Laser angioplasty is likely to reduce the rate of restenosis compared to conventional balloon dilatation by rather removing then only displacing atherosclerotic material. Animal studies [21] and recent larger clinical studies [15, 22] supported this theory. Sanborn reported a significant reduction of recurrence for femoropopliteal stenosis and short (≤ 3 cm) obstructions [22]. In our group the long term success rates of patients treated for femoropopliteal lesions by combined laser and balloon angioplasty (76% within a mean follow up of 19.7 months) are at least comparable to those reported for conventional balloon dilatation [10, 23]. Further studies in a larger group of patients are necessary to prove these initial impressions. The follow-up time for patients treated by sole laser therapy is to short (12.2 months) to prove an increased patency rate compared to balloon angioplasty, nevertheless, until now there is no case of recurrence in this group.

Meanwhile, other laser sources and energy transmitting devices have been developed for clinical laser angioplasty, especially the excimer laser systems are regarded to have some advantages over thermal lasers. Future studies using 'cold' excimer laser energy will demonstrate the importance of this new tool for transluminal angioplasty [8, 12].

References

1. Abela GS, Seeger JM, Fenech A, Pepine CJ, Conti CR (1985) Laser recanalization of peripheral arteries in man: a preliminary report. *Circulation* 72, Suppl III: 303.
2. Choy DSJ, Stertzer S, Rotterdam HZ, Sharrock N, Kaminow IP (1982) Transluminal laser catheter angioplasty. *Am J Cardiol* 50: 1206–1208.
3. Cumberland DC, Sanborn TA, Tayler DI, Moore DJ, Welsh CL, Greenfield AJ, Guben JK, Ryan TJ (1986) Percutaneous thermal laser angioplasty: initial clinical results with a laser probe in total peripheral artery occlusion. *Lancet* i, 1457–1459.
4. Datena S, McCready R, Siderys H, Pittman J, Herod G, Halbrook H, Beckman D, Stephenson S, Kuehr S, Hawk A, Fehrenbacher J (1989) Six months arteriographic follow-up of argon laser-assisted balloon angioplasty of the ower extremities. Laser and Stent Therapy in vascular disease, International Congress II, *Abstract-book*: 106.
5. Geschwind HJ, Teisseire B, Boussignac G, Vieilleden C (1986) Laser angioplasty of arterial stenoses. *Cardiovasc Intervent Radiol* 9: 313–317.
6. Ginsburg R, Kim DS, Guthaner D, Toth J, Mitchel RS (1984) Salvage of an ischemic limb by laser angioplasty: description of a new technique. *Clin Cardiol* 7, 54–58.
7. Ginsburg R, Wexler L, Mitchell RS, Profitt D (1985) Percutaneous transluminal laser angioplasty for treatment of peripheral vascular disease. *Radiology* 156: 619–624.
8. Grundfest WS, Litvack IF, Goldenberg T, Sherman T, Morgenstern L, Carroll R, Fishbein M, Forrester J, Margitan J, McDermid S, Pacala TJ, Rider DM, Laudenslager JB (1985) Pulsed ultraviolet lasers and the potential for safe laser angioplasty. *Am J Surg* 150: 220–226.
9. Heintzen MP, Neubaur T, Klepzig M, Richter EI, Zeitler E, Strauer BE (1988) Clinical experiences in Nd:YAG laser angioplasty in the periphery, in: Biamino G, Müller GJ (eds), *Advances in Laser Medicine I: First German Symposium on Laser Angioplasty*, pp. 103–113. Landsberg: Ecomed.
10. Heintzen MP, Neubaur T, Klepzig M, Zeitler E, Strauer BE (1988) Nd:YAG laser angioplasty of peripheral arteries in humans: acute results and follow-up. *Eur Heart J* 9, Suppl I: 332.
11. Heintzen MP, Neubaur T, Klepzig M, Strauer BE (1989) Laser angioplasty of iliac and femoropopliteal obstructive lesions, in: Höfling B, v. Pölnitz A (eds), *Interventional Cardiology and Angiology* pp. 153–161. Darmstadt: Steinkopff.
12. Isner JM, Fortin-Donaldson R, Deckelbaum LI, Clarke RH, Laliberte SM, Ucci AA,

Salem DN, Konstam MA (1985) The excimer laser: gross, light microscopic and ultra-structural analysis of potential advantages for use in laser therapy of cardiovascular disease. *J Am Coll Cardiol* 6: 1102–1109.

13. Katzen BT, Kaplan JO, Schwarten DM, v Breda A (1988) Complications of 'hot-tip' laser assisted angioplasty. *Circulation* 78, Suppl II: 417.

14. Klepzig M, Neubaur T, Stellwaag M, Strauer BE (1986) Nd-YAG laser angioplasty: vascular effects, catheter development and in vivo application. *Circulation* 74, Suppl II: 203.

15. Lammer J, Karnel F (1988) Percutaneous transluminal laser angioplasty with contact probes. *Radiology* 168: 733–737.

16. Lee G, Ikeda RM, Theis JH, Chan MC, Stobbe D, Ogata C, Kumugai A, Mason DT (1984) Acute and chronic complications of laser angioplasty: vascular wall damage and formation of aneurysms in the atherosclerotic rabbit. *Am J Cardiol* 53: 290–293.

17. Lee G, Chan MC, Ikeda RM, Rink RL, Lee MH, Dukich J, Reis RL, Mason DT (1985) Intravascular laser-heated metal cautery cap in dissolution of human atherosclerotic disease. *Am Heart J* 110: 1304–1306.

18. Lee G, Ikeda RM, Chan MC, Lee MH, Rink JL, Reil RL, Theis JH, Low R, Bommer WJ, Kung AH, Hanna ES, Mason DT (1985) Limitations, risks and complications of laser recanalization: a cautious approach warranted. *Am J Cardiol* 56: 181–185.

19. Neubaur T, Klepzig M, Strauer BE (1988) Perkutane transluminale Laserangioplastie bei peripherer arterieller Verschlußkrankheit—Entwicklung eines neuen Laserkatheter-systems. *Z Kardiol* 77: 245–250.

20. Neubaur T, Klepzig M, Heintzen MP, Richter EI, Zeitler E, Strauer BE (1989) Peripheral percutaneous laser angioplasty in man: in vitro investigations and clinical results with a novel laser catheter system. *Clin Cardiol* 12: 313–320.

21. Sanborn TA, Faxon DP, Haudenschild CC, Gottman SP, Ryan TJ (1986) Laser thermal angioplasty: reduced restenosis compared to balloon angioplasty. *Circulation* 74, Suppl II: 6.

22. Sanborn TA, Cumberland DC, Greenfield AJ, Welsh CL, Guben JK (1988) Percutaneous laser thermal angioplasty: initial results and 1-year follow-up in 129 femoropopliteal lesions. *Radiology* 168: 121–125.

23. Schneider E, Grüntzig A, Bollinger VA (1983) Long-term patency rates after percutaneous transluminal angioplasty for iliac and femoropopliteal obstructions, in: Dotter CT, Grüntzig AR, Schoop W, Zeitler E (eds) *Percutaneous Transluminal Angioplasty* pp. 175–180 Berlin: Springer.

24. Seyfert W, Ernsting M, Grosse-Vorholt R, Zeitler E (1983) Complications during and after percutaneous transluminal angioplasty, in Dotter CT, Grüntzig AR, Schoop W, Zeitler E (eds), *Percutaneous Transluminal Angioplasty* pp. 161–169. Berlin: Springer.

25. Strauer BE, Neubaur T, Klepzig M, Heintzen MP, Zeitler E, Richter EI (1988) Perkutane periphere Laserangioplastie: erste klinische Ergebnisse. *Z Kardiol* 77: 29–35.

20. Preliminary experience with the implantation of Strecker-stents in peripheral arteries

H.-H. OSTERHUES, M. VOGELPOHL, C. FELDER, M. KOCHS
and V. HOMBACH

Summary

The aim of implanting vascular endoprothesis is to avoid acute complications and restenosis after percutaneous transluminal angioplasty. The
Strecker stent is a new development, based on the principle of balloon-
expandable endoprothesis.

We treated 7 patients (5 male, 2 female) aged 48 to 84 years (average 68
years) with Strecker stents in the iliac and femoropopliteal region. The
indications for the implantion of stents were restenosis, reocclusion, recoiling
and kink stenosis. Also acute complications as dissection or intimal flaps
after PTA were stented.

The implantation of the Strecker stents was in every case without technical complications. The condition of 3 patients suffering from a stage III
according to Fontaine's classification improved to stage IIa after treatment.
In 3 out of 4 patients with a stage IIb clinical symptoms were changed to stage
IIa after stenting. One patient had an acute thrombosis during the intervention,
which could not be solved by local thrombolysis. The Doppler sonographic
index raised after treatment to an average of 0.31.

The follow-up-period up to 6 months showed persistent clinical improvement. Intimal hyperplasia with stent occlusion or thrombo embolic occlusions
were not observed.

The Strecker stent is a technically unproblematic system, which is qualified for endoprothetic therapy of the iliac and femoropopliteal region.

Introduction

The use of vascular endoprothesis is a new method for the therapy of
stenosis and occlusion in peripheral arterial disease. With regard to recurrences of long stenosis and occlusions in the femoropopliteal region after
percutaneous transluminal angioplasty (PTA) [6, 8] this new method seems
to be an improvement of the therapy. Further indications for vascular

V. Hombach et al. (eds), Interventional Techniques in Cardiovascular Medicine, 169–179.

endoprothesis are recoiling and kink stenosis. In case of acute complications of peripheral transluminal angioplasty, such as dissection and intimal flaps, the implantation of stents might prevent further thrombo embolic complications.

At the moment different types of vascular endoprotheses are in use. Spring loaded stents are made of tempered stainless steel alloys. Other types of stents are expanded in a controlled manner, reaching the diameter imposed by a coaxial balloon, that bends the stent members beyond the elastic limit of the metal. The Palmaz stent as a balloon expandable intraluminal stent is based on this mode of action. Depending on the expansion of this prothesis, which has an universal size, a shortening of the stents after expansion takes place [5, 7, 12, 13].

A new type of balloon expandable stents is the 'Strecker-stent', which differs from the introduced Palmaz stent. We report about preliminary experience in using the Strecker stent in the iliacal and femoropopliteal region for various indications.

Method

We used the Strecker stent, a woven tantalwire stent. Earlier studies using this material showed excellent biocompatibility of tantal [17]. On the other hand tantal has a high x-ray absorption, which provides good recognition of the implanted stent. The prothesis is elastic, with longitudinal flexibility, so that the implantation in bending vessels is also possible. In contrast to the Palmaz stent, which is crimped manually over any commercially available balloon system, the Strecker stent is pre-set on a carrier balloon. Each stent has its own size: diameters between 4 and 8 mm, by a length of 40 or 80 mm are available.

In our study the diameter of the implanted stent was chosen according to the angiographic vessel diameter. The introduction of the Strecker stent takes place over a 8 F sheath. After placement at the target site the expansion of the carrier balloon was performed. When the balloon is deflated the stent remains in the vessel wall by its own expanding force. There is no shortening of the stents, which enables an exact positioning of the device.

In our study group the occlusion or stenosis was recanalised and/or dilatated after angiography by peripheral balloon angioplasty or low speed rotational angioplasty (Rotacs system). In connection with this manoeuvre the elected implantation of the stent, or the implantation as a consequence of acute complication of PTA took place. In cases of long stenosis or occlusions several stents were implanted in an overlapping manner. Finally a control angiography was performed.

During the treatment 5,000–10,000 i.E. Heparin were infused intra-arterially. After treatment the patients were full dose heparinised for 48 hours. Marcumarisation or low dose ASS was chosen as long-term medical therapy before discharge of patients.

Patients

7 patients, 5 men and 2 women, aged 48 to 84 years (medium 68 years) were selected. All patients suffered from iliacal and femoropopliteal stenosis or occlusions: 3 patients had iliacal lesions (2x common iliac artery, 1x external iliac artery), 4 patients had stenosis or occlusion in the femoropopliteal region. Most patients also suffered from lesions in other regions as e.g. lower limbs.

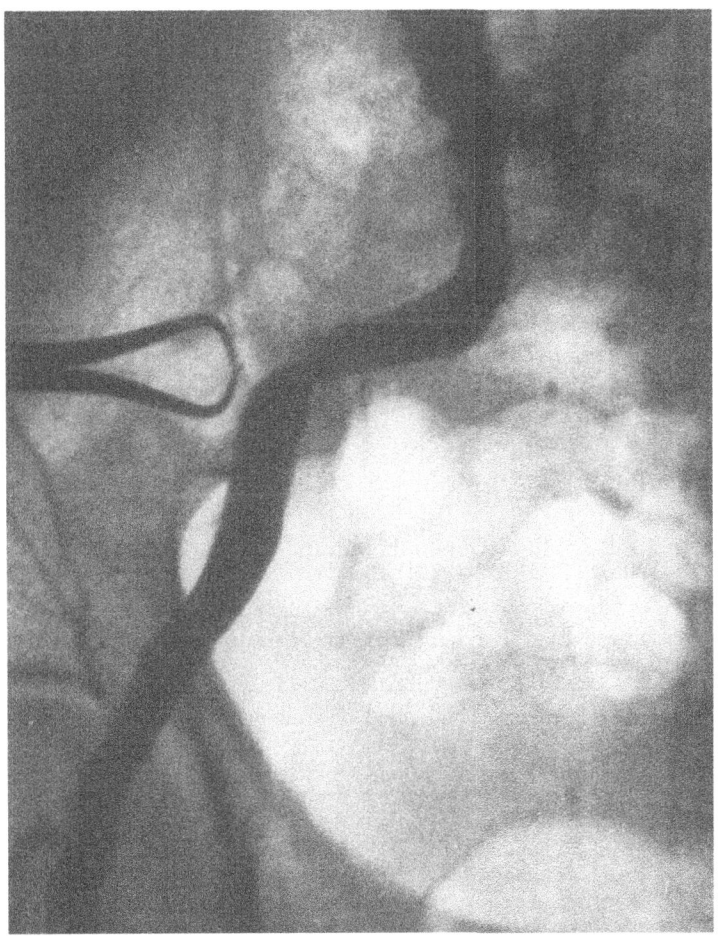

Fig. 1(a)

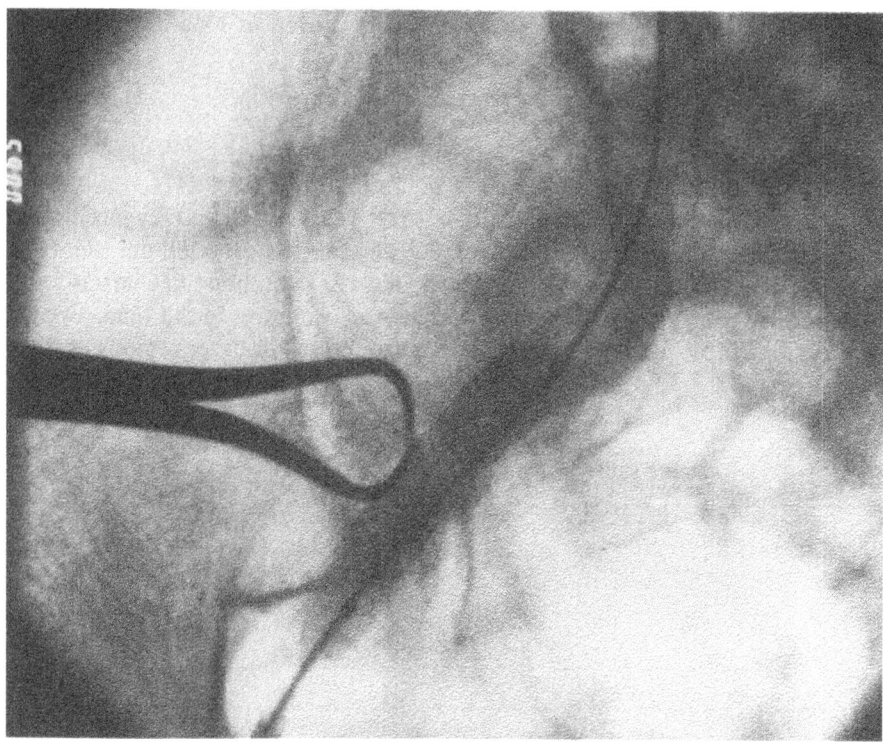

Fig. 1(b)

According to the Fontaine classification 4 patients represented a stage IIb and 3 patients a stage III. The indications for implantation were 2 kink stenosis, 1 recoiling stenosis, 1 restenosis and 1 reocclusion (in each case there has been PTA carried out in the past). There were acute complications after PTA, which were treated by stenting: 1 patient with a dissection, 1 intimal flap. Depending on the length of lesions the numbers of

Table 1. Vessel treated and stage according to the Fontaine classification (before therapy). Indications and number of stents implanted.

Pts	Stage	Vessel	Indication	Number of stents
1	IIb	Ext. iliac a.	Kink stenosis	1
2	III	Sup. femoral a.	Restenosis	2
3	IIb	Sup. femoral a.	Reocclusion	3
4	III	Sup. femoral a.	Intimalflap	1
5	IIb	Sup. femoral a.	Dissection	3
6	III	Com. iliac a.	Recoiling	1
7	IIb	Com. iliac a.	Kink stenosis	1

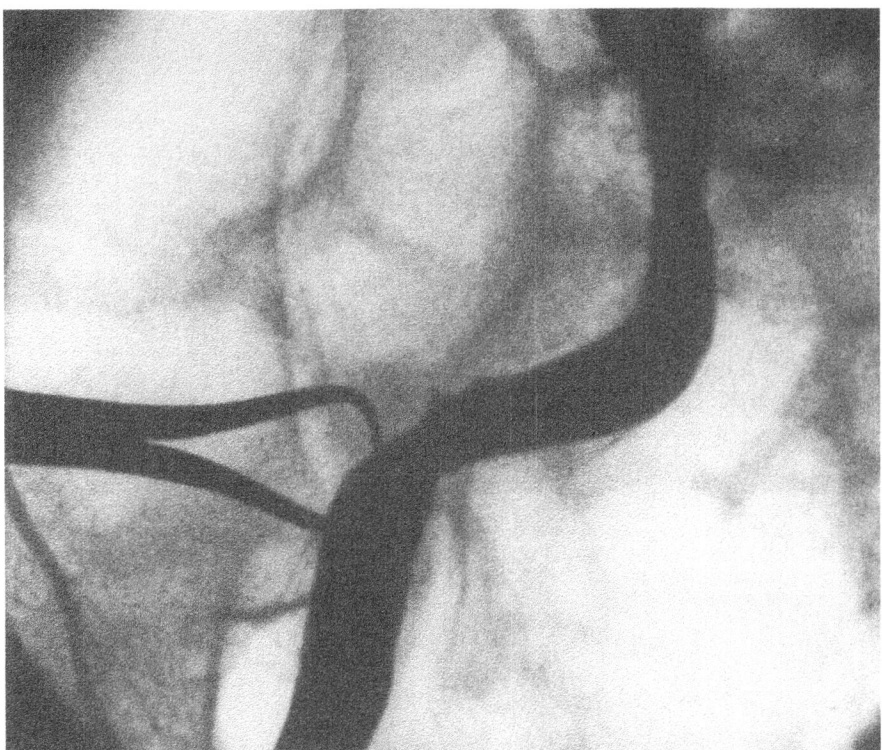

Fig. 1(c)

Figure 1.   Patient with an iliac stenosis (a) before treatment; (b) stent in situ; (c) final result.

stents changed from 1 stent in the iliac region to 3 stents in the femoral region (Table 1).

Results

There was no technical complication when the stents were implanted. Positioning of the prothesis was exact without dislocation by drawing back of the carrier balloon. Immediate angiographic control showed successful expansion of the vessel lumen. Control angiography revealed that side branches of the main vessel remained patent, which is possible by the mash-structure of the stents.

The length of treated lesions varied from 10 to 100 mm. The number of implanted stents varied from 1 to 3 stents (maximal stented distance of 110 mm). In the iliac region diameters up to 9 mm were chosen, in the femoropopliteal region the maximum was 5 mm (Figure 1).

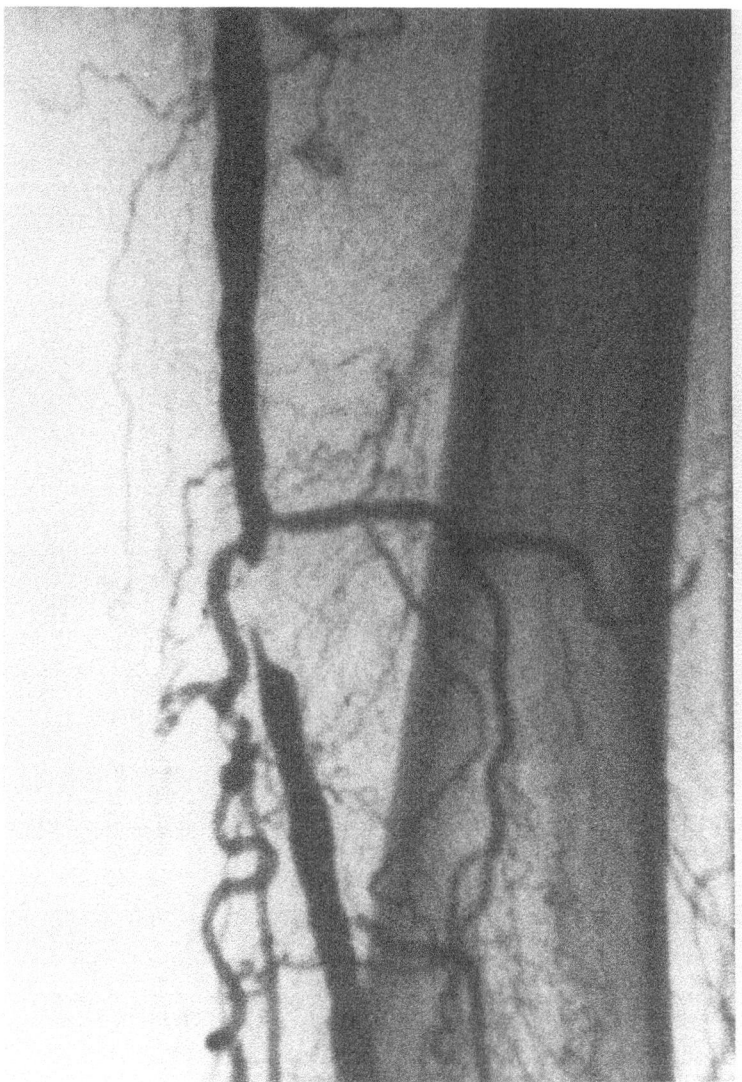

Fig. 2(a)

3 patients with stage III of Fontaine changed to stage IIa after the therapy. In 3 out of 4 patients in stage IIb clinical state improved to stage IIa. It is important to notice that no patient suffered from an isolated stenosis in one region, in most cases more than one region was affected. One patient, who had a long restenosis, which made the implantation of three stents necessary, developed a thrombosis during treatment. Performance of local thrombolysis failed to recanalise the vessel. Surgical treatment was carried out successfully.

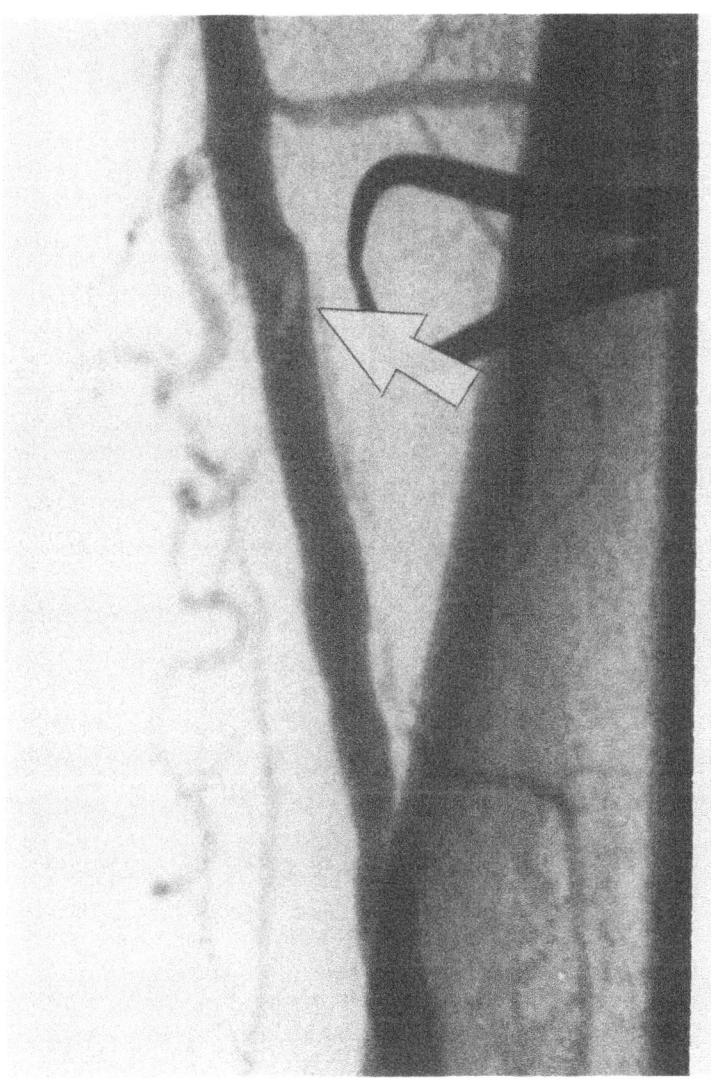

Fig. 2(b)

The Doppler sonographic index before implantation varied from 0.20 to 0.62, average 0.48. After stenting the index ranged from 0.60 to 0.95, average 0.88. In this calculation the patient with immediate stent occlusion was included. Apart from this case the Doppler sonographic index increased after the therapy to an average of 0.31.

The period of follow-up varies from 10 weeks to 6 months. All initally successful implantations showed persistent clinical improvement and patency of the stents. 3 patients improved their walking distance. Transstenotic

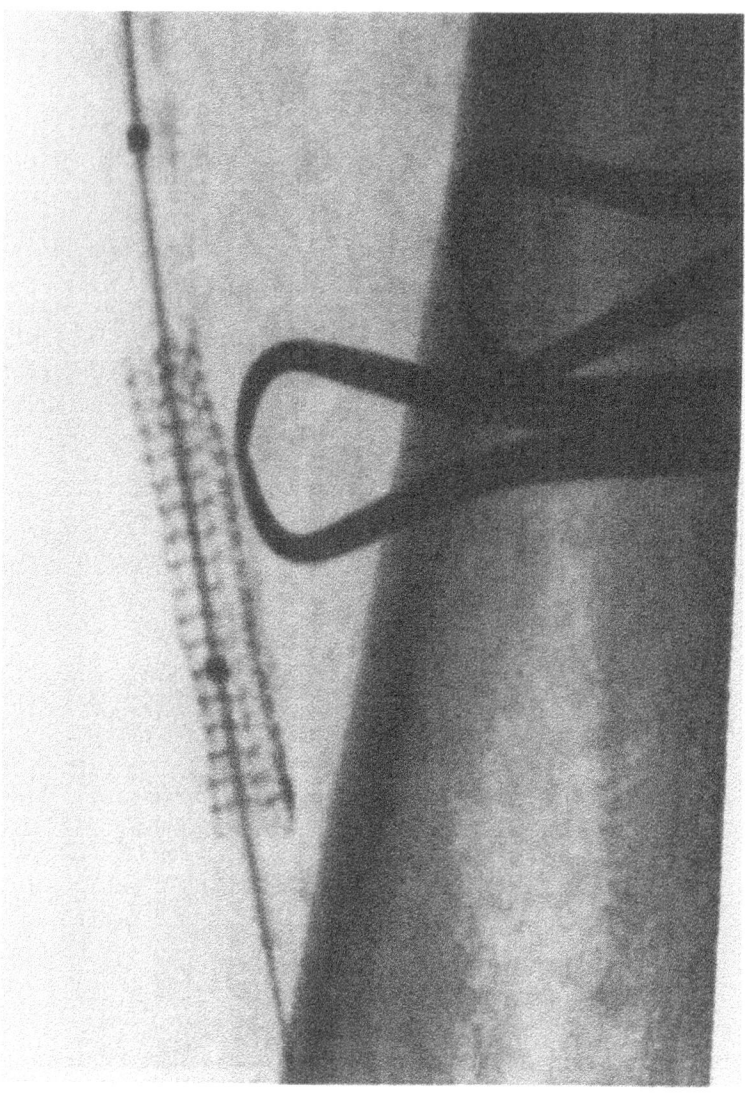

Fig. 2(c)

pressure measurements were performed in only one patient with significant reduction of the gradient. Peripheral pressure pulses were not recorded as a rule.

Discussion

Implantation of vascular endoprotheses is a method whose performance does not need great technical experience. Conventional PTA is proven as a

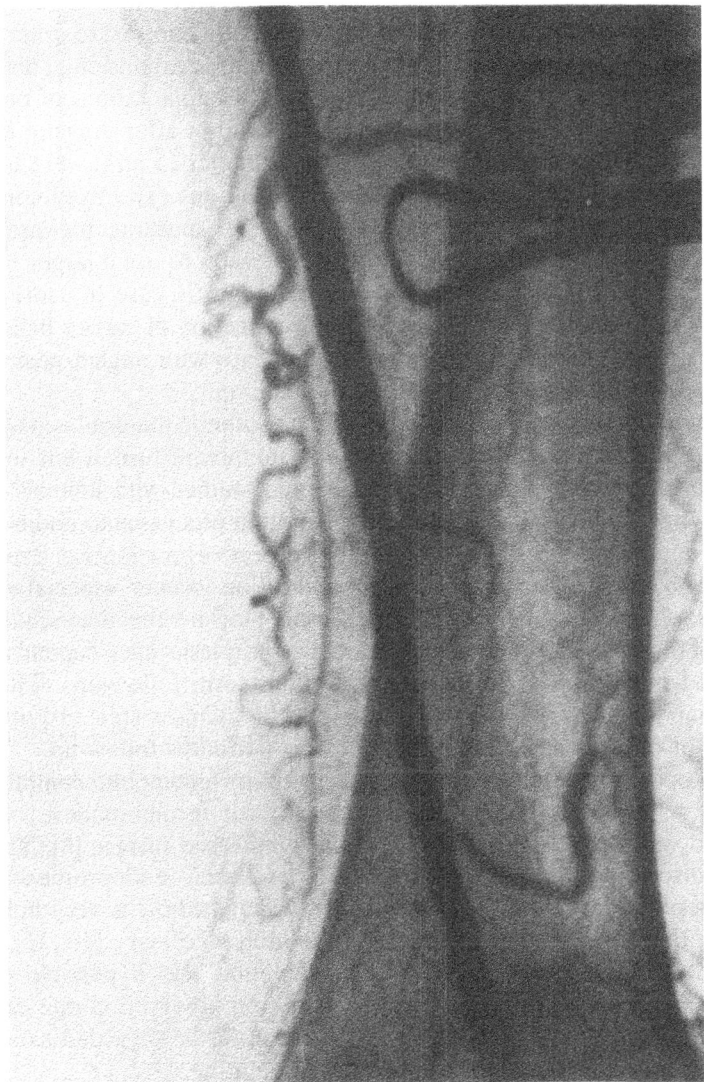

Fig. 2(d)

Figure 2.   Patient with an occlusion of the superficial femoral artery (a) before treatment; (b) after low speed rotational angioplasty and PTA (—> Intimaflap); (c) stent in situ; (d) final result.

successful treatment of short, concentric stenoses and occlusions. In cases of long lesions and excentric stenoses the results are moderate. In these situations additional treatment by implanting a vascular prothesis might improve the therapy. On the other hand stenting may avoid thrombo embolic occlusions of acute complications after PTA (Figure 2). [1, 2, 4, 6, 9, 19].

In our patient cohort we used the Strecker stent, which belongs to the group of balloon expandable intravascular stents. In contrast to other systems of this kind, there is no shortening of the stent after expansion. This enables optimal positioning of the prothesis [10, 16]. All implantations of our group were exact and successful. There was no dislocation after drawing back the carrier balloon. Even when stents with low diameter (5 mm) were used, the withdrawal could be managed without complications. The fixed connection between stent and carrier balloon allows a safe pushing forward of the prothesis through an 8 F sheath. There is no reason to use a larger or longer sheath (e.g., 10 F), so that an exchange of sheath in case of acute complications is not necessary. In our group the connection of carrier balloon and stent was always fixed. Even in cases of a sheath with angled position, the stent position remained unchanged on the balloon.

The most important aspect by implanting synthetic material is its biocompatibility. The Strecker stent fabricated by tantalwire turned out to have a good biocompatibility [11, 17]. Experimental studies with animals showed the growing of a neointima after the implantation of a vascular endoprothesis [13]. A complication of this proliferative process is an intimal hyperplasia followed by stent occlusion. This complication occurs especially in the femoropopliteal region [3, 18]. One reason may be the inadequate distal outflow [14, 17]. The question if intimal hyperplasia also depends on the implanted material, has to be proven by long-term follow-ups. This might imply that tantalwire is more favourable than stainless steel. In our group we did not observe any hyperplasia during a 6 months follow-up.

Early occlusion after stenting is caused by thromembolic complications. Blood flow and run-off are important factors of thrombokinesis, which is increased when it gets in contact with the synthetical surface [8]. Therefore critical discussion of indications by using vascular endoprothesis in the femoropopliteal region is necessary. A sufficient run-off is very important. On the other hand anticoagulation is absolutely necessary [10, 15]. In our study group all patients received anticoagulation and if possible cumarin derivates. Immediate thrombo embolic occlusion observed in one case took place during stent implantation, so that this cannot be regarded as a typical complication, such as early thrombosis after stenting.

Our investigations show that the Strecker stent system is an uncomplicated device, which can be used in the iliac and femoropopliteal region. Future prospective studies will be necessary to compare this system with other balloon expandable systems.

References

1. Gallino A, Mahler F, Probst P, Nachbur B (1984) Percutaneous transluminal angioplasty of the arteries of the lower limbs: 5 year follow-up. *Circulation* 4: 619–623.
2. Günther RW (1989) Laserangioplastie und Gefäßendoprothesen. *Dtsch med Wschr* 114: 435.

3. Günther RW, Vorwerk D, Bohndorf K, El-Din, Peters I, Messmer BJ (1989) Perkutane Implantation von Gefäßendoprothesen (Stents) in Becken- und Oberschenkelarterien. *Dtsch med Wschr* 114: 1517–1523.

4. Johnston KW, Rae M, Hogg-Johnston S, Loapinto RF, Walker PM, Baird RJ, Sniderman KW, Kalman P (1987) 5-year results of prospective study of percutaneous transluminal angioplasty. *Ann Surg* 206: 403–413.

5. Maass D, Zollikofer CL, Largiader F, Senning A (1984) Radiological follow-up of transluminally inserted vascular endoprothesis: an experimental study using expanding spirals. *Radiology* 152: 659–663.

6. Murray RR, Hewes RC, White RI, Mitchell SE, Auster M, Chang R, Kadir S, Kinnison ML, Kaufmann SL (1987) Long-segment femoropopliteal stenosis. Is angioplastie a boon or a bust? *Radiology* 162: 473–476.

7. Palmaz CP (1988) Balloon-expandable intravascular stent. *AJR* 150: 1263–1269.

8. Palmaz JC, Richter GM, Nöldge G, Kauffmann GW, Wenz W (1987) Die intraluminale Stentimplanatation nach Palmaz. *Radiologe* 27: 560–563.

9. Palmaz JC, Richter GM, Nöldge G, Schatz RA, Robinson PD, Gardiner GA, Becker GJ, McLean GK, Denny DF, Lammer J, Paolini RM, Rees CR, Alvarado R, Heiss HW, Root HD, Rogers W (1988) Intraluminal stents in atherosclerotic iliac artery stenosis: preliminary report of a multicenter study. *Radiology* 168: 727–731.

10. Palmaz JC, Sibbitt RR, Tio FO, Reuter SR, Peters JE, Garcia F (1985) Expandable intraluminal vascular graft: a feasibility study. *Surgery* 99: 199–205.

11. Rabenseifer L, Küssweter W, Wünsch PH, Schwab M (1984) Ist die Knochenbruchheilung bei den gewebsverträglichen Implantatwerkstoffen Tantal und Niob gegenüber Stahlimplantaten verändert? *Z Orthop* 122: 349.

12. Rollins N, Wright KC, Charnsangavej, Wallace S, Gianturco C (1987) Self-expanding metallic stents. Preliminary evaluation in an atherosclerotic model. *Radiology* 163: 739–742.

13. Rousseau H, Puel J, Joffre F, Sigwart U, Duboucher CH, Imbert CH, Knight CH, Kropf L, Wallsten H (1987) Self-expanding endovascular prothesis: an experimental study *Radiology* 164: 709–714.

14. Schatz RA, Palmaz JC, Tio FO, Garcia F, Garcia O, Reuter SR (1987) Balloon-expandable intracoronary stents in the adult dog. *Circulation* 76: 450–457.

15. Sigwart U, Puel J, Mirkovitch V, Joffre F, Kappenberger L (1987) Intravascular stents to prevent occlusion and restenosis after transluminal angioplasty. *New Engl J Med* 316: 701–706.

16. Strecker EP, Romaniuk P, Schneider B, Westphal M, Zeitler E, Wolf HRD, Freudenberg N (1988) Perkutan implantierbare, durch Ballon aufdehnbare Gefäßendoprothese. *Dtsch med Wschr* 113: 538–542.

17. Strecker EP, Berg G, Weber H, Bohl M, Schneider B (1987) Experimentelle Untersuchungen mit einer neuen perkutan einführbaren und aufdehnbaren Gefäßendoprothese. *Fortschr Röntgenstr* 147: 669.

18. Triller J, Mahler F, Do D, Thalmann R (1989) Die vaskuläre Endoprothese bei femoropoplitealer Verschlußkrankheit. *Fortschr Röntgenstr* 150: 328–334.

19. Zeitler E, Richter EI, Roth FJ, Schoop W (1983) Results of percutaneous transluminal angioplasty. *Radiology* 156: 69–72.

21. Angioplasty of peripheral vessels: surgical aspects

J. F. VOLLMAR and S. CYBA-ALTUNBAY

Introduction

Any type of interventional technique on peripheral vessels includes a certain risk of complications which afford immediate or delayed surgical repair [1]. The main indications for a surgical intervention are listed in Table 1. Not every hematoma at the puncture side affords a surgical control. But surgery is indicated in the presence of a *pulsating hematoma* which results frequently in the formation of a false aneurysm. The best diagnostic approach is a *duplex scan investigation*.

Table 1. Complications in interventional vascular techniques

1. Hematoma
2. Perforation with excessive bleeding
3. Local thrombosis
4. Embolisation
5. Dissection of the arterial wall

Another complication is a *local thrombosis* of the artery induced by external vascular compression due to the hematoma but more frequently caused by a local dissection of the arterial wall.

The classical signs of an acute ischemia (6 × Ps) herald the inflow stop of the extremity. An identical clinical picture may be caused by *arterial emboli* dislodged in the distal arterial tree.

Small emboli may be asymptomatic and escape the clinical diagnosis; other can induce an ascending or descending arterial thrombosis threatening the affected limb. In such cases an *emergency embolectomy* is mandatory to prevent irreversible ischemic limb damage or amputation.

In a consecutive series 528 PTAs for the repair of stenotic lesions at the renal arteries [2], the aorto-iliac and femoropopliteal segment 20 complications have been registrated necessitating surgical repair: there were 2 patients

181

V. Hombach et al. (eds), Interventional Techniques in Cardiovascular Medicine, 181–183.

Table 2. Surgical treatment of complications following PTA (n = 520)

	1978–1988
Dissection	7
Embolisation	6
Local thrombosis	5
Wall perforation with critical bleeding	2
Summary	20

with life threatening *bleeding* due to vessel perforation with extensive retroperitoneal bleeding (Table 2).

Local thrombosis in 5 were mostly restricted to the puncture site. There were 6 *peripheral arterial emboli* which caused pronounced ischemia of the leg.

7 patients needed surgery for localized or lengthy *intimal dissection* by intramural passage of the guide wire and the catheter. This most frequently seen surgical complication happened especially in arteriosclerotic diseased arteries.

The *diagnosis* of arterial wall dissection may be asymptomatic for several days or weeks. Symptomatic patients with a pronounced narrowing of the true lumen or a secondary thrombosis may be recognized immediately or early by Duplex-scan or more exactly by a secondary arteriogram. If the infrarenal aorta is included in the dissecting process a transperitoneal approach is necessary for surgical repair. The *method of choice* is the total removement of the dissected intimal core between two or three arteriotomies.

Conclusions

From a surgical point of view three aspects should be taken into consideration:

1. Selection of patients for interventional therapy should be done in close cooperation with a vascular surgeon. Concerning clinical indication there is still a field of disagreement between both specialities which should be overcome.
2. For interventions on renal or visceral arteries a surgical stand-by is recommended as a routine.
3. Diagnosis of surgical complications should be realized immediately, i.e., without any delay for surgery.

Under these prerequisites the mortality and morbidity of interventional therapy can be best kept in a very low range justifying these procedures as an alternative approach to a primary surgical reconstruction which includes especially in high risk patients a higher level of morbidity and mortality.

References

1. Menger MD, Jager S, Scherer K, Walter P, Kramann B (1989) Die Bedeutung der gefäßchirurgischen Behandlung von Komplikationen nach perkutaner transluminaler Angioplastie der unteren Extremitäten. *VASA* 18: 215–220.
2. Menges H–W, Jaschke W, Trede M (1988) Percutaneous transluminal angioplasty: the surgeon's role. *World J Surg* 12: 788–797.

PART THREE

Balloon valvuloplasty

22. Balloon pulmonary valvoplasty

M. TYNAN, S. ARAB, S. QURESHI, E. BAKER, R. dos ANJOS,
J. PARSONS and A. HAYES

Introduction

It is over 40 years since Brock [1] introduced closed pulmonary valvotomy
for the treatment of valvar pulmonary stenosis and extended the technique
to the palliation of the tetralogy of Fallot. Since that time open valvotomy
using cardiopulmonary bypass has become the prefered surgical treatment
for valvar stenosis, whilst systemic to pulmonary shunts are generally used in
the tetralogy. Despite effective surgical treatment cardiologists soon attempted catheter interventions as a substitute for surgery. In 1955 Rubio
Alvarez et al. [2] reported an attempt to 'saw' through the stenosed
pulmonary valve with a catheter mounted guide wire. It is difficult to tell
whether or not they effected any improvement. The field of catheter
interventions in this condition remained fallow for the next 30 years until the
introduction of balloon angioplasty catheters, experimental work indicated
the feasibility of the application of this technology to pulmonary valvar
stenosis [3]. Then in 1982 Kann and her colleagues demonstrated that this
could be done successfully in the human patient [4]. The use of balloon
valvoplasty spread rapidly from the United States throughout the world
[5–10]. Recently in the United Kingdom, in Liverpool [11] and subsequently
at Guy's Hospital, extension of the use of balloon dilation to the right
ventricular outflow tract in the tetralogy of Fallot has been explored and,
together with balloon pulmonary valvoplasty, deserves mention.

Technique

The technique used varies somewhat from unit to unit. There is also
variation according to the age of the patient. We will describe the methods
we use since they appear to be successful.

The procedure is performed under local anaesthesia with ketamine
sedation, intubation and general anaesthesia are only used in very anxious
patients or in haemodynamically unstable neonates. The diagnostic cardiac

V. Hombach et al. (eds), Interventional Techniques in Cardiovascular Medicine, 187–193.
© 1991 *Kluwer Academic Publishers.*

catheterization is performed using the percutaneous femoral venous approach, a femoral artery monitoring line is also introduced. Following measurement of pressures and oxygen saturations a right ventricular angiogram is performed. The diameter of the pulmonary artery root ('ring') is measured in the lateral projection. The size of balloon is selected to be 1.2 to 1.4 times the diameter of pulmonary 'ring'. The indications to procede to balloon valvoplasty are; a right ventricular systolic pressure greater than 50 mm/Hg with a transvalvular systolic pressure gradient of more than 25 mm/Hg when the arterial duct is closed, as is usually the case in patients older than one month. When the duct is patent, as is often the case in the neonatal period, the gradient is of less importance and the procedure is indicated when the right ventricular pressure is elevated and the right ventricular angiogram demonstrates valvar pulmonary stenosis. The valve is then crossed once again with a cardiac catheter and a suitable guide wire is introduced to the periphery of the left pulmonary artery and the catheter withdrawn. A balloon catheter of appropriate size is then introduced over the wire to straddle the pulmonary valve and inflated and deflated as quickly as possible. Observation of a waist in the mid portion of the balloon due to the constriction produced by the stenosed valve confirms correct position. Elimination of this waist indicates successful dilatation. Two or three inflations, in good position, are usually made. The balloon catheter is then withdrawn, leaving the wire in situ, a cardiac catheter is then introduced over the wire and final withdrawal pressures are recorded.

There are several modifications of the technique which are particularly applicable in the neonate. When difficulty in crossing the pulmonary valve is anticipated, for example, in critical pulmonary stenosis in the newborn, no attempt is made to enter the pulmonary artery until after a right ventricular angiogram has been performed so that, having crossed the valve, the catheter can be withdrawn leaving a guide wire in place. In such cases the initial passage across the valve can often only be achieved using a small, 0.018 or 0.020, floppy steerable wire. Ideal guide wire position is with the tip in the periphery of the left pulmonary artery, however, in neonates, this may not be stable or may not be achievable. When this is the case the wire may be advanced through the arterial duct to the aorta. When the orifice in the valve is too small to allow passage of a valvoplasty catheter of the ideal balloon diameter then progressive dilation may be indicated. We have used up to four balloon catheters; starting with a 3 mm coronary balloon progressing to, for example, a 10 mm balloon. Conversely when the valve 'ring' is large two balloons may be needed side by side, we have not yet had to employ the double balloon technique.

The basic technique for palliation of the tetralogy of Fallot is similar but a larger balloon to 'ring' ratio is employed approaching 1.5 : 1. Also, more inflations are performed since it is necessary to position the balloon separately for dilation of the valve and for dilation of the subvalve region.

Results

The safety of balloon pulmonary valvoplasty is attested by the fact that in a registry of valvuloplasty and angioplasty in congenital cardiac anomalies (VACCA), recording the immediate results from several centers from 1982 to 1986, there were only two deaths in 818 patients a mortality rate of 0.24%, this includes the learning curve of the procedure. In the same group of patients non fatal complications occurred in 25 patients or 0.33%. The valvoplasty was not performed i.e. there was technical failure in 1.7% of patients.

In our own experience at Guy's Hospital from 1983 to 1989 73 patients, including three who had prior surgical valvotomy, had 87 attempted procedures. The ages ranged from one day to 20 years. Three patients have died. All were infants, only one was related to the procedure or to pulmonary stenosis, the remaining two died of congenital hepatic anomalies. Non fatal complications occurred in six of 87 procedures or 6.7%. These are listed in Table 1. The procedure was not performed in 9 of 87 attempts. There were four failures in the 73 attempted first valvoplasty all were neonates and were in the early part of our experience. Failures at repeat procedures were mainly due to failure to obtain venous access.

Table 1. Balloon pulmonary valvoplasty, non fatal complications in 87 procedures

Arrythmias	1	1.1%
I.V.C. occlusion	2	2.2%
Guide wire fracture	2	2.2%
RV perforation	1	1.1%

Table 2. Balloon pulmonary valvoplasty, immediate haemodynamic results

69 technically successful first procedures

	Before	After	
RV systolic pressure mm/Hg	86+/−24	54+/−25	p < 0.0001
RV/systemic pressure ratio	0.93+/−0.38	0.59+/−0.31	p < 0.0001
RV-PA gradient mm/Hg	63+/−24	29+/−22	p < 0.0001

2 patients had a rise in RV pressure due to infundibular shut down.

Abbreviations: RV = right ventricle; PA = pulmonary artery.

Haemodynamic results following a first dilation are shown in Table 2. There was a significant reduction of right ventricular systolic pressure (RVP), of right ventricle to systemic arterial systolic pressure ratio (RV: S ratio) and of right ventricle to pulmonary artery systolic pressure gradient (RV-PA gradient). There were individual failures to improve these indices due to the use of too small a balloon or due to the valve being dysplastic.

Repeat valvoplasty was attempted on one further occasion in 12 patients and was accomplished in eight. In these eight significant improvement was demonstrated in the group as shown in Table 3. There were too few patients having a third procedure for any conclusions to be drawn.

Table 3. Balloon pulmonary valvoplasty, haemodynamic results after a second procedure in 8 patients

	Before	After	
RV systolic pressure mm/Hg	77+/−13	62+/−18	p < 0.0001
RV/systemic pressure ratio	0.74+/−0.20	0.57+/−0.13	p < 0.0001
RV-PA gradient mm/Hg	51+/−11	40+/−17	p < 0.0001

Abbreviations: RV = right ventricle; PA = pulmonary artery.

Failure to perform the procedure or a result deemed unsatisfactory lead to nine patients being referred for surgery.

The effect of balloon size on the immediate result was sought using the balloon to 'ring' ratio. The only differences found were that balloons more than 1.2 times the diameter of the 'ring' were associated with a greater percentage reduction in RVP and RV : S ratio than smaller balloons, the differences were statistically significant at the 5% level.

Follow up was by Doppler echocardiographic estimation of the RV/PA gradient; patients referred for surgery were not included. Follow up data were available on 43 patients one month to 6.3 years after the completion of their therapy, in 24 the duration was longer than one year. The group as a whole had significantly lower gradients at follow up than prior to valvoplasty although a small rise from the immediate post valvuloplasty was common. There appeared to be no statistically significant difference associated with duration of follow up.

The results of balloon dilation of the right ventricular outflow in palliation of the tetralogy of Fallot are preliminary but, briefly stated they are as follows. In a 13 month period from March 1988 to April 1989 the procedure has been attempted in 12 patients in the first two years of life. The indications were cyanotic 'spells' or severe hypoxaemia with polycythaemia, in other words the same indications as for surgery. There has been one failure to accomplish the dilation. One death occurred in an infant with multiple congenital anomalies, the CHARGE syndrome. This occurred after surgery for tracheo-oesophageal fistula. The outcome in the remaining 10 was that three have now had corrective surgery and five are awaiting it, three after a second dilation. Two patients, deemed uncorrectable, have had elective palliative shunts.

Conclusion

Undoubtedly, balloon pulmonary valvoplasty for congenital valvar pulmonary stenosis is a safe procedure. The low mortality and complication rates must be taken in the context that they include the earliest cases performed and also the initial extension of the method to critical pulmonary stenosis in the new born period. In fact the mortality from the procedure, in our institution, is confined to this age group. The other deaths in our series were due to non cardiac anomalies; multiple congenital anomalies are particularly common in symptomatic newborns. Furthermore failure to accomplish the valvoplasty is also confined to the young infant; with the introduction of small gauge steerable guide wires, more appropriately sized balloon catheters and modifications of technique, such as progressive dilation, we would not now expect to fail to perform the dilation at any age. The low risk and efficacy of the procedure should not blind one to the difficulties that can be encountered particularly in young infants [12] and in this age group only experienced units should attempt the procedure.

The recognition that oversized balloons can be used with safety in the right ventricle and pulmonary outflow tract [13, 14] has lead to the elimination of one source of haemodynamic failure, the use of too small a balloon catheter. However, to show any difference in the results, related to balloon size, balloon: 'ring' ratios of greater than 1.2 : 1 must be used. This ratio is the one usually recommended, perhaps the recommendation should be in the region of 1.4 : 1.

Pulmonary regurgitation has not been dealt with in this study but, although it can occasionally be detected on auscultation and can often be seen on Doppler echocardiography, we have never encountered it as a clinically or haemodynamically significant problem. This is probably due to the fact that the most frequent mechanism of relief of stenosis is splitting of the commissures. Although avulsion of a valve leaflet can occur, such information as there is suggests that this is uncommon [15, 16].

Three other problems have not been discussed. Firstly, post valvoplasty infundibular shut down. By this is meant the appearance of a new subvalvar obstruction after successful valvoplasty [17]. It has also been reported following surgical valvotomy [18]. Usually it is a self limiting phenomenon but occasionally beta blockers or even surgery have been used. We have not encountered this complication as a clinical problem and have only recognized its possible occurrence on two occasions. It may be that the routine use of ketamine sedation has some protective role. Secondly, there is the problem of the dysplastic valve. Such valves are thick with nodules on them. They can obstruct pulmonary outflow because they are space occupying, then relief cannot be obtained by balloon dilation; surgery, with an outflow patch or excision of all or part of the valve, is necessary [19, 20]. But dysplasia is relative. All stenosed valves are, to some extent affected. We must resist the temptation to call dysplastic all valves which have apparently not responded to balloon valvoplasty. Too small a balloon is a more usual reason for failure. Thirdly, transient prolongation of the QT interval [21] has been reported after balloon valvoplasty and it has been suggested that there may be a risk of serious arrythmias following these procedures. This does not appear to be a problem in practice. We continue to discharge our children 24 hours after the procedure with no apparent ill effects.

Balloon dilation in the palliation of the tetralogy offers an alternative to early surgery. Shunt operations are not always successful in young infants and, even when they work, distortion of the anatomy of the pulmonary arteries is a recognized complication. Balloon dilation, when prosecuted aggressively, even if it needs to be repeated, is worthy of further investigation.

Today no patient with valvar pulmonary stenosis should be operated upon unless optimal balloon valvoplasty, by an experienced operator, has unequivocally failed. Tomorrow, perhaps, no infant should have palliative surgery for the tetralogy. A two stage approach consisting of transcatheter palliation during the first year of life with the first operation being total correction promises to be the pattern of the future.

References

1. Brock RC (1948) Pulmonary valvulotomy for the relief of congenital pulmonary stenosis. *Brit Med J* 1: 1121–1126.
2. Rubio-Alvarez V, Limon Lason R, Soni J (1953) Valvotomias intraccardiacas por medio de un catheter. *Arch Inst Cardiol Mexico* 23: 183–192.
3. Kan JS, Anderson JH, White RI Jr (1982) Experimental basis for balloon valvoplasty congenital pulmonary valvar stenosis. *Proc Sect Cardiol Am Acad Ped*, New York, October: 101A.
4. Kan JS, White RI Jr, Mitchell SE, Gardener TJ (1982) Percutaneous balloon pulmonary valvoplasty: a new method for treating congenital pulmonary valve stenosis. *N Engl J Med* ·307: 540.
5. Kann JS, White RI Jr, Mitchell SE, Anderson JH, Gardener TJ (1984) Percutaneous transluminal balloon valvuloplasty for pulmonary valve stenosis. *Circulation* 69: 554–560.
6. Lababidi Z, Wu J (1983) Percutaneous balloon pulmonary valvuloplasty. *Am J Cardiol* 52: 560–562.
7. Rocchini AP, Kveselis DA, Crowley D, Dick M, Rosenthal A (1984) Percutaneous balloon valvuloplasty for the treatment of pulmonary valvular stenosis in children. *J Am Cardiol* 3: 1005–1012.
8. Tynan M, Baker EJ, Rohmer J, Jones ODH, Reidy JF, Joseph MC, Ottencamp J (1985) Percutaneous balloon pulmonary valvuloplasty. *Br Heart J* 53: 520–524.
9. Rey C, Marache P, Matina D, Mouly A (1985) Percutaneous transluminal valvuloplasty of pulmonary stenosis. Report of 24 cases. *Arch Mal Coer* 78: 703–710.
10. Fontes VF, Eduardo J, Sousa MR, Silva VD, Esteves CA, Pontes SC (1986) Percutaneous transluminal balloon valvuloplasty for pulmonic valve stenosis, in Doyle EF, Engle MA, Gersony WM, Rashkind WJ, Talner NS (eds), *Pediatric Cardiology*, pp. 326–330. New York: Springer-Verlag.

11. Qureshi SA, Kirk CR, Lamb RK, Arnold R, Wilkinson JL (1988) Balloon dilatation of the pulmonary valve in the first year of life in patients with tetralogy of Fallot: a preliminary study. *Brit Heart J* 60: 332–335.

12. Piechaud JF, Voshtani H, Kachener J, Sidi D, Gay F, Lebidois J, Villain E (1987) Problémes posés par la valvuloplastie pulmonaire percutanée chez l'enfant. *Arch Mal Coeur* 80: 413–419, 425.

13. Ring JC, Kulik TJ, Burke BA, Lock JE (1984) Morphologic changes induced by dilatation of the pulmonary valve annulus with overlarge balloons in normal newborn lambs. *Am J Cardiol* 55: 210–214.

14. Radtke W, Keane JF, Fellows KE, Lang P, Lock JE (1986) Percutaneous balloon valvotomy of congenital pulmonary stenosis using oversized balloons. *JACC* 8: 909–915.

15. Ettedgui JA, Ho SY, Tynan M, Jones ODH, Martin RP, Baker EJ, Reidy JF (1987) The pathology of balloon pulmonary valvoplasty. *Int J Cardiol* 16: 285–294.

16. Benson LN, Smallhorn JS, Freedom RM, Trusler G, Rowe RD (1985) Pulmonary valve morphology after dilatation of pulmonary valve stenosis. *Catheterization and Cardiovascular Diagnosis* 11: 161–166.

17. Ben-Shachar G, Cohen MH, Sivakoff MC, Portman MA, Riemenschneider TA, VanHeeckeren DW (1985) Development of infundibular obstruction after percutaneous pulmonary balloon valvoplasty. *JACC* 5: 754–756.

18. Griffith BP, Hardesty RL, Siewers RD, Lerberg DB, Ferson PF, Bahnson HT (1982) Pulmonary valvotomy alone for pulmonary stenosis: results in children with and without muscular infundibular hypertrophy. *J Thorac Cardiovasc Surg* 83: 577–383.

19. Watkins L, Donahoo JS, Harrington D, Haller JA, Neill CA (1977) Surgical management of congenital pulmonary valve dysplasia. *Ann Thorac Surg* 24: 498–502.

20. Vancini M, Roberts KD, Silove ED, Singh SP (1980) Surgical treatment of pulmonary stenosis due to dysplastic leaflets and small valve anulus. *J Thorac Cardiovasc Surg* 79: 464–468.

21. Martin GR, Stanger P (1985) Transient prolongation of the QTc interval after balloon valvuloplasty and angioplasty in children. *Am J Cardiol* 58: 1233–1235.

23. Mitral valvuloplasty

U. U. BABIC

Introduction

In the last 7 years, the interventional cardiology has extended its domain to stenotic heart valves. All 4 heart valves have become amenable to balloon dilation. While the technique for pulmonary valvuloplasty used is more or less the same in all centers there are attempts to use different approaches for aortic and numerous variations for mitral valvuloplasty. The subject of this report is the single author experience in two main techniques for mitral balloon valvuloplasty (transvenous-Inoue [1], transarterial [7]).

Patient population

Transarterial mitral valvuloplasty was performed in 247 patients and transvenous mitral valvuloplasty was performed in 76 pts. The patients were between 15 and 75 years old (mean $37+/-7$), and there was no difference in age of patients of both groups. Female/male ratio was 289/34. Patients were selected for mitral dilation according to the echocardiographic and/or catheterization data as well as the symptoms. Even asymptomatic females in generative period who desired pregnancy in the near future were accepted and recommended to balloon valvuloplasty. The approach was choosen arbitrarely, i.e., there were no criteria for transvenous or transarterial technique to be used in a patient. Depending on availability of balloons in our center the transvenous or transarterial approach were used (Table 1).

Table 1. Population

N	323 Patients
F/M	289/34
Age	$15-76$ ($37+/-7$)
Transarterial	247 Patients
Transvenous	76 Patients

V. Hombach et al. (eds), Interventional Techniques in Cardiovascular Medicine, 195–202.

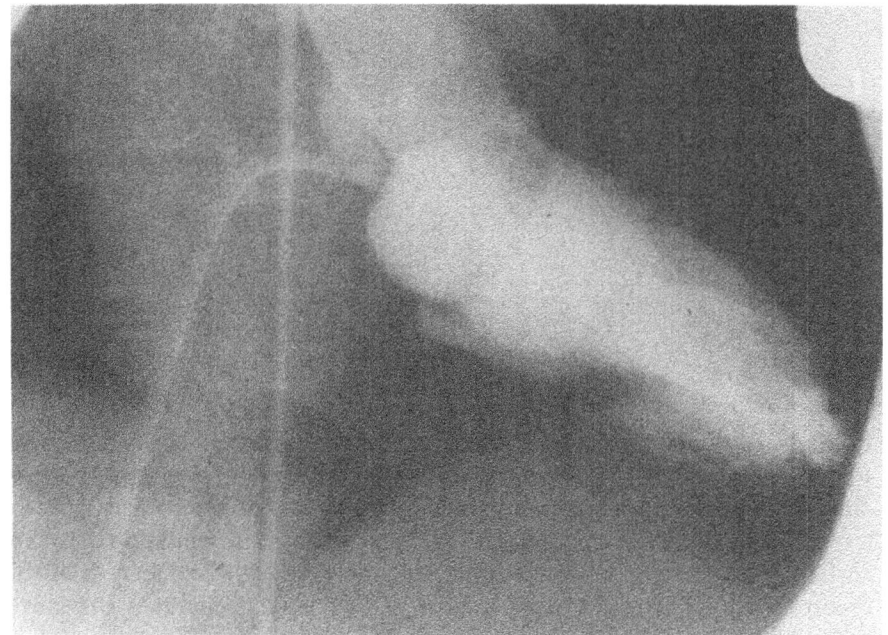

Figure 1.   Left ventriculography during the inflation of the Inoue balloon across the mitral valve.

Technique

Original transarterial technique [7] was performed (Figure 1) using either a bifoil 2 × 19 mm (Schneider Europe) or 2 balloons of 2 × 18, 2 × 20, 18 + 20 mm in diameter (Medi-Tech). Left atrial angiography was regularly performed during balloon inflation in order to properly visualize the correct position of the balloons across the valve (Figure 2).

Patients in atrial fibrillation received whenever possible coumadin at least 1 months prior to dilation. After the valvuloplasty all patients received coumadin at least 6 months.

Results

The results are outlined in Table 2. There were no differences in achieved mitral valve area between the two techniques. The time needed for the accomplishment of the transvenous valvuloplasty with the Inoue balloon was shorter than that needed for the transarterial approach (40 min versus 52 min). In 2 patients the Inoue balloon could not be advanced across the stenotic mitral valve and the transarterial technique had to be used to accomplish the dilation.

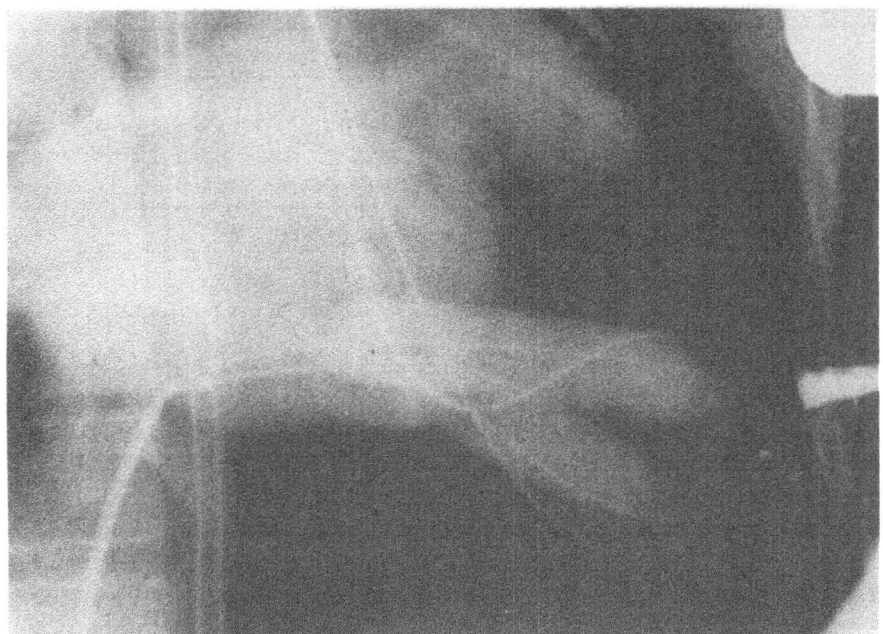

a

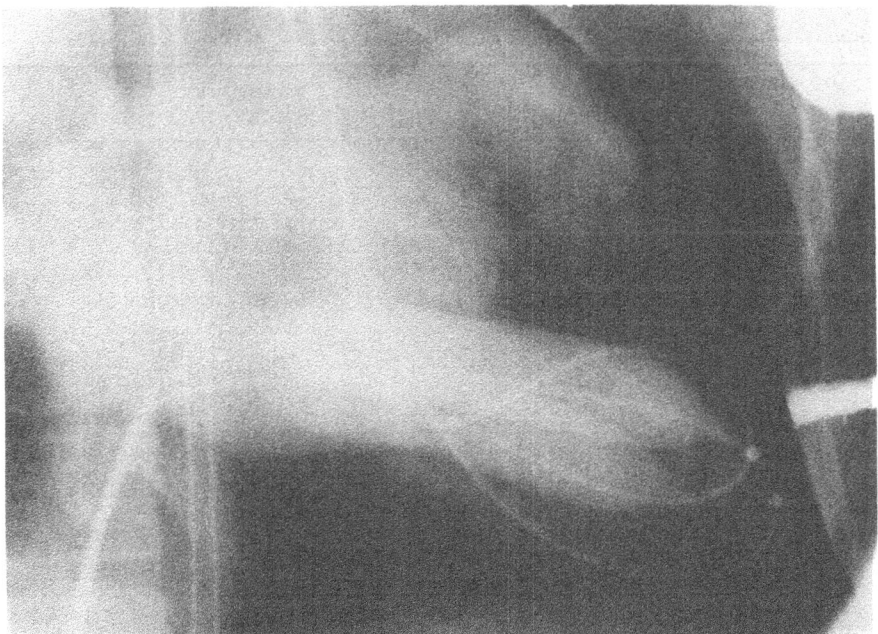

b

Figure 2. Left atrial direct angiography during inflation of 2 balloons across the mitral valve.

Table 2. Results of transarterial MBV versus transvenous MBV

	Transarterial	Transvenous	
MVA cm^2			
Pre	1.1	1.2	p > 0.05
Post	1.9	2.0	p > 0.05
Time Needed	52+/− 14 min	40+/− 7 min	p > 0.01

MVA = mitral valve area; MBV = mitral balloon valvuloplasty.

Complications

Complications are outlined in the Table 3. Of 247 patients who underwent the transarterial valvuloplasty 2 died due to embolic events (0.8%). There were no deaths among the patients treated with Inoue technique (n = 76).

Incidence of stroke was similar in both groups (2.4% vs. 2.6%).

Although the transarterial technique had more vascular problems (2.4% versus 1.3%), none of patients had any chronic circulatory sequelae to the legs. Mitral regurgitation was more frequently produced after transvenous approach (21% versus 12.9%). Angiographically and/or oximetrically detected ASD (atrial septal defect) was found in 11% of patients after transvenous and in none of patients after transarterial technique.

Table 3. Complications

	Transarterial n = 247		Transvenous n = 76	
Stroke	6(2.4%)	2(2.6%)		
MR IV	3(1.2%)		2(2.6%)	
III		4(1.2%)	1(1.3%)	
II		8(3.3%)	7(9.2%)	
I		17(6.8%)	6(7.8%)	
I–IV	34(12.9%)		16(21%)	p < 0.01
Death	2(0.8%)		0	
Vascular	6(2.4%)		1(1.3%)	
ASD	0		9(11%)	
		Qp/Qs > 1.5	3(3.9%)	

Abbreviations: ASD = atrial septal defect; MR = mitral regurgitation; QP/QS = pulmonary to systemic flow ratio.

Surgery after mitral balloon valvuloplasty

Two patients underwent immediate surgery because of acute mitral regurgitation grade 4 (1 after transarterial and 1 after transvenous approach). One of these patients developed pulmonary edema, hemopthysis and cardiogenic

shock. The hemodynamic stabilization was achieved by the use of percutaneous left atrial-aortic bypass with a roller pump [13] at the catheterization
laboratory and the patient was transported to the operating room while the
roller pump was driven manually. In both patients a rupture of the anterior
mitral leaflet was found intraoperatively. One patient underwent surgical
suture of the perforation site of the left ventricular apex (after transarterial
approach). Table 4 shows the cause, number of patients and the time
surgery was performed after valvuloplasty.

Table 4. Surgery after MBV (n = 323)

Cause	n	Time post MBV
MR	2	Immed. post
	3	1–2 years
Restenosis	3	2–4 years
La thromb	1	2 years
Endocarditis	1	3 months
Pseudomonas		

MR = mitral regurgitation.

Reusability of the balloon catheters

Due to financial problems in our country we could not afford using the
expensive balloons only once. After the use the balloon catheters were
vigorously flushed with the detergicide solution, cleaned and dried. Before
the reuse, the catheters were immersed into the detergicide solution for 1
hour. In average, the Medi-Tech balloons were used 3–4, Schneider bifoil
balloons 5–7, and Inoue balloons 3–5 times. We noticed no adverse effects
of the balloon catheters reuse. One patient was found to have a pseudomonas endocarditis 3 months post dilation.

Follow up

Patients treated with transvenous technique were followed up of from 3 to
18 months. Restenosis defined as a loss of more than 50% of the achieved
gain in valve area or the absolute valve area less than 1.5 cm^2 was not found
in any patient (according to ech-doppler data 65 patients, to recatheter-
ization 29 patients).

Two hundred patients who underwent transarterial mitral valvuloplasty
were followed up for at least 1 to maximally 4.5 years. Restenosis was found
in 6 patients (3%) (2 patients developed restenosis after 2 years and 4
patients after 3 years). Three of these patients underwent surgery and 3
repeat valvuloplasty with balloon. One patient underwent surgery because
of the left atrial thrombus 2 years post dilation, and one patient required
surgery because of pseudomonas endocarditis 3 months post dilation.

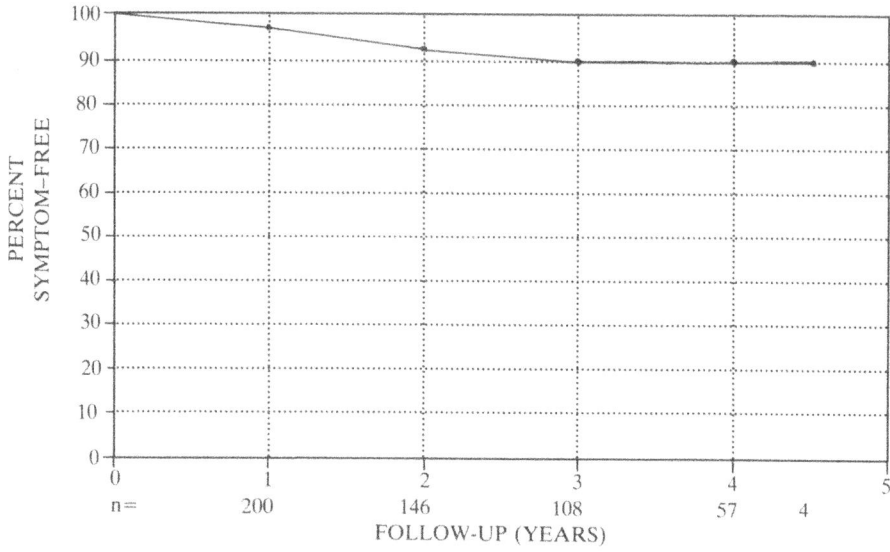

Figure 3.   Redo-free percent in 200 patients followed up 1–4.5 years.

In addition, 3 patients required surgery because of worsening of mitral regurgitation, 1, 2, 2 years post dilation. One patient died 2 months post dilation (cause not known).

Symptom free percent was 96%, 93%, 90%, 90%, and the 'redo' free percent was 99%, 96%, 94.5%, 94.5%, 1, 2, 3, 4 years respectively (Figures 3 and 4).

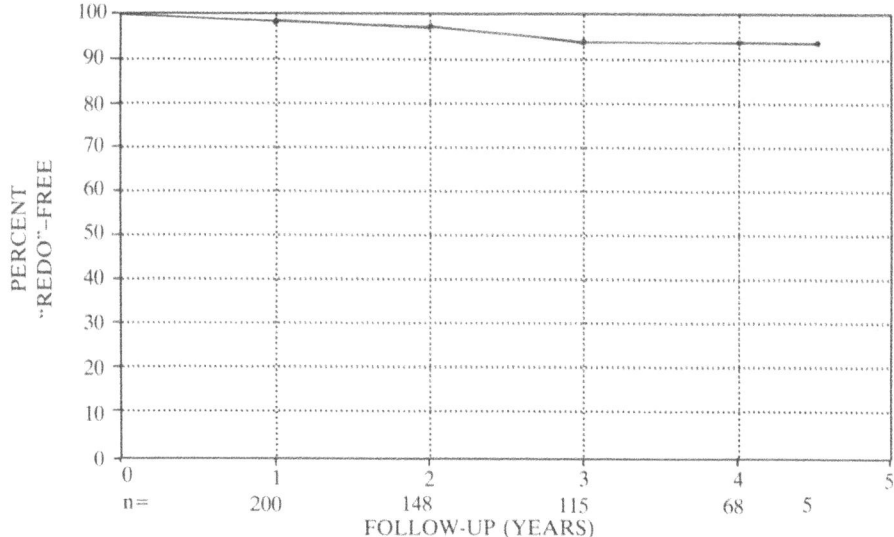

Figure 4.   Symptom-free percent in 200 patients followed-up 1–4.5 years.

Discussion

In contrast to the enthusiasm for balloon valvuloplasty of the calcified aortic stenosis, which is being more and more attenuated, the mitral balloon valvuloplasty has found its approval even by surgery. Good intermediate-term results and low restenosis rate encourage the cardiologists to use this principle in the majority of patients with mitral stenosis and to search for various approaches to the mitral valve [1–8, 11, 12].

The hitherto experience with numerous techniques seems to justify some general considerations:

1. Independently of the technique used the achieved valve area is approximately the same.
2. After transvenous valvuloplasty there is a poor correlation between echo-doppler and hemodynamic data immediately post dilation [9, 10], also the reported restenosis rate after transvenous technique is unusually high −24% [8]. Both features could possible be explained through a mis-calculation of the hemodynamic values due to the created hole on the atrial septum immediately after transseptal valvuloplasty.
3. In order to avoid injury to the subvalvular apparatus, the route which will be taken by the dilating balloon catheter must be created by a floating catheter first for both transvenous and transarterial techniques.
4. The time needed for the accomplishment of the procedure seems to be the shortest for Inoue technique.
5. Mitral balloon valvuloplasty may create an acute mitral insufficiency requiring urgent surgery or mechanical circulatory support [13]. Because of this the procedure should be performed only in centers where this kind of emergency treatment is available.

References

1. Inoue K, Owaki T, Kitamura F, Miymoto N (1984) Clinical application of transvenous mitral commissurotomy by a new balloon catheter. *J Thorac Cardiovasc Surg* 87: 394–402.
2. Babic UU (1985) Percutaneous transarterial balloon valvuloplasty for mitral valve stenosis: a new technique, in: Vucinic M (ed), *Yugoslav-French International Seminar on Cardiac Surgery*, Belgrade, June 20–22, pp. 17–25. Belgrade: Studio Plus.
3. Lock EJ, Khalilullah M, Shrivastava S, Bahl V, Keane J (1985) Percutaneous catheter commissurotomy in rheumatic mitral stenosis. *N Engl J Med* 313: 1515–1518.
4. Zeibag AM, Kasab AS, Ribeiro AP, Fagih AM (1986) Percutaneous double balloon mitral valvotomy for rheumatic valve stenosis. *Lancet* I: 756–761.
5. Vahanian A, Michel PL, Cormier B et al. (1988) Perkutane transluminale Valvuloplastie der Mitralklappe. *Herz* 13: 84–87.
6. Stefanadis Ch, Kourouklis C, Stratos C, Pitsavos Ch, Toutouzas P (1989) Retrograde left atrial catheterization using a new steerable cardiac catheter. *Eur Heart J* 10: 102, suppl.
7. Babic UU, Dorros G, Pejcic P, Djurisic Z, Vucinic M, Lewin R, Grujicic S (1988) Percutane mitral valvuloplasty: retrograde transarterial double-balloon technique utilizing the transseptal approach. *Cath and Cardiovasc Diagn* 14: 229–237.

8. Serra A, Bonan R, Cequier A, Dyrda I, Crepeau J (1989) Restenosis after mitral valvuloplasty. *Eur Heart J* 10: 33g, suppl.
9. Reid CL, McKay CR, Chandraranta PAN et al. (1987) Mechanism of increase in mitral valve area and influence of anatomic features in double balloon, catheter balloon valvuloplasty in adults with rheumatic mitral stenosis: an echocardiographic-doppler study. *Circulation* 76: 628–636.
10. Rahimtoola HS (1989) Perspective on valvular heart disease: an update. *JACC* 14: 1–23.
11. Vahanian A, Michel PL, Cormier B et al. (1989) Percutaneous balloon valvotomy in mitral stenosis: a report on 300 cases. *European Heart J* 10: 339, suppl.
12. Inoue K (1989) Efficacy of percutaneous transvenous mitral commissurotomy by Inoue-Balloon. *European Heart J* 10: 95, suppl.
13. Babic UU, Pejcic P, Djurisic Z, Vucinic M, Popovic Z, Grujicic S (1989) Percutaneous left atrial-aortic bypass with nonpulsatile flow: experience in 4 patients. *European Heart J* suppl 10: 18.

24. Balloon aortic valvuloplasty

A. CRIBIER and R. KONING

Introduction

Balloon aortic valvuloplasty (BAV) has been introduced 4 years ago as a palliative treatment in elderly patients with severe aortic stenosis. After an experience of 4 years and more than 450 patients treated, we better know in 1989 the advantages, indications and limits of the procedure.

Clinical experience

From September 1985 up until December 1988 our experience can be divided into 3 phases. A preliminary series of 40 cases where we were in our learning phases, and 2 comparable series of 180 patients, Group 1 (May 86—September 1987) and Group 2 (September 1987—December 1988). In Group 1 standard balloon catheters were used and several exchange procedures were needed. No sheat could be used for femoral insertion of the balloon catheter and a manual control of bleeding was necessary. In Group 2 we used a new device with a double size balloon limiting the exchange procedures. Further more the low profile pigtail catheter could be inserted through a 14 French introducer and allowed aortic pressure and gradient measurements through a third lumen. This improved technique has considerably decreased the duration of the procedure to 38 minutes in average instead of 2 hours before, an important point in the case of very elderly patients.

However, the results in the two series remained grossly comparable: same reduction of the peak gradient (73 to 28 mmHg p < 0.001) and slight improvement of the final post procedure valve area in Group 2 if compared to Group 1 (1,01 vs 0,92 cm² p < 0.01). With more experience and using new devices the valve area could be opened to above 1 cm² in 47% of the patients instead of 34% before, when the less good results, a valve area below 0,7 cm² decreased to 12% (Group 2) when it was 22% before (Group 1), results significantly different (p < 0.01). The increase in aortic valve

203

V. Hombach et al. (eds), Interventional Techniques in Cardiovascular Medicine, 203–204.

area can generally be expected to be in the range of 0.4 cm^2 whatever may be the severity of the decrease before dilatation.

Major complications were rare in Group 2 especially death (1 patient) and stroke (1 patient) as well as severe aortic insufficiency (2 patients). The main problem was the complication rate at the femoral artery entry site. In Group 2, it remained 12% with need for femoral repair in 4%. However, over the last year and with the use of an arterial introducer, these complications have almost disappeared. The total intra and post-procedure mortality decreased from 5% to 3% which is an acceptable rate especially when considering the old age and the bad clinical condition of most of these patients.

Balloon aortic valvuloplasty is an efficient, well tolerated and low risk procedure. However, in 1989 we definitely know the two major limits of the method: the usual persistance of a less severe degree of aortic stenosis, and the high mid term restenosis rate which has been demonstrated to be in the range of 50% to 70% at one year follow-up on Echo Doppler studies, in our experience as well as in the literature.

Our data suggest that elderly patients are likely to benefit the most from valvuloplasty. However, age per se cannot be considered as the only criterion for selecting patients either for BAV or surgery. Physiologic age is often different from chronologic age. Some elderly patients, even in their eighties, remain very healthy active persons, strong enough to survive major heart surgery. On the other hand, some septuagenerians or younger patients with advanced cardiac failure of associated disease can be poor surgical candidates or even non operable but they can always be considered for BAV. In all cases, valve replacement can still be discussed in case of insufficient BAV results or restenosis.

In very old patients or in case surgery is contraindicated or definitely refused, a second BAV can always be performed.

Valvuloplasty will never be competitive with valve replacement whose benefit and long term results are well established. At the opposite, it will likely remain a technique of choice in all cases where surgery carries a very high risk or is contraindicated. This is particularly true in elderly patients, those patients who in their vast majority can resume normal activities for their age after a relatively simple and safe procedure requiring only local anesthesia and a brief hospitalization stay.

25. Surgical aspects of balloon valvuloplasty (BVP)

H. DALICHAU, K. L. NEUHAUS and U. TEBBE

Introduction

Serious complications (except valvular injuries) which have to be treated operatively as an emergency rarely occur during balloon valvuloplasty (BVP). For this reason a surgical stand-by during the procedure is not mandatory as a routine. That is why the surgeon's involvement in BVP is not identical with that in coronary angioplasty. Consequently, the discussion about surgical aspects of BVP can be directed only to the question which part in fact this new interventional technique may play in the treatment of valvular stenoses in general in the present state from a surgeon's point of view. It is, however, extremely difficult to answer this question, because for any comparison with surgical results so far only short-term experiences with BVP are available. Moreover, as both techniques are applied to various entities of patients not only with regard to the topographical location of the valve but also to their pathomorphology one cannot deal with this issue as a whole.

According to the publications on BVP its seems, however, to be quite obvious that this procedure will not become an alternative to surgical treatment in general, but the therapy of first choice at best or a complementary method for selected groups of patients with critically diseased cardiac valves. However, this will have to be discussed in more detail with a view to the following questions:

1. How effective is BVP in comparison to surgical therapy in the treatment of severe valvular stenoses applied to the different cardiac valves?
2. Is BVP a temporary or a definite therapeutic procedure for valvular stenosis?
3. How far will the results obtained by BVP influence the indications for operative treatment of stenotic valves?

205

V. Hombach et al. (eds), Interventional Techniques in Cardiovascular Medicine, 205–212.
© 1991 *Kluwer Academic Publishers.*

BVP for congenital valvular malformations

Pulmonic stenosis

Isolated pulmonic stenosis seems to be the best defined indication for performing BVP as the therapy of first choice. As most patients affected are young and the stenosis is mostly congenital rather than acquired the procedure usually can be applied without relevant technical problems, with a low risk of major complications and mortality and obviously with comparable good early and medium term results as with open valvulotomy [11]. Furthermore, one can expect an identically low incidence of valvular restenosis as after operative treatment because the therapeutical results will hardly be influenced by progressive degenerative changes and/or calcification of the valve. For this reason, BVP may be the appropriate and possibly curative therapy for pulmonic stenosis in children and adolescents which can be attempted on a less traumatic way than thoractomy does (Table 1).

Table 1. Present status of pulmonic valvuloplasty

Indication identical as for surgical treatment
Gradient decreased to 20–30%
Low complication rate
Excellent immediate effects (> 90% improved)
Excellent long-term results (no restenosis)

Since BVP was introduced into clinical therapy patients with isolated pulmonic stenoses have been transferred to the surgeon for operative treatment only rarely.

For infants with complex congenital lesions including pulmonic stenosis, however, dilatation of the valve can be only a palliative procedure in most cases, because often the pulmonic valve is extremely dysplastic in such cases and the effect of BVP is additionally limited due to a hypoplastic valvular ring. But even under these circumstances the procedure may be indicated, as otherwise an emergency palliative surgical intervention with a higher risk has to be performed as an alternative.

Aortic stenosis

Part of what has been said of the pulmonic stenosis may also be true for the congenital aortic stenosis with the restriction, however, that the effect of BVP is palliative and therefore rather temporary than curative as a rule. This is due to the fact that stenotic aortic valves are mostly dysplastic and residual gradients across the valve or resulting regurgitation are of greater importance than at the pulmonic valve at long-term follow-up. For the majority of infants, however, these problems can be accepted primarily, because one has to take into account that even with early operative treatment in those individuals only a surgical palliation with a high complication rate can be performed. These observations justify the application of BVP even in critically ill infants despite of the high risk [13]. Sometimes, however, the stenotic aortic valve orifice can not be passed with the balloon catheter and primary operative intervention will become unavoidable.

BVP for acquired valvular lesions

Mitral stenosis

Mitral stenosis is rheumatic for the majority of patients. The most striking feature normally appears to be commissural fusion. In uncalcified valves this typical morphologic alteration can usually be treated successfully by mechanical separation of the fused leaflets. In the past this has been achieved mainly by applying closed instrumental transventricular commissurotomy which in principle has worked at the same way as BVP does nowadays. The excellent short- and long-term results which have been reached with mitral commissurotomy in the majority of patients should therefore be also obtainable with BVP. This refers to the increase of valve opening area due to dilatation as well as to the incidence of valvular restenosis at follow-up. As far as medium-term observations after BVP of pure uncalcified mitral stenosis are available this certainly is true [1, 6].

One also would expect that BVP can be performed with a lower risk of operative mortality and morbidity because the surgical approach requires a thoracotomy. But as a matter of fact, this does not seem to be true. According to the literature the early mortality of BVP and closed surgical commissurotomy is nearly equal. Furthermore, the number and incidence of early complications after BVP are relatively high (Table 2). This refers to cerebrovascular embolism, cardiac tamponade, resulting mitral incompetence and left-to-right shunt caused by the balloon introduction via the atrial septum as well [14].

Table 2. Early complications of mitral valvuloplasty (according to literature)

Early mortality	0–1%
Cerebral embolism	1–3%
Myocardial infarct	~ 1%
Pericardial tamponade	1–3%
Mitral incompetence	2–10%
Atrial septal defect	0–40%

As far as late results are concerned there is no evidence up to now that BVP is prior to closed commissurotomy. According to the literature 80% of the patients are clinically and hemodynamically improved 6–14 months after

Table 3. Late results of mitral commissurotomy

Follow up (yrs)	Death (%)	Valve repl. (%)
1	1	2
5	10	9
10	20	25
20	40	60

n = 267 pats; Op 1960–64; Op mort. 2,6%; Follow-up 43 yrs; Holmes et al., Mayo Clinic ACC, 1989.

BVP of course, but on the other hand 1.5 to 9% of the patients died during the same period of time. In contrast, Holmes and coworkers have reported in 1989 on 267 patients after closed mitral commissurotomy operated at the Mayo Clinic from 1960 to 1964 with a 5 and 10 years survival rate of 90 and 80 percent respectively (Table 3).

From the surgeon's point of view yet another aspect will have to be mentioned. Reviewing the past 2 decades it becomes quite obvious that the indications to treat mitral stenosis have changed significantly. While at the beginning of that period of time a certain part of patients with mitral stenosis could be treated by either closed or at least open commissurotomy, in the majority of patient which have been transferred to surgery nowadays only difficult reconstructive procedures or even valve replacement can be performed because of the severity of valvular and subvalvular alterations.

BVP for mitral stenosis should be indicated only in those individuals in which no calcification of the valve is present and leaflet movement can still be observed at echocardiography. Patients with heavy calcification, valvular incompetence of major degree or evidence of left atrial thrombi and recent thromboembolic events should be considered as candidates for surgical treatment (Table 4).

Table 4. Contraindications to mitral valvuloplasty

Heavy valve calcification
Mitral incompetence > II°
Left atrial thrombosis
Recent thromboembolic events

As emergency interventions for mitral stenoses rarely become necessary urgent BVP is not often indicated. It may become the treatment of choice when valve replacement is contraindicated for cardiac reasons (poor left ventricular function, untreatable coronary artery disease) or because of the presence of other severe illness (malignancy f.e.).

Otherwise, BVP is justified only

1. in patients with pure uncalcified mitral stenosis; and
2. if the risk of an urgently indicated noncardiac operation should be reduced.

Aortic stenosis

Acquired aortic stenosis has certainly been the main indication to apply BVP during the last years including patients with severely calcified valves and those of the older age group. The leading argument for the attempt to treat aortic stenoses by a nonsurgical approach refers to the lower risk of BVP especially in elderly individuals. This opinion, however, does not reflect the real facts (Table 5). Early mortality (defined as death rate within

Table 5. Complications of aortic valvuloplasty (n > 1.100)

Death during procedure	1% (0–3%)
Hospital mortality	8% (5–10%)
Late mortality (up to 12 mo.)	15% (9–43%)
Cerebrovascular injury	2%
Myocardial infarct	«1%
Pericardial tamponade	1–2%
Vascular injury/bleeding	11%

According to Spielberg et al. [12].

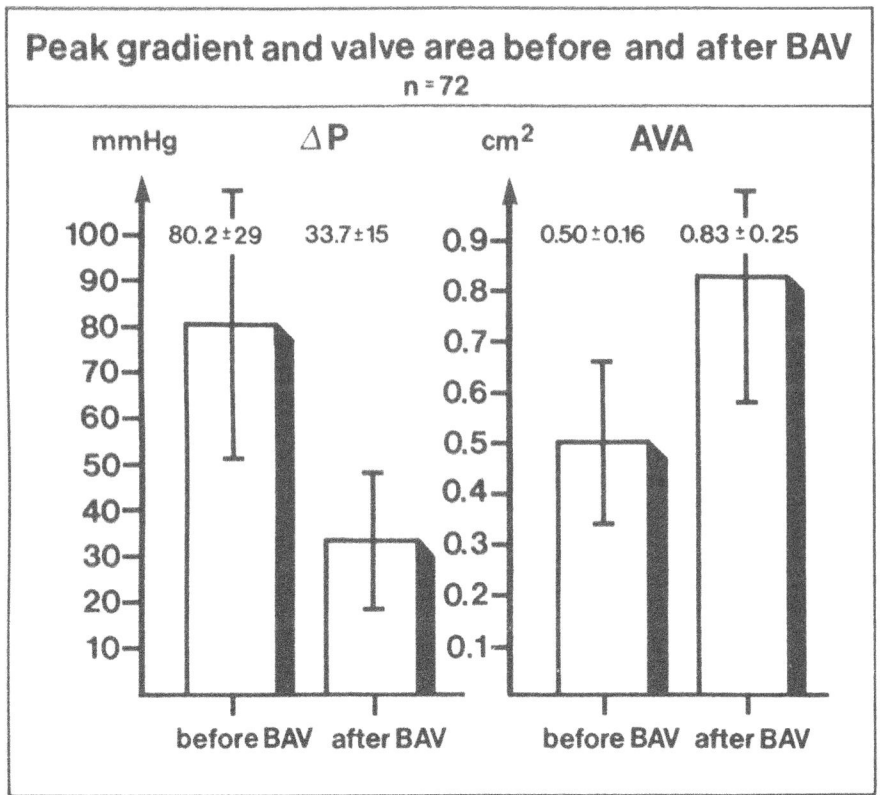

Figure 1.

Table 6. Comparison of results of aortic valvuloplasty (BVP) and aortic valve replacement (AVP) in elderly patients

	BVP	AVR
Early mortality	1–5%	3–15%
'Late' mortality	high (> 10%)	low (< 5%)
Restenosis	50–100%	< 5%
Thromboembolism	0	2%
Clinical improvement	moderate	good
Functional result	moderate	optimal

30 days after the intervention) after aortic valve replacement might be slightly earlier in the older population, especially when compared with earlier statistical data. But the outcome of these patients after long-term follow-up is absolutely superior to that who underwent valvuloplasty (Table 6). This is primarily due to the fact that BVP cannot achieve the same hemodynamic improvement as valve replacement does. This refers to the reduction of pressure gradient across the valve as well as to the increase of valve opening area which rarely exceeds 1 square centimeter after BVP [2, 3, 9, 10, 12, 13] (Figure 1). The effect of BVP must be temporary in most of the patients therefore, and restenosis may occur very early after the dilatation. According to recent reports the same degree of valvular stenosis as before BVP can be established in the majority of patients 7–12 months later already. Late mortality after BVP due to hemodynamic deterioration for this reason is significantly higher than following aortic valve replacement [2, 5]. (Table 7).

Table 7. Follow-up after aortic valvuloplasty according to publications in 1988

Author	Year	Hospital mortality	Months follow-up	Late mortality	Valve replaced
Cribier	1988	4.6%	8	16%	–
Safian	1988	3.5%	9	15%	11%
Erdmann	1988	5.6%	6	11%	11%
Scherer	1988	5.8%	9	14%	31%
Spielberg	1988	9.0%	11	24%	30%
Vogt	1988	0.0%	14	10%	36%

These observations just favour to consider patients with severely damaged and calcified valves as candidates for primary valve replacement even when they belong to the older age group. Similar to the treatment of mitral stenosis, however, BVP is still justified in patients with cardiac or noncardiac contraindications to valve surgery and in those with an extreme surgical risk due to other cardiac or noncardiac diseases [4, 8, 9] (Table 8).

Furthermore, BVP may be applied prior to other surgical procedures in

Table 8. Indications for valvuloplasty in calcified aortic stenosis

Contraindications to valve replacement (COPD, malignancy, stroke, AMI)
High surgical risk (physiologic age > 80y, renal or liver disease, poor LV function, advanced CAD)
Urgent need for non-cardiac surgery

patients with severe congestive heart failure in the presence of aortic stenosis to achieve cardiac recompensation [3].

Conclusion

While coronary angioplasty has become an accepted procedure in the treatment of coronary artery disease in the meantime, BVP did not reach a similar therapeutical importance for stenotic valve lesions. According to world-wide experience BVP is far from being an alternative approach to valvular surgery in general (Table 9).

Table 9. Indications for BVP—present status

Pulmonic stenosis		Therapy of first choice
Mitral stenosis		Therapy of first choice (?) in selected patients
Aortic	Congenital	Therapy of first choice (?)
stenosis	Acquired	Valve replacement contra-indicated or with entreme risk

Isolated *congenital pulmonic stenosis* is the classical indication nowadays for performing BVP as the therapy of choice as results are comparable to those of operation [7].

It may also be primarily indicated for the treatment of *noncalcified mitral stenosis* in that group of patients in which comissurotomy was performed in the past. Patients presenting left atrial thrombi or having suffered from recent or recurrent embolic episodes, however, are therefore no candidates for BVP.

As an initial therapeutic approach BVP may be also indicated in selected infants and children with *congenital aortic stenosis* despite the fact that most of those individuals will need definite operative treatment later on.

For *acquired aortic stenosis*, however, BVP is contraindicated and should be attempted only if valve replacement cannot be performed. In case that valve replacement should be indicated BVP should not be considered.

References

1. Babic UU, Pejic P, Djurisic Z, Vucinic M, Grujicic SM (1986) Percutaneous transarterial balloon valvuloplasty for mitral stenosis. Am J Cardiol 57: 1101–1104.
2. Cribier A, Savin T, Berland I, Rocha P, Mechmeche P, Saoudi N, Behar P, Letac B (1987) Percutaneous transluminal balloon valvuloplasty of adult aortic stenosis: report of 92 cases. J Am Coll Cardiol 9: 381–386.
3. Erdmann E (1989) Die dekompensierte Aortenklappenstenose — Valvuloplastie als Noteingriff. Internist 30: 77–81.
4. Lewin RF, Dorros G, King JF, Mathiak L (1989) Percutaneous transluminal aortic valvuloplasty: acute outcome and follow-up of 125 patients. J Am Coll Cardiol 14: 1210–1217.
5. Litvack F, Jakubowski AT, Buchbinder NA, Eigler N (1988) Lack of sustained clinical improvement in an elderly population after percutaneous aortic valvuloplasty. Am J Cardiol 62: 270–275.
6. Mc Kay RG, Lock JE, Safian RD, Come PC, Diver DJ, Baim DS, Berman AD, Warren SE, Mandell VE, Royal HD, Grossman W (1987) Balloon dilatation of mitral stenosis in adults: post-mortem and percutaneous mitral valvuloplasty studies. J Amer Coll Cardiol 9: 723–731.
7. Rao PS (1989) Balloon pulmonary valvuloplasty: a review. Clin Cardiol 12: 55–74.
8. Roth RB, Palacios IF, Block PC (1989) Percutaneous aortic balloon valvuloplasty: its role in the management of patients with aortic stenosis requiring major noncardiac surgery. J Am Coll Cardiol 13: 1039–1041.
9. Safian RD, Berman AD, Diver DJ, Mc Kay LL, Come PC, Riley MF, Warren SE, Cunningham MJ, Wyman RM, Weinstein JS, Grossman W, Mc Kay RG (1988) Balloon aortic valvuloplasty in 170 consecutive patients. N Engl J Med 319: 1225–1230.
10. Scherer HE, Hörmann E, Engel HJ (1987) Ballondilatation verkalkter Aortenstenosen. Dtsch med Wschr 112: 1694–1697.
11. Schmaltz AA, Bein G, Grävinghoff L, Hagel K, Hentrich F, Hofstetter R, Lindinger A, Kallfelz HC, Kramer HH, Mennicken U, Mocellin R, Pfefferkorn JR, Redel D, Rupprath G, Sandhage K, Singer H, Sebening W, Ulmer H, Vogt J, Wessel A (1989) Balloon valvuloplasty of pulmonary stenosis in infants and children — co-operative study of the German Society of Pediatric Cardiology. Eur Heart J 10: 967–971.
12. Spielberg Ch, Kruck I, Linderer Th, Schröder R (1989) Die Ballon-Valvuloplastie der kalzifizierten Aortenstenose ist keine realistische Alternative zur Operation: klinische und invasive Ergebnisse 17 Monate nach 1. oder evtl. 2. Dilatation. Z Kardiol 78: 86–94.
13. Vogt A, Rupprath G, Tebbe U, Neuhaus KL (1988) Verlaufsbeobachtungen nach Dilatation angeborener und erworbener Aortenstenosen. Dtsch med Wschr 113: 1956–1959.
14. Yoshida K, Yoshikawa I, Akasaka T, Jamaura Y, Shakudo M, Hozumi T, Fukaya T (1989) Assessment of left-to-right atrial shunting after percutaneous mitral valvuloplasty by transesophageal color doppler flow-mapping. Circulation 80: 1521–1526.

PART FOUR

Catheter ablation of tachycardias

26. DC-ablation of the atrioventricular conduction system in patients with supraventricular tachyarrhythmias

G. STEINBECK

Introduction

In general, the occurrence of the various forms of supraventricular tachy-arrhythmias is associated with a benign prognosis. Antiarrhythmic drug therapy, if necessary at all, is and will remain the cornerstone of therapy in these patients. Nevertheless, in a small, selected subgroup of these patients alternative, more aggressive therapy is needed in case antiarrhythmic drug therapy is ineffective, associated with untolerable side effects and the arrhythmia poorly tolerated hemodynamically. For these patients, Gallagher and Scheinman clinically introduced in 1982 the method of ablation of the atrioventricular conduction system by DC energy from defibrillators via percutaneously introduced standard electrode catheters [1, 2].

Method

The method is schematically illustrated in Figure 1. After positioning of the tip of a standard electrode catheter close to the His bundle under fluoro-scopic control (large A and His bundle spike), the distal electrode is connected to the cathode of a standard defibrillator, the anode of the defibrillator being connected with a large paddle in the back of the patient.

With a temporary pacing wire placed in the right ventricle for stimulation in case complete AV block is achieved, and under general anesthesia then a synchronous DC shock of high energy (200–400Ws) is delivered (see original recording in Figure 2. In case a third degree block can be achieved and persists during the following two to four days, a permanent pacemaker has to be implanted.

Indications

If one of the following supraventricular tachyarrhythmias is associated with a rapid ventricular response with anti-arrhythmic drugs either being ineffec-

V. Hombach et al. (eds), Interventional Techniques in Cardiovascular Medicine, 215–220.

HIS BUNDLE ABLATION

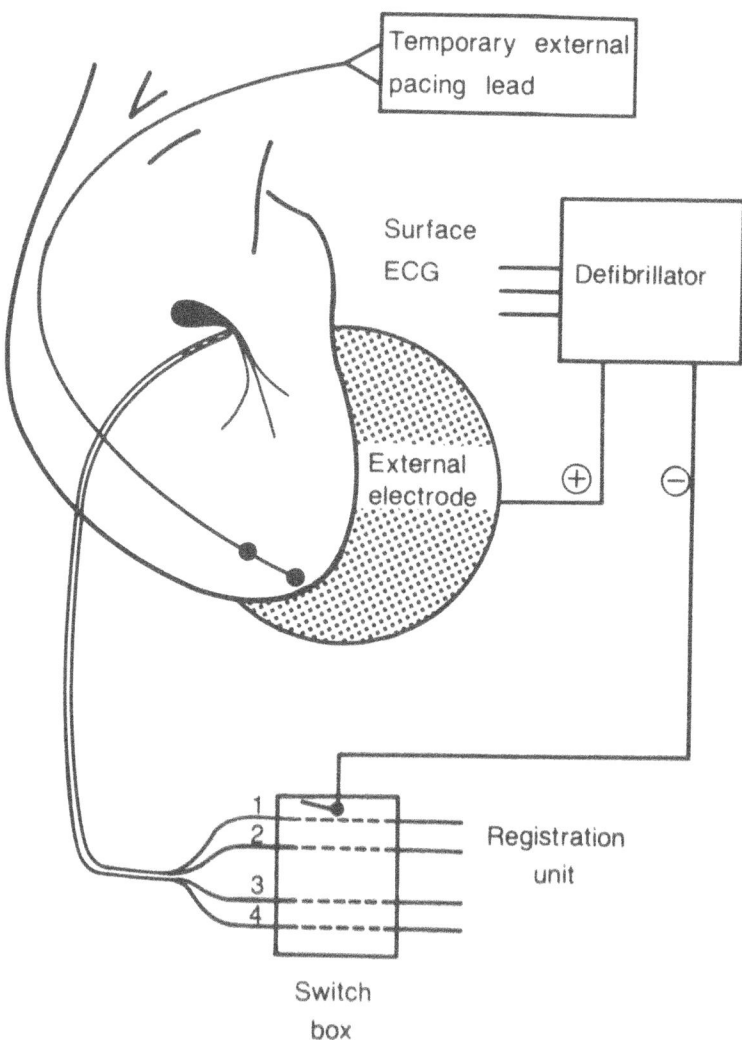

Figure 1.   Scheme of the method of DC ablation of the atrioventricular conduction system (see text). A switch box is used in order to allow quick application of DC energy after correct positioning of the electrode catheter guided by His bundle recordings.

tive or associated with side effects, the following arrhythmias may be treated by DC catheter ablation of the normal artrioventricular conduction system:

– atrial fibrillation;
– atrial flutter;

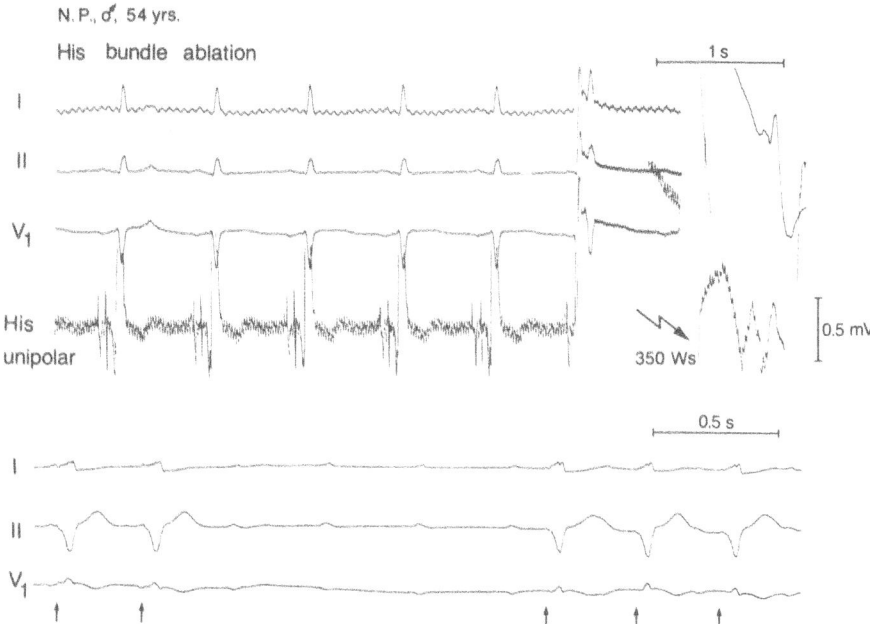

Figure 2.   Original recordings (I, II, V₁ unipolar His bundle recording) in a 54 year-old
patient with a history of recurrent atrioventricular reentry tachycardia.
Upper panel: Sinus rhythm, application of an R-synchronized DC-shock (350Ws).
Lower panel: Ventricular pacing. After temporary termination of pacing, complete AV-block is
apparent.

- atrial tachycardia;
- AV nodal reentry;
- atrioventricular reentry due to WPW-syndrome [3].

Only a few patients with WPW-syndrome appear to be suitable for DC-
ablation of the normal atrioventricular conduction system, mainly in those in
whom reciprocating atrioventricular reentry tachycardia with antegrade conduction via the normal AV conduction system is the only clinically occurring
tachycardia mechanism and in whom the accessory pathway is not able to
conduct in the antegrade direction [4]. Also in a few cases of permanent
junctional tachycardia due to a slowly conducting posteroseptal accessory
pathway in the retrograde direction, DC catheter ablation of the atrioventricular conduction system has been attempted to cure the arrhythmia.

Recently it has been tried to ablate the area of the arrhythmia substrate
itself responsible for the various forms of supraventricular tachyarrhythmias
(such as the accessory pathway, the retrogradely conducting pathway close
or within the AV node in AV nodal reentry, the reentry circuit responsible
for atrial flutter or the focus in atrial tachycardia) instead of ablation of the
normal arterioventricular conduction system, in order to avoid the dis-

advantage of permanent pacemaker implantation in these patients. Experience in this field is limited and is discussed elsewhere in this book.

Results of DC catheter ablation of the atrioventricular conduction system

Both the long term result as well as early and late complications of the method are described in a final report of the Percutaneous Cardiac Mapping and Ablation Registry based on a total of 552 patients [3].

The success rate in these patients is given in Figure 3, complications are listed in Tables 1 and 2. As can be seen therefrom, the arrhythmia is cured in the vast majority of patients, however, at the expense of pacemaker dependence in most of these patients.

The major problems arising from the application of DC catheter ablation include the occurrence of ventricular arrhythmias, the possibility of negative inotropic hemodynamic consequences during the long term, and those associated with pacemaker implantation. Of great concern is the small, but definite number of patients dying suddenly and dying in heart failure after

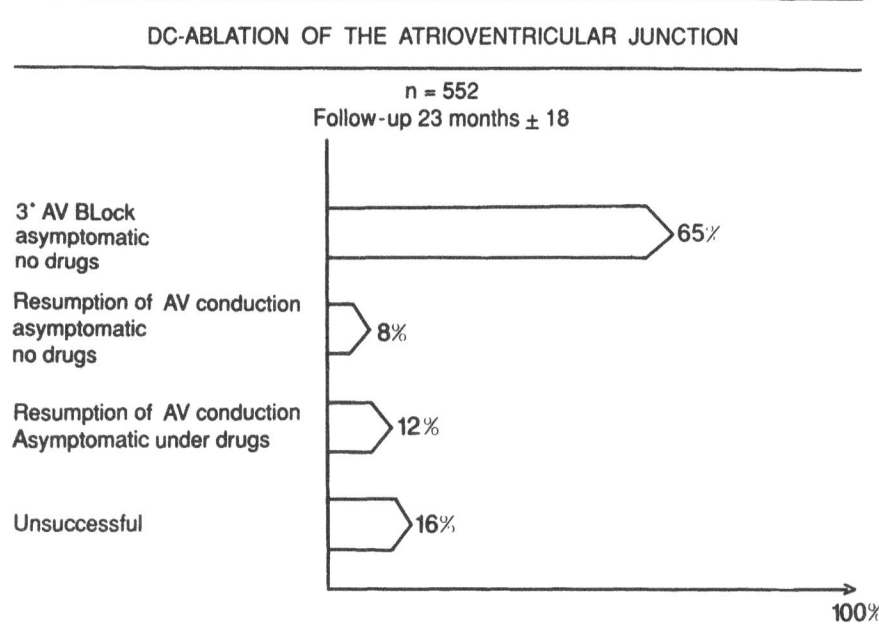

Figure 3.   Clinical long-term results of DC catheter ablation of the atrioventricular conduction system in 552 patients.

Table 1. Early complications

n = 552	
Hypotension	n = 8
Perforation/tamponade	n = 6
Embolization	n = 3
Sepsis	n = 10
Pericarditis	n = 9
Hemothorax	n = 2
NSVT	n = 21
VT/VF	n = 7

PCMAR, 1988.

Table 2. Late complications

n = 552	
Total deaths	n = 46 (8.3%)
procedure-related	n = 2
sudden death	n = 10 (1.8%)
acute myocardial infarction	n = 2
congestive heart failure	n = 10
other cardiac deaths	n = 4
non-cardiac deaths	n = 16
unknown	n = 1
Stroke	n = 2
Pacemaker problems	n = 23

PCMAR, 1988.

application of this method. Very few studies exsist which have investigated the long term hemodynamic consequences of DC catheter ablation. In a recently presented study on 47 patients, functionally evaluated one to six years after DC ablation, 40% reported on the occurrence of exertional dyspnoea; measurement of maximal oxygen uptake showed a distinct reduction as indication of reduced exercise capacity both in patients in whom AV conduction resumed (normal heart rate response to exercise) and in patients with persistent 3° AV block in whom standard VVI or rate adaptive VVI pacemakers had been implanted [5]. Clinical follow up observations of patients undergoing DC catheter ablation of the atrioventricular conduction system and the latter study suggest that hemodynamic impairment might occur.

Future directions

Because of the various disadvantages of DC catheter ablation, several improvements of the method are currently under investigation in various groups. A modification of DC energy delivery has been suggested [6], and other energies such as radiofrequency or laser energy have been studied. While with application of radiofrequency energy, the clinical success rate to obtain control of the arrhythmia by impairing oder interrupting atrioventricular conduction is clearly less in preliminary reports, this mode of energy offers several advantages versus DC energy, since the delivery of energy can be better controlled, there seems to be a close relationship between energy dose and effects on the myocardium, no general anesthesia is needed and hemodynamic impairment appears not to be a problem. It is hoped that with further developments such as temperature-controlled delivery of radiofrequency energy and specially designed electrode catheters the clinical success rate of this method can be substantially improved [7].

Also, the method of transcoronary chemical ablation of the atrioventricular conduction system [8] needs further evaluation.

It is hoped that in the near future DC catheter ablation of the atrioventricular conduction system will be stepwise replaced by more specific interventions aimed to attack the arrhythmia substrate instead of ablation of the normal atrioventricular conduction system in the various forms of drug-refractory supraventricular tachyarrhythmias.

References

1. Gallagher JJ, Svenson RH, Kasell JH, German LD, Bardy GH, Broughton A, Critelli G (1982) Catheter technique for closed-chest ablation of the atrioventricular conduction system. A therapeutic alternative for the treatment of refractory supraventricular tachycardia. *N Engl J Med* 306: 194.
2. Scheinman MM, Morady F, Hess DS, Gonzalez R (1982) Catheter-induced ablation of the atrioventricular function to control refractory supraventricular arrhythmia. *JAMA* 248: 851.
3. PCMAR (1988) The percutaneous cardiac mapping and ablation registry: final summary of results. *Pace* 11: 1621.
4. Steinbeck G, Bach P, Haberl R, Markewitz A (1986) Ventricular pre-excitation following catheter ablation of the His bundle in concealed WPW syndrome. *Eur Heart J* 7: 444.
5. Clementy J, Coste P, Douard H, Bricaud H (1989) Functional evaluation of patients one to six years after transvenous ablation of artrioventricular conduction. *Eur Heart J* 10: 147, abstr.
6. Cunningham D, Rowland E, Rickards AF (1986) A new low energy power source for catheter ablation. *PACE* 9: 1384.
7. Hoffmann E, Dainat C, Mattke S, Dorwarth U, Steinbeck G (1989) Optimized radiofrequency catheter ablation by temperature-controlled bipolar-asymmetrical coagulation. *Eur Heart J* 10: 221, abstr.
8. Brugada P, de Swart H, Bar F, Smeets J, Janssen J, Wellens H (1989) Transcoronary chemical ablation of atrioventricular conduction. *Eur Heart J* 10: 148, abstr.

27. Localization and catheter ablation of accessory atrioventricular pathways

Y. BASHIR and A. J. CAMM

Introduction

Surgical interruption of accessory atrioventricular pathways was first reported more than twenty years ago [1]. Improvements in technique have resulted in a success rate approaching 100% with extremely low mortality in the best centres [2, 3], and surgical ablation is now the standard treatment for drug-refractory tachycardia and for patients who are prone to life-threatening arrhythmias. Transcatheter delivery of high energy electrical discharges was initially used to ablate the atrioventricular junction [4, 5] but was also successfully applied to accessory pathways [6, 9]. The attractiveness of a closed-chest technique as an alternative to major cardiac surgery is self-evident, and over the last five years catheter ablation of accessory pathways has been extensively evaluated and refined. This has been linked with efforts to improve the accuracy of pathway localization during electrophysiological mapping as a necessary prelude to any attempt at ablation. Recent developments in these important areas are reviewed and the current status of catheter ablation in the management of accessory pathway tachycardias is discussed.

Localization of accessory pathways

Before any form of ablative therapy can be considered it is essential to accurately localize the accessory pathway and demonstrate its functional properties and participation in the observed arrhythmia. Identification of multiple accessory pathways (present in approximately 10% of patients with the Wolff-Parkinson-White syndrome) is also important but may not always be possible prior to ablation. When there is manifest pre-excitation on the surface electrocardiogram, it may be possible to localize the accessory pathway by a simple algorithm [10]. Numerous methods have been proposed or are currently being evaluated to try to improve non-invasive localization, including nuclear phase imaging [14], body surface potential mapping [11],

V. Hombach et al. (eds), Interventional Techniques in Cardiovascular Medicine, 221–232.

dynamic CT scanning [12], high-resolution magnetocardiographic mapping [13] and echocardiography during transoesophageal atrial stimulation [15]. Although some of these techniques show great promise, they can only complement and not replace a preliminary electrophysiology study with accurate endocardial mapping, which is needed for positioning of the electrode catheter prior to attempted ablation. Nevertheless, developments in this field might be of value, for example, if it were possible to reliably identify the presence of multiple accessory pathways prior to the intracardiac study [15].

Standard electrophysiological mapping techniques

Various intracardiac electrophysiological methods are available for local- izing the anomolous pathway [16]. The simplest approach is to study the retrograde sequence of atrial activation during orthodromic tachycardia; ideally, the earliest area of retrograde atrial activation is 'bracketed' between later areas of activation. The left atrioventricular ring can be conveniently accessed via the coronary sinus using multipolar catheters but mapping of the right atrioventricular junction is more difficult and requires a special curved rotatable catheter. Precision can be improved by using smaller interelectrode distances and unipolar rather than bipolar recordings [17]. Changes in the ventriculo-atrial interval with bundle branch block aberration may also provide useful localizing information, particularly for differen- tiating antero- and postero-septal pathways [18]. If orthodromic tachycardia cannot be induced the retrograde atrial activation pattern can be studied with resonable accuracy during ventricular pacing [19] although this is less satisfactory because of atrial fusion due to retrograde activation through the atrioventricular node. If the pathway is only capable of antegrade con- duction, atrial pacing at various sites around the artrioventricular ring can be used for localization. Pacing close to the pathway should produce the shortest stimulus-delta interval and the greatest degree of pre-excitation. At the same site it may be possible to record the earliest ventricular potentials relative to onset of the delta wave.

The presence of multiple pathways may be suspected from spontaneous changes in the pattern of pre-excitation during atrial fibrillation, the presence of pre-excited reciprocating tachycardia or the results of differential atrial pacing, but at present the only reliable approach is to repeat the electro- physiological study immediately after successful ablation of the primary pathway.

Direct recording of accessory pathway potentials

Standard electrophysiological techniques for localizing accessory pathways depend on deductive analysis rather than on direct recordings of the con- nections themselves. However, in the last few years it has become possible to record electrograms due to activation of the accessory pathway [20, 21]. These present as high frequency deflections of low amplitude (usually less than 1 mV) between the atrial and ventricular electrograms when recording from the atrioventricular ring in the vicinity of the pathway. These accessory pathway (AP) potentials can be dissociated from local atrial and ventricular activation by programmed stimulation techniques [21, 22]: for example, atrial pacing and premature stimuli resulting in loss of pre-excitation and the AP potential without a change in atrial activation (block at the atrial-AP interface) excludes a late atrial potential. Similarly, dissociation of local ventricular activation could be demonstrated by inducing block at the ventricular-AP interface during ventricular pacing. In some cases it may be necessary to demonstrate resetting of the AP potential by atrial extrastimuli introduced during ventricular pacing or orthodromic tachycardia. If the pathway is close to the atrioventricular junction, His bundle activation also needs to be excluded, either by demonstrating a constant relationship of the AP potential to the onset of the QRS complex during atrial fibrillation with varying degrees of pre-excitation, or by demonstrating non-decremental conduction in response to atrial pacing.

There is some interest in exploiting AP potentials as electrophysiological markers to guide catheter ablation of accessory pathways. Using standard multipolar catheters with a 5 mm interelectrode distance, Warin has been able to record and verify AP potentials in approximately half of his patients prior to catheter ablation [22]. This may be one reason for the outstanding success rate reported by his centre (see below) [23]. In an attempt to improve direct recording of the AP potential, Jackman has developed an orthogonal electrode catheter for mapping in the coronary sinus [24]. This catheter has groups of four electrodes spaced evenly around its circumference and selecting two adjacent electrodes provides a closely spaced recording dipole oriented perpendicular to the axis of the catheter and the atrioventricular groove. Mapping with this orthogonal catheter, they were able to record and verify AP potentials from 42 out of 45 'accessible' left free wall pathways [25]. Using a 2 mm spaced octapolar electrode to simultaneously map the tricuspid annulus, they also obtained AP potentials in 19 out of 23 posteroseptal pathways. Quite apart from this remarkable success rate in recording AP potentials, the technique can also provide important information about the orientation of the pathway and the site of conduction block. For left-sided accessory pathways, conduction block in response to programmed stimulation usually develops at or near the ventricular insertion [26] and this is probably the site at which conduction can be most reliably interrupted by ablation. However, the sequence of AP activation in successive electrode groups suggests that most left freewall pathways follow an oblique course, with up to 30 mm lateral excursion of the ventricular insertion [24, 25]. Thus, if catheter ablation were guided solely by the site of earliest retrograde atrial activation, the chances of success might be significantly reduced. Clearly these excellent preliminary results with the orthogonal catheter need to be confirmed by other groups, but potentially the technique may enable routine identification and mapping of AP activation. Although the orthogonal catheter itself is unsuitable for ablation it could be used to plan the optimum site for delivery of the shock and this might improve overall success rate.

Catheter ablation of accessory pathways

Catheter ablation involves localized destruction of myocardial tissue and is achieved by delivery of high-energy pulses from an external power source to the endocardial surface through a transvenous electrode. Published data is now available on over 150 patients with accessory pathways treated by catheter-based techniques. Most of these ablations have been performed using direct-current electrical shocks but alternative energy sources are being developed to overcome some of the limitations associated with the capacitor discharge technique.

Systems for energy delivery

The standard method of ablation uses high energy, electrical discharges from a conventional defibrillator: shocks are delivered under general anaesthesia via an ordinary electrode catheter to the vicinity of the pathway as predetermined by endocardial mapping. Abolition of accessory pathway conduction typically requires a cumulative energy of 400–800 Joules. The electrical discharge produces a variety of physical effects at the catheter tip including high voltage and current, heat and arcing (fulguration) with the associated high-pressure disturbance or barotrauma [27]. The resultant myocardial lesion is approximately 1 to 2 cm in diameter but may contract with the resolution of local oedema, underlining the need for precise localization [28]. Available evidence suggests that of the physical changes at the catheter tip, voltage is the most important mediator of local tissue damage probably due to dielectric breakdown of cell membranes [29]. Explosive barotrauma is thought to be responsible for many of the adverse effects, in particular rupture of the coronary sinus with cardiac tamponade [27, 30]. In principle, the safety margin of DC ablation could be improved without sacrificing therapeutic efficacy by the development of systems capable of delivering high voltages without arcing, although this presupposes that barotrauma is not required for successful ablation. Cunningham et al. at the National Heart Hospital have introduced a modified capacitor power source which discharges over a shorter period of time than the Lown defibrillator, achieving higher voltages for much less energy delivered in total [31]. This results in reduced gas formation by electrolysis and dis-courages arcing. The arcing threshold can be further elevated by using a specially designed electrode catheter with a more uniform electric field density and anodal configuration [31]. Self-fixation electrodes have also been suggested as a means of lowering the energy required for ablation [32]. Preliminary results with nonfulgurative DC ablation are encouraging, but the validity of this approach remains to be confirmed by ongoing clinical trials.

Apart from the risks of barotrauma, the major limitation of direct-current ablation is lack of control over the size of lesion or 'titratability'. There is now considerable interest in developing safer methods of energy delivery such as radiofrequency current and laser photocoagulation, which are not associated with barotrauma and may allow more controlled endocardial ablation. Radiofrequency ablation depends on delivery of high frequency alternating-current which causes resistive heating and thermal necrosis of tissue around the tip of the catheter [33]. Power density falls off very rapidly around the electrode [34] producing a discrete lesion, the volume of which is a complex function of tip temperature, electrode design and energy dose [34–36]. Unlike DC ablation, radiofrequency energy is delivered over a relatively long period of time and can be controlled by monitoring current, voltage and tip temperature [36]. New systems equipped for continuous feedback control of tip temperature are currently being evaluated and may improve precision and reduce the risk of deleterious effects of thermal injury. Preliminary clinical experience has confirmed that radiofrequency techniques can be used to ablate the atrioventricular junction and accessory pathways [37–41] and this includes a number of patients successfully treated via the coronary sinus [39]. As yet there have been too few cases to make a meaningful comparison with DC ablation as regards efficacy and complication rate, but radiofrequency ablation seems to be a safer, more controllable energy source and has the extra advantage of not requiring general anaesthesia.

Catheter-based laser systems are also being considered as an energy source for transvenous ablation [42]. Intraoperative endocardial resection of arrhythmia substrates including accessory pathways by laser irradiation is well established [43] and transcatheter laser systems have already been extensively developed for use in angioplasty [44]. Although there remain major technical problems particularly as regards a satisfactory catheter-guidance system, preliminary studies on animals suggest that this approach is feasible and may enable much greater precision [45]. Finally, selective intracoronary injection of ethyl alcohol has recently been reported as a non-energy based technique for ablation of ventricular tachycardia and AV nodal conduction [46, 47], but it is unlikely that the blood supply of an accessory pathway could be reliably targeted with an acceptable degree of selectivity.

Methods

Experimental studies on dogs [30] and early clinical reports [48] emphasised the serious risk of rupture and cardiac tamponade if DC shocks are delivered from within the coronary sinus [48]. As a result, most groups have concentrated almost exclusively on posteroseptal pathways mapped close to the ostium of the coronary sinus so that the tip of the ablation catheter can be stabilized in the sinus but the electrodes positioned to deliver the shock close to or even outside the ostium, allowing dissipation of the pressure wave [49–51]. Others including Warin [23, 52] have advocated a direct approach to the atrioventricular ring completely avoiding the coronary sinus in spite of the problems that this causes with catheter stability: these groups have been able to tackle pathways at all sites including left-sided tracts reached via a patent foramen ovale, transseptal puncture or retrograde catheterisation.

Electrical shocks are usually delivered between the endocardial catheter and a large surface electrode. Recently, Kuck et al. have proposed using two electrode catheters in an 'endocardial-epicardial' configuration across the mitral annulus (coronary sinus and left ventricle) to achieve more precise delivery of ablative energy [39]. So far, this technique has only been used in a few patients undergoing radiofrequency ablation, but it may assume greater importance if there is a trend towards accurate mapping of ventricular insertion site prior to attempted ablation of the accessory pathway (see above).

Results of catheter ablation

The results from five recent series all using high energy DC ablation are summarized in Table 1. Overall, complete ablation of the accessory pathway was achieved in approximately 74% of cases. Clinical success (i.e., abolition of symptomatic tachycardia off all drug therapy) was slightly higher at 82% after including patients in whom accessory pathway conduction was only modified but who remained arrythmia-free and were not advised to have surgery on prognostic grounds. Although these figures look encouraging, the overall success rate has been heavily weighted by the exceptional results achieved by Warin et al. in their series of 70 patients (63 pathways ablated and 68 patients symptomatically controlled) [23]. Their relative success is

Table 1. Results of catheter ablation of accessory pathways by direct-current electrical shock in five published series

	Patients (%)	Complete ablation (%)	Clinical success
Ruder et al. [49]	12	4 (33)	7 (58)
Bardy et al. [50]	19	13 (68)	13 (68)
Weber et al. [52]	6	5 (83)	6 (100)
Morady et al. [51]	48	28 (61)	32 (67)
Warin et al. [23]	70	63 (90)	68 (97)
	155	113 (74)	126 (81)

unlikely to have been due to selection bias (in fact they treated a wider range of patients) and presumably reflects differences in technique. Unlike all the other groups, they routinely tried to record the accessory pathway potential and were able to use this to direct ablation in 33 cases (47%). The other distinct feature of their methodology was the direct approach to the atrioventricular ring including transseptal or retrograde catheterisation for left-sided pathways. The only other workers to use this approach were Weber et al. [52] who ablated 5 out of 6 pathways and successfully modified the other. It will be of considerable interest to see if others can match this excellent success rate by adopting a similar protocol.

Complications

Potential complications of transcatheter DC ablation that need to be considered are coronary sinus rupture with cardiac tamponade, injury to coronary arteries, diffuse myocardial damage, permanent atrioventricular block and other arrhythmias [23, 49–52]. The most worrying immediate complication is cardiac tamponade due to coronary sinus rupture which often requires emergency surgical drainage and has resulted in death [48, 54]. Among the first 26 accessory pathway ablations reported to the Percutaneous Catheter Mapping and Ablation Registry (PCMAR) there were 4 cases of pericardial tamponade including one fatality [53] but fortunately, this disturbingly high incidence has only been seen in one of the recent series (Table 2). Bardy et al. reported tamponade in 3 out of 9 cases requiring emergency surgery and there were 5 other patients with asymptomatic pericardial effusions detected echocardiographically possibly due to self limiting tears [50]. Although all ablations were performed at or near the ostium of the coronary sinus, the problem may have been partly related to using catheters of too large a diameter. Using a similar technique, Ruder et al. had no cases of tamponade in their 12 patients [49]. Morady et al. reported only 1 case of tamponade and 3 asymptomatic effusions in a series

Table 2. Incidence of pericardial tamponade and asymptomatic pericardial effusion following DC ablation of accessory pathways

	Patients	Tamponade	Asymptomatic effusion
PCMAR [53]	26	4	ns
Coronary Sinus Technique			
Fisher et al. [48]	8	1	ns
Ruder et al. [49]	12	0	ns
Bardy et al. [50]	19	3	5
Morady et al. [51]	48	1	3
Direct Approach			
Weber et al. [52]	6	0	0
Warin et al. [23]	70	0	0

of 48 patients [51]. They routinely used angiography to define the ostium before finally positioning the ablating catheter: in their first 12 patients they had the two electrodes straddling the ostium and one patient developed tamponade but subsequently they did 36 uncomplicated cases with both electrodes outside the ostium. However, using the same technique, Linker et al. reported a case of fatal coronary sinus rupture in which the sinus was found to be unusually large and ectatic at post-mortem [54]. By contrast, neither Warin [22] nor Weber [52] reported any cases of tamponade or subclinical effusion in a combined total of 76 cases using a direct approach to the aterioventricular ring. Thus, it would appear that this serious complication can be avoided in most cases.

Hartzler has demonstrated that coronary artery spasm can occur following DC ablation [55] and experimental studies have raised the possibility that intimal hyperplasia can develop later near the site of the shock [56]. Bardy recommends routine coronary angiography and exclusion of any patients with major vessels close to the accessory pathway but even so there was one patient in his series of 19 who developed a small posterior infarct probably due to spasm of a branch of the right coronary artery [50]. None of the series reported any abnormality on follow up coronary angiography [23, 51] but only a minority of patients were studied and in any case it may be too soon to rule out any long-term deleterious effects on the coronary vasculature. Diffuse myocardial injury does not seem to have been a major problem although as expected, all groups reported a modest rise in the creatinine kinase MB fraction [23, 49–52].

Transient atrioventricular block occurs almost invariably but permanent damage requiring an antibradycardia pacemaker was rare and only developed in 1 of 48 patients in Morady's series [51] and 2 of 70 patients in Warin's [23]. Only Warin reported ventricular fibrillation at the time of ablation (in spite of using synchronized shocks) in 4 cases. Benign ventricular arrhythmias not requiring treatment were found in some patients by ambulatory monitoring but resolved within 72 hours and to date there have been no reports of clinically significant delayed ventricular arrythmias [23, 49–51]. However, late sudden death has occurred after catheter ablation of the atrioventricular junction, and must be regarded as a cause for concern until longer follow up data is available. Bardy and Morady both reported cases of ectopic atrial tachycardia developing after ablation, but in all three patients this resolved and there were no recurrences after the first few months [50, 51]. Another question is whether a failed ablation attempt increases the difficulty of subsequent surgery. Although Ruder et al. commented on abnormal local atrial electrograms and difficulty with intraoperative mapping, surgery was successful in all 5 patients following failed ablation [49] and this problem was not encountered by others [50, 51].

In summary, DC catheter ablation of accessory pathways seems to be associated with an acceptable immediate and medium-term safety record. There were no deaths amongst the 155 patients in these five series although one fatality was reported to the PCMAR [53] and there have been other isolated case reports [54]. It seems likely that the most serious complication of cardiac tamponade could be largely eliminated by avoiding catheterisation of the coronary sinus or at least positioning the electrodes outside the ostium and the risks of the procedure may be further decreased by the introduction of safer energy sources. Recently two groups have published preliminary reports on radiofrequency ablation in small series of patients. Borggrefe et al. attempted radiofrequency ablation on 14 patients with right-sided or posteroseptal bypass tracts [41]: conduction was abolished in 6 cases and modified in another and all 7 patients (50%) remained free of tachycardia off antiarrhythmic therapy. No acute complications were mentioned. Kuck et al. used a bipolar configuration of electrodes in the coronary sinus and left ventricle to apply radiofrequency energy across the mitral annulus in 8 patients with left-sided bypass tracts but conduction was only abolished in two cases and prolonged in two others [39]. Nevertheless, their data suggests that it may be feasible and safe to use radiofrequency energy from within the coronary sinus. It is to be expected that the success rate of this technique will improve as experience accumulates and further results are awaited with interest.

Catheter ablation or surgery for accessory pathway tachycardia?

Catheter-based techniques for accessory pathway ablation offer the potential for curative therapy without the need for major cardiac surgery. If an attempt is unsuccessful, it can be repeated and the option of surgical treatment is still available for persistent failures. On the other hand the procedure is often lengthy and uncomfortable for the patient. Since surgery in good centres is now extremely reliable and safe [2, 3], should catheter ablation be recommended as an alternative first-choice treatment for patients with drug-refractory of life-threatening accessory pathway tachycardia? Available data indicates a satisfactory short and intermediate term safety record and this may improve with the introduction of safer power sources. The other key issue is success rate but here the literature reveals a striking dichotomy. The centres from the United States using the coronary sinus technique have all reported a success rate of around 65% and have only treated the subset of patients with posteroseptal pathways [49–51]. Based on this experience, catheter ablation could only be recommended for the minority of patients with posteroseptal pathways who are prepared to accept a 30–40% risk or failure rather than opting for surgical treatment directly. By contrast, Warin and others have achieved an overall success rate for all locations of approaching 100% using the direct approach [22, 52]. If these sort of results could be achieved consistently, it would be hard to ever justify open heart surgery as first line treatment.

Until a more general picture emerges it will be necessary for each centre to adopt an individualised policy on catheter ablation depending on their own performance with the technique. Certainly it should only be practised by cardiologists with a specific interest in interventional electrophysiology and with routine surgical standy. For the moment, catheter ablation should probably be confined to patients with a definite indication although in the future it may be considered in some symptomatically controlled patients as an alternative to lifelong antiarrhythmic therapy. Management of failed surgical ablation may represent another potential use of the technique.

References

1. Cobb FR, Blumenschein SD, Sealy WC et al. (1968) Successful surgical interruption of the bundle of Kent in a patient with Wolff-Parkinson-White syndrome. *Circulation* 36: 644–662.
2. Cox JL, Cain ME (1986) Surgery for pre-excitation syndromes, in: Benditt DG, Benson DW (eds), *Cardiac Pre-Excitation Syndromes*, pp. 527–534 Boston: Martinus Nijhoff Publishing.
3. Guiraudon GM, Klein GJ, Sharma AD et al. (1988) Surgery for Wolff-Parkinson-White syndrome using the epicardial approach. *JACC* 11: 110A.
4. Scheinman MM, Morady F, Hess DS, Gonzales R (1982) Catheter-induced ablation of the atrioventricular junction to control refractory supraventricular arrhythmias. *JAMA* 248: 851–855.
5. Gallagher JJ, Svenson RH, Kasell J et al. (1982) Catheter technique for closed chest ablation of the atrioventricular conduction system. *N Eng J Med* 306: 194–200.
6. Weber H, Schmitz L (1983) Catheter technique for closed-chest ablation of an accessory pathway. *N Eng J Med* 308: 653–654.
7. Morady F, Scheinman MM (1984) Transvenous catheter ablation of a postero-septal accessory pathway in a patient with the Wolff-Parkinson-White syndrome. *N Eng J Med* 310: 705–770.
8. Bardy GH, Poole JE, Coltorti F et al. (1984) Catheter ablation of a concealed accessory pathway. *Am J Cardiol* 54: 1366–1368.
9. Nathan AW, Davies DW, Creamer JE et al. (1984) Successful catheter ablation of abnormal atrioventricular pathways in man (abstr.) *Circulation* 70 (suppl II): 11–99.
10. Milstein S, Sharma AD, Guiraudon GM, Klein GJ (1987) An algorithm for the electro-cardiographic localization of accessory pathways in the Wolff-Parkinson-White syndrome. *Pace* 10: 555–563.
11. Liebman J, Olskansky B, Cohen M et al. (1988) Correlation of body surface potential mapping with electrophysiological study and surgical mapping (abstr.) *Circulation* 78.
12. Abbott JA, Bokrinick EH, Scheinman ED (1988) Noninvasive localization of accessory pathways (abstr.) *Circulation* 78: suppl. II, 978.
13. Makijarvi M, Nenone J, Toivonen L et al. (1989) Localization of accessory pathways in Wolff-Parkinson-White syndrome by high-resolution magnetocardiographic mapping (abstr.) *Pace* 12: 1155.
14. Johnson IL et al. (1986) Phase analysis of gated blood pool scintigraphy images to localize bypass tracts in Wolff-Parkinson-White syndrome. *J Am Coll Cardiol* 8: 67–75.
15. Blomstrom P, Caidahl K, Wallentin I, Blomstrom-Lundqvist C (1989) Echocardiography during transoesophageal atrial stimulation — a new method for localizing single and multiple bypass tracts (abstr.) *Pace* 12: 1155.
16. Gallagher JJ (1978) Accessory pathway tachycardia: techniques of electrophysiological study and mechanisms. *Circulation* 75; Suppl. III–31–36.

17. Blomstrom P, Edvardsson N, Blomstrom-Lundqvist C, Olsson SB (1987) Precision of preoperative electrophysiological study in predicting the intraoperatively defined location of single left-sided accessory pathways. *Eur Heart J* 8: 510–520.
18. Kerr CR, Gallagher JJ, German LD (1982) Changes in ventriculoatrial interval with bundle branch block aberration during reciprocating tachycardia in patients with accessory atrioventricular pathways. *Circulation* 66: 196–204.
19. Crossen KJ, Lindsay BD, Cain ME (1987) Reliability of retrograde atrial activation patterns during ventricular pacing for localizing accessory pathways. *JACC* 9: 1279–1287.
20. Jackman WM, Friday KJ, Scherlag BJ et al. (1983) Direct endocardial recording from an accessory atrioventricular pathway: localization of the site of block, effect of antiarrhythmic drugs and attempt at non-surgical ablation. *Circulation* 68: 906–916.
21. Winters SL, Gomes A (1986) Intracardiac electrode catheter recordings of atrioventricular bypass tracts in Wolff-Parkinson-White syndrome: techniques, electrophysiologic characteristics and demonstration of concealed and decremental propagation. *JACC* 7: 1392–1403.
22. Warin JF, Haissaguerre M, Lemetayer P et al. (1988) Catheter ablation of accessory pathways with a direct approach. *Circulation* 78: 800–815.
23. Warin JF, Haissaguerre M, (1989) Fulguration of accessory pathways in any location: report of seventy cases. *Pace* 12: 215–218.
24. Jackman WM, Friday KJ, Yeung-Lai-Wah JA et al. (1988) New catheter technique for recording left free-wall accessory atrioventricular pathway activation. *Circulation* 78: 598–610.
25. Jackman WM, Friday KJ, Fitzgerald DM et al. (1989) Localization of left free-wall and posteroseptal accessory atrioventricular pathways by direct recording of accessory pathway activation. *Pace* 12: 204–214.
26. Kuck KH, Kunze KP (1987) Site of conduction block in accessory pathways — explanation for absence of right-sided concealed accessory pathways? (abstr.) *Circulation* 76: (suppl IV)–IV–176.
27. Bardy GH, Coltorti F, Ivey TD et al. (1986) Some factors affecting bubble formation with catheter-mediated defibrillator pulses. *Circulation* 73: 525–538.
28. Lerman BB, Weiss JL, Bulkley BH, Becker LC, Weisfeld MC (1984) Myocardial injury and induction of arrhythmias by direct shock delivered via endocardial catheter in dogs. *Circulation* 69: 1006–12.
29. Ahsan AJ, Cunningham AD, Rowland ER et al. (1988) Characteristics of energy delivery during catheter discharges in man: the primary role of voltage in successful ablation (abstr.) *Br Heart J* 59: 627.
30. Coltorti F, Bardy GH, Reichenbach D et al. (1985) Catheter mediated electrical ablation of the posterior ventricular septum via the coronary sinus: electrophysiological and histological observations in dogs. *Circulation* 72: 612–622.
31. Ahsan AJ, Cunningham D, Rowland E, Rickards AF (1989) Catheter ablation without fulguration: design and performance of a new system. *Pace* 12: 131–133.
32. Holt P, Boyd EGCA, Crick J, Sowton E (1985) Low energies and Helifix electrodes in the successful ablation of atrioventricular conduction. *Pacing Clin Electrophysiol* 8: 639–645.
33. Marcus I (1987) The use of radiofrequency energy for intracardiac ablation: historical perspectives and results of experiments in animals, in: Breithardt D, Borggrefe M, Zipes DP (eds), *Nonpharmacological Therapy of Tachyarrhythmias*, pp. 213–219. Mount Kisco: Futura Publishing Company.
34. Franklin JA, Langberg JJ, Oeff M et al. (1989) Catheter ablation of canine myocardium with radiofrequency energy. *Pace* 12: 170–176.
35. Blouin LT, Marcus FI (1989) The effect of electrode design on the efficiency of delivery of radiofrequency energy to cardiac tissue in vitro. *Pace* 12: 136–143.
36. Haverkamp W, Hindricks G, Gulker H et al. (1989) Coagulation of ventricular myocardium using radiofrequency alternating current: biophysical aspects and experimental findings. *Pace* 12: 187–195.

37. Kuck KH, Kunze KP, Geiger M, Schluter M (1988) Modulation of AV nodal conduction in man by radiofrequency (abstr.) *Pace* 11: 909.
38. Borggrefe M, Budde T, Podczeck A, Breithardt G (1987) High frequency alternating current ablation of an accessory pathway in humans. *J Am Coll Cardiol* 10: 576–582.
39. Kuck KH, Kunze KP, Geiger M, Schluter M (1989) Attempted ablation of left-sided accessory pathways by radiofrequency current (abstr.) *J Am Coll Cardiol* 13: 168A.
40. Naccarelli GV, Rinkenberger RL, Dougherty AH et al. (1989) Successful radiofrequency catheter ablation of right anteroseptal accessory atrioventricular connection (abstr.) *J Am Coll Cardiol* 13: 176A.
41. Borggrefe M, Martinez-Rubio A, Budde T et al. (1989) Radiofrequency ablation of accessory pathways (abstr.) *Pace* 12: 644.
42. Saksena S (1989) Catheter ablation of tachycardias with laser energy: issues and answers. *Pace* 12: 196–203.
43. Saksena S, Hussain SM, Gielikinski I et al. Intraoperative mapping-guided argon laser ablation of supraventricular tachycardia in Wolff-Parkinson-White syndrome. *Am J Cardiol* 60: 196.
44. Sanborn TA, Faxon DP, Kellett MA et al. (1987) Percutaneous coronary laser thermal angioplasty with a metallic capped fiber (abstr.) *J Am Coll Cardiol* 9: 104A.
45. Curtis AB, Abela GS, Griffin JC et al. (1989) Transvascular argon laser ablation of atrioventricular conduction in dogs: feasability and morphological results. *Pace* 12: 347–357.
46. Brugada P, de Swart H, Smeets JLRM, Wellens HJJ (1989) Transcoronary chemical ablation of ventricular tachycardia. *Circulation* 79: 475–82.
47. Brugada P, de Swart H, Bar F et al. (1989) Transcoronary chemical ablation of atrioventricular conduction. *Eur Heart J* 10: 148 (abstr-suppl).
48. Fisher JD, Brodman R, Kim SG et al. (1984) Attempted nonsurgical electrical ablation of accessory pathways via the coronary sinus in the Wolff-Parkinson-White syndrome. *J Am Coll Cardiol* 4: 684–694.
49. Ruder MA, Mead RH, Gaudiani V et al. (1988) Transvenous catheter ablation of extranodal accessory pathways. *J Am Coll Cardiol* 11: 1245–1253.
50. Bardy GH, Ivey TD, Coltorti F et al. (1988) Developments, complications and limitations of catheter-mediated electrical ablation of posterior accessory atrioventricular pathways. *Am J Cardiol* 61: 309–316.
51. Morady F, Scheinman MM, Kou WH et al. (1988) Long-term results of catheter ablation of a posteroseptal accessory atrioventricular connection in 48 patients. *Circulation* 79: 1160–1170.
52. Weber H, Schmitz L (1989) Catheter technique for ablation of accessory atrioventricular pathway: long-term results. *Br Heart J* 10: 388–399.
53. Percutaneous catheter mapping and ablation registry. Final summary of results. (1988) *Pace* 11: 1621–1626.
54. Linker NJ, Ward DE, Davies MJ, Camm AJ (1989) Fatal coronary sinus rupture following attempted catheter ablation of an accessory pathway. *J Electrophysiol* 3: 2–6.
55. Hartzler GO, Giorgi LV, Diehl AM, Hamaker WR (1985) Right coronary artery spasm complicating electrode catheter ablation of a right lateral accessory pathway. *J Am Coll Cardiol* 6: 250–253.
56. Brodman R, Fisher JD (1983) Evaluation of a catheter technique for ablation of accessory pathways near the coronary sinus using a canine model. *Circulation* 67: 923–929.

28. Radiofrequency ablation of supraventricular and atrioventricular tachyarrhythmias

M. BORGGREFE, G. HINDRICKS, W. HAVERKAMP,
A. MARTINEZ-RUBIO, U. KARBENN, Th. BUDDE and
G. BREITHARDT

Introduction

Most symptomatic supraventricular and atrioventricular tachyarrhythmias can be treated with antiarrhythmic drugs. Especially with the use of newer antiarrhythmic agents such as flecainide, propafenone and amiodarone a significant number of patients can be effectively treated. However, some patients can not be controlled by antiarrhythmic drug therapy or do not accept life-long therapy. Over the past ten years, electrode catheters mostly used for diagnostic tools have been introduced for therapeutic purposes.

The technique for which most experience is available is catheter ablation of the atrioventricular junction. Almost 10 years ago the first clinical application of catheter ablation was to create complete heart block in patients with supraventricular tachycardia using high energy defibrillator impulses [18]. This technique has now been used with considerable success in more than 500 patients [14]. More recently, transcatheter application of radiofrequency alternating currents as an alternative energy source for catheter ablation has been introduced [2–4, 6, 8, 10, 13, 19, 20, 22, 23, 25, 26, 29, 30, 31, 38, 41]. The purpose of this chapter is to provide a brief perspective on the current role of radiofrequency catheter ablation techniques in the treatment of supraventricular and atrioventricular tachyarrhythmias.

Historical aspects

The use of alternating current for cutting and coagulation in surgical medicine has been practised for many years. The first use of RF-current to cut living tissue was published by Cark in 1911 [11]. Following these observations, RF-current for surgery came into clinical practice after the pioneering work of H. Cushing and W. T. Bovie [12]. In contrast to surgical knives, electrical cutting devices simultaneously provide precise cutting and coagulation effects depending on the parameters used. This means that RF-current is not only able to exactly separate two parts of tissue but, at the

233

V. Hombach et al. (eds), Interventional Techniques in Cardiovascular Medicine, 233–244.

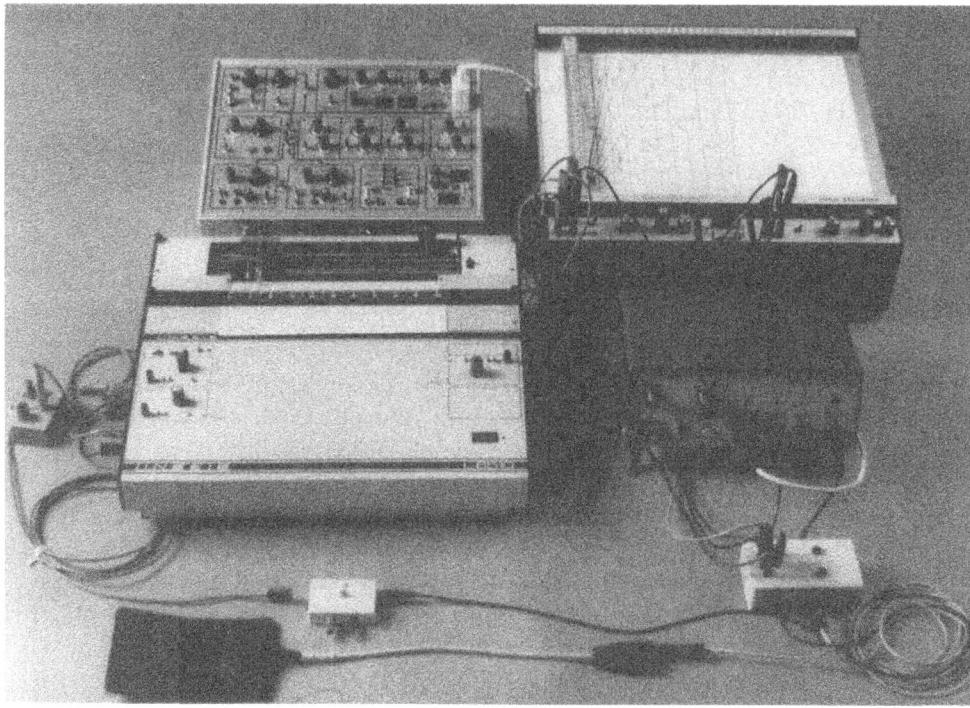

Figure 1.   Technical equipment for transcatheter radiofrequency ablation; the radiofrequency generator (HAT 100, Dr. Osypka, Grenzach Whylen, Germany, F.R.) is connected to a digital timer (1) for precise preselection of pulse duration. A X/T (2) and a X/Y recorder are connected to the device registrations of current, voltage and catheter tip temperature and display of delivered power and impedance, respectively.

same time, is able to stop profuse tissue bleeding at the site of cutting. For these reasons, the method has been applied first in general surgery to cut muscular or connective tissue, resect vascular tissue and tumors or stop bleeding in parenchymatous organs. Indications have then been extended to other fields of medicine. Nowadays, electrical cutting by the use of radio-frequency is a routine method in gynecology, neurology, dental surgery or other fields. Recently, with technical improvements the method has also been used for endoscopic interventions, e.g., the resection of small tumors or to stop bleeding from ulcers in gastroenterology. The latest approach has been to use the principle of radiofrequency alternating current application to improve catheter ablation techniques (Figure 1).

Biophysical aspects

The biophysical and technical aspects of radiofrequency alternating current application for catheter ablation are discussed in detail elsewhere in this book (see Breithardt et al., p. 279). In brief, high frequency- or radiofrequency (RF) alternating currents are defined as an electrical current of changing polarities in frequencies ranging between 30 kHz–300 MHz (DIN 40 015). Several types of radiofrequency currents with disparate properties can be generated: the so-called modulated RF-current that is preferentially used for surgical cutting and the unmodulated RF-current that can be applied for the coagulation of biological tissue [43]. Since transcatheter radiofrequency application should result in the formation of coagulation necrosis unmodulated RF-current is used for ablation of cardiac tissue.

In general, the mechanism of action of RF-currents can be attributed to three effects: (1) electrolytic effects, (2) faradic effects; and (3) conversion of electrical energy into heat.

When radiofrequency alternating current flows through tissue, ions in solution are accelerated and resistive heating occurs [43]. A precondition for the flow of any electrical current is the existence of a closed electrical circuit which, in case of radiofrequency current application for cardiac ablation, consists of the radiofrequency generator, the connecting leads, the so-called 'active' and 'passive' electrode (in case of mono- or unipolar current delivery) or two 'active' electrodes (in case of bipolar coagulation) and, the tissue to be coagulated in between the electrodes. In such a circuit, heating occurs where current density is high and electrical conductivity is relatively low [43]. Both factors are achieved at the contact point of the 'active' electrode(s) and the tissue surface. Maximal heat develops at the tissue electrode interface and decreases as a function of current density. The extent of tissue injury depends on multiple variables that govern the effects of radiofrequency energy at the point of transition between 'active' electrode(s) and tissue surface. Some variables cannot be considered as static components. They dynamically influence each other during each specific coagulation procedure [15].

Radiofrequency ablation of the sinus node

Ablation or modification of the sinus node pacemaker activity has so far only been investigated in experimental animals. Recently, Chorra and coworkers reported an attempt of radiofrequency ablation of the sinus node in 8 dogs [10]. Radiofrequency currents (600 kHz, 5–10 Watt) were applied for up to 60 seconds to the sinus node area. In 6 out of 8 animals the sinus rhythm was abolished after application of 8–21 radiofrequency impulses. These findings show that the sinus node can be effectively destroyed by radiofrequency currents. Catheter ablation of the sinus node may be of clinical value and superior to ablation the AV conduction system in the setting of drug refractory sinus node tachycardia. However, further experimental investigations are necessary to outline the efficacy and risk profile as well as the long-term stability of electrophysiologic effects following radiofrequency ablation of the sinus node.

Radiofrequency ablation of atrial tissue

Several experimental studies investigated the feasibility of radiofrequency alternating current for ablation of atrial tissue [40]. Since atrial tissue is usually very thin, the risk of perforation has to be considered. Published data and own observations (unpublished data) indicate, that atrial lesions induced by RF-energy are often transmural. However, the risk of perforation seems to be relatively low [40]. The only available clinical observation has been reported by our group [5]. However, in 2 patients undergoing RF-ablation none could be successfully managed [5]. Further studies are needed to investigate the usefulness of RF application in ablating ectopic atrial tachycardia foci.

Ablation of the AV-junction

Ablation of the AV-junction has been performed in experimental studies as well as in a growing number of patients. The first series of animal experiments was performed by Huang et al. who reported a more than 80% success rate in producing complete heart block [29]. Subsequent animal investigations supported the initial findings of Huang et al., showing that the procedure is effective and not associated with severe complications [41].

After these encouraging experimental results, several groups have used RF-energy for transcatheter ablation of the AV-junction in the setting of

Table 1.   Clinical results of attempted radiofrequency ablation for drug-refractory supraventricular and atrioventricular tachyarrhythmias

	No of pts.	Success	Failure
1. Ablation of AV-junction			
Langberg [38]	10	5	5
Lavergne [39]	12	9	3
Budde [9]	13	6	7
Huang [28]	6	5	1
Saksena [44]	1	1	–
Goy [19]	3	1	2
2. Modification of AV-junction for the treatment of AV-nodal reentrant tachycardia			
Kunze [36]	6	6	–
3. Ablation of ectopic atrial tachycardia			
Borggrefe [5]	2	0	2
4. Ablation of right*- and left**-sided accessory pathways			
Goy* [19]	3	1	2
Borggrefe* [3]	14	7	7
Naccarelli* [42]	1	1	–
Kuck** [34]	8	4	4

drug-refractory supraventricular tachyarrhythmias (see Table 1) [8, 19, 28, 28, 39, 44]. The first clinical application on ablation of the AV-junction has been performed by our group [7]. In our experience, long-term complete AV-block or sufficient modification of the AV-conduction by RF-current application can be achieved in about 50%–70% of patients. In our patients acute success rate of ablation or modification of the AV-junction was 69%. In patients, who developed complete AV block, accelerated junctional rhythms always proceeded complete heart block. During long-term follow up AV-conduction resumed in 3 patients, reducing the success rate to 46% [8]. One patient, however, in whom modification of the AV-junction was acutely achieved, developed III° AV block during a follow-up period of 3 months following the ablation session [9]. Thus, due to the observed long-

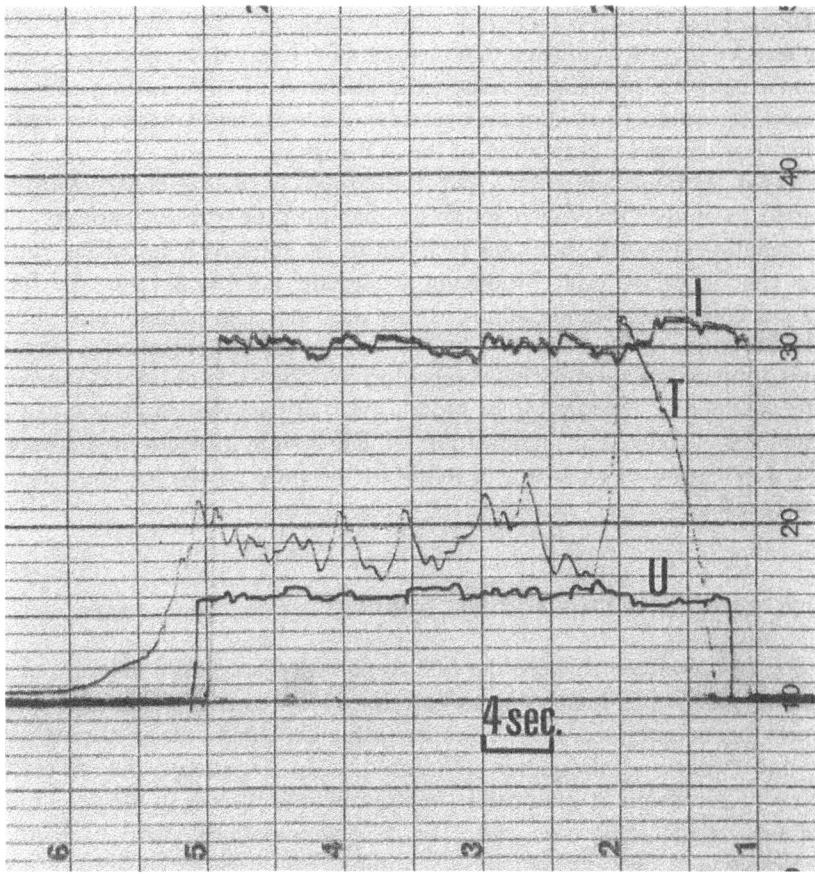

Figure 2. Registration of current (U), voltage (I) and catheter tip temperature (T) during ablation of the AV -conduction system. With the onset of energy delivery catheter tip temperature sharply increased indicating a good electrode–tissue contact. After approximately 4 seconds, temperature suddenly decreased due to dislocation of the electrode catheter. Note that the time course of current and voltage did not indicate catheter dislocation.

term changes of AV-conduction after RF-ablation, pacemaker implantation is recommended, even for patients in whom only modification of AV-conduction properties (e.g., AV-block I°) is acutely induced.

The most critical factor, that governs the success of the procedure, is the contact of the ablation catheter to the tissue surface (see Figure 2). The ability to achieve an adequate wall contact of the coagulation electrode depends in part on individual anatomical features. In our experience, if we were not able to affect the AV-conduction with a total of 10 discharges using different catheters and power settings, application of additional discharges was also ineffective. Although large His-bundle potentials (> 500 microvolts) were obtained, we were not able to affect the AV-conduction in some patients. As the purpose of RF-ablation to ablate the AV node, we were applying the energy at the proximal position of the AV conduction system as evidenced by a long AH interval and a large A : H ratio. Data from Langberg et al. also indicate that a long HV interval suggesting a more proximal catheter position increases the likehood of AV-junction ablation success [38]. Table 1 provides an overview of the currently available clinical results of attempted RF-ablation of the AV-region.

It is of particular interest, that the group of Kunze and coworkers intended to modify the AV-junction conduction properties in patients with symptomatic AV-nodal reentrant tachycardia by selectively impairing retrograde conduction without producing antegrade AV-block [36]. We have observed comparable modulations in our patients. The feasibility of modifying AV-conduction properties by application of RF-currents in experimental animals has recently been reported by Marcus et al. [41]. However, whether complete interruption or modification of the AV-conduction can be reproducibly achieved by application of RF-current remains to be established. Furthermore, long-term stability of the induced changes remains to be observed.

Radiofrequency ablation of accessory pathways

In 1987, Borggrefe et al. were the first to publish a successful ablation of an accessory pathway in man using radiofrequency energy [2]. This experience has now being extended to 14 patients with right-sided accessory pathways who underwent radiofrequency-ablation [3]. In 9 patients the accessory pathway was located at the postero-septal region, whereas in the remaining 5 patients at the right free wall. The accessory pathway was successfully interrupted in 6 patients and modification of the accessory pathway conduction, resulting in a significant increase of accessory pathway refractory period was achieved in another patient. Thus, 50% of the patients could be successfully managed using RF-energy. Naccarelli et al. [41] also reported a successful ablation of a right sided anteroseptal accessory pathway.

RF-ablation via the coronary sinus has stimulated a lot of research in experimental animals. The feasibility of two different electrode configurations for radiofrequency ablation of left-sided accessory pathway has been investigated: Langberg et al. [37] and Huang and coworkers [39] showed the feasibility of unipolar energy application between the coronary sinus catheter ('active' electrode) and a large chest-wall electrode ('passive' electrode). Recently, Jackman and Kuck [32] introduced a bipolar 'epi-endocardial' catheter electrode configuration. One catheter is placed within the coronary sinus and a second catheter beneath the mitral valve, high against the annulus, and directly opposite the coronary sinus electrode. One advantage of bipolar 'epi-endocardial' coagulation compared to unipolar electrode configuration seems that the current field is focussed through the mitral annulus encompassing the usual course of left free wall accessory atrioventricular pathways (Figure 3) [16]. Our own experimental series using this approach confirmed the initial findings of Jackman and Kuck (Figure 4)

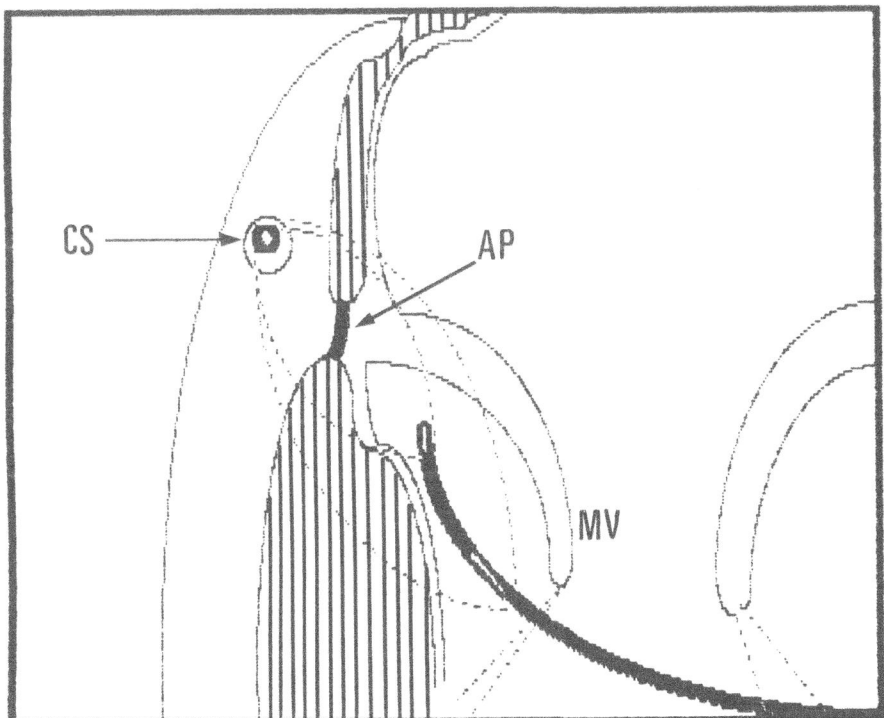

Figure 3   Schematic plot of catheter positioning of radiofrequency ablation of left sided accessory pathways (AP) using the 'epi-endocardial' electrode configuration as introduced by Kuck and coworkers The energy field is build up between two catheters, one in the coronary sinus (CS), one the underneath mitral valve (MV) in the left ventricle Current field is focussed through the mitral annulus encompassing the usual course of left sided accessory pathways

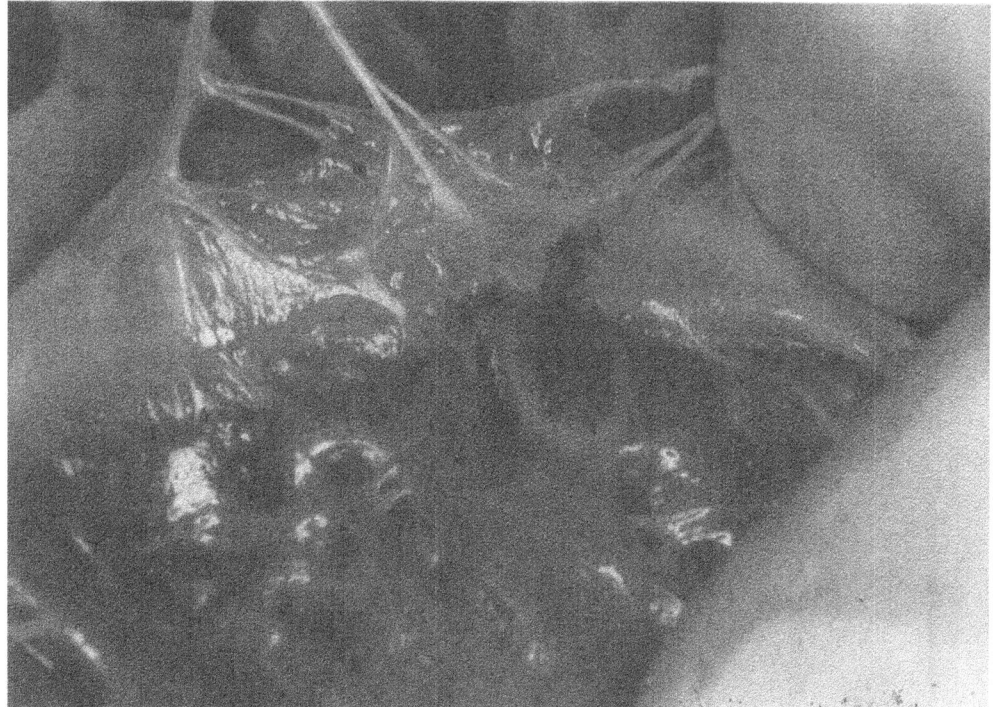

Figure 4.   Macroscopic aspect of ventricular tissue injury high at the mitral annulus induced by radiofrequency energy using 'epi-endocardial' electrode configuration.

[33]. Recent reports also showed the clinical feasibility of the procedure in a very limited number of patients [34, 35]. The clinical usefulness and safety of this approach, however, remains to be established.

Radiofrequency ablation vs. DC ablation for supraventricular tachyarrhythmias

Currently available clinical data reveal that DC-electrical ablation for the treatment of drug refractory supraventricular and atrioventricular tachy-arrhythmias seems to be more effective compared to radiofrequency alter-nating current ablation [7, 14, 45]. Based on investigations made by others and our own experimental and clinical experience with both ablation tech-niques it seems likely to assume that the target tissue has to be more precisely localized and most importantly the contact of the ablation catheter onto the target tissue has to be better for successful radiofrequency ablation [21, 23, 25, 27]. During radiofrequency ablation a close contact of the 'active' catheter electrode is necessary to guarantee flow of energy to the tissue, whereas during DC-shock ablation tissue effects can be induced due to the development of barotrauma even when there is no stable contact to the target tissue. In addition, the fact that during radiofrequency ablation energy is delivered over a longer period of time (5–90 sec compared to approx. 10 ms during DC ablation) further explains the importance of a good electrode–tissue contact to induce tissue necrosis.

One mayor advantage of radiofrequency ablation techniques compared to DC-electrical ablation is that energy delivery is usually not painful for the patient and therefore no general anaesthesia is required during the ablation procedure. However, two patients of our series developed intense chest pain during radiofrequency application and general anaesthesia was necessary in these cases (unpublished data).

DC-catheter ablation is associated with a significant incidence of procedure related complications [14, 17, 24]. This is of major importance especially for ablation of accessory pathway using DC-shocks (i.e., when DC shock delivery inside the coronary sinus [1, 17]). Although the clinical experience with radiofrequency ablation is still limited, it seems that the incidence of procedure related complications is lower compared to DC-techniques. So far we have not seen any significant complication in our patients. This includes the occurrence of arrhythmias, hemodynamic complications, ischemia as well as thrombotic or embolic complications. However, by taking theoretical aspects of RF-current delivery and experimental findings into consideration there is a procedure related potential of severe side effects (see also Breithardt et al., p. 279), and further experience is needed to delineate the risk profile of the technique. To avoid significant complications during radiofrequency ablation measurements of biophysical parameters (current, voltage, impedance, catheter tip temperature) are necessary to improve the controlability of the coagulation process.

Current status and future perspectives

The results of experimental and clinical studies on the use of radiofrequency alternating currents reported so far indicate that the procedure is feasible and relatively safe. Compared to the most widely used DC-fulguration technique, radiofrequency ablation seems to have both potential theoretical and practical advantages particularly with respect to unwanted side effects and procedure-related complications.

Ablation or modification of the AV-junction and right-sided accessory pathways using radiofrequency energy have been successfully performed already in man. There is evidence that with growing experience the application and steerability of transcatheter radiofrequency energy for ablation purposes can be improved and that modification of the conduction system instead of total ablation is possible. This would be of particular importance for catheter modification of the AV conduction system. However, further studies are needed to ascertain the efficacy and safety of this new procedure.

Since the experimental and clinical experience on the use of RF-current for ablation of atrial tachyarrhythmias and left-sided accessory pathways is limited, the procedure has still to be considered experimental.

References

1. Bardy GH, Ivey D, Coltorti F, Stewart RB, Johnson G, Greene HL (1988) Developments, complications and limitations of catheter-mediated electrical ablation of posterior accessory atrioventricular pathways. Am J Cardiol 61: 309–1316.
2. Borggrefe M, Budde T, Podczeck A, Breithardt G (1987) High frequency alternating current ablation of accessory pathway in humans. J Am Coll Cardiol 10: 576–582.
3. Borggrefe M, Karbenn U, Haverkamp W, Hindricks G, Breithardt G (1989) Radio-frequency ablation of accessory pathways. Pace 12: 644.
4. Borggrefe M, Budde Th, Podczeck A, Breithardt G (1987) Hochfrequenzablation der atrioventrikulären Überleitung und akzessorischer Leitungsbahnen — erste klinische Erfahrungen. Z Kardiol 76 (Suppl. 1): 59 (abstr).
5. Borggrefe M, Budde Th, Podczeck A, Breithardt G (1987) Application of transvenous radiofrequency alternating current ablation in humans. Circulation 76 (Suppl. IV: IV–406 (abstr).
6. Budde Th, Borggrefe M, Podczeck A, Jacob B, Langwasser J, Frenzel H, Breithardt G (1987) Radiofrequency ablation: an improvement of ablation techniques in comparison to direct-current delivery? in: Breithardt G, Borggrefe M, Zipes DP (eds), Non Pharmacological Therapy of Tachyarrhythmias pp. 221–241. Mount Kisco: Futura Publishing Company.
7. Budde Th, Breithardt G, Borggrefe M, Podczeck A, Langwasser J (1987) Erste Erfahrungen mit der Hochfrequenzstromablation des AV-Leitungssystems beim Menschen. Z Kardiol 76: 204–211.
8. Budde Th, Borggrefe M, Martinez-Rubio, Karbenn U, Haverkamp W, Hindricks G, Breithardt G (1989) Ergebnisse der Hochfrequenz-Katheterablation des AV-Überleitungssystems beim Menschen. Z Kardiol 78 (Suppl 1): 18 (abstr).
9. Budde Th, Borggrefe M, Martinez-Rubio A, Karbenn U, Breithardt G (1989) Late occurrence of total AV-block after initially only partial destruction of the AV-conduction system with catheter ablation. 4th European Symposium on Cardiac Pacing, Stockholm, May 28th–31st 1989, Abstract-Book: 138.
10. Chorro FJ, Sanchis J, Lopez-Perino V, Musoles S, Burguera M, Gil F, Cerda M (1989) Closed chest ablation of the sinus node in dogs with radiofrequency energy. Europ Heart J 10: 221 (abstr).
11. Clark W (1911) Oscillatory desiccation in the treatment of accessible malignant growth and minor surgical conditions. J Adv Therap 29: 169.
12. Cushing H, Bovie WT (1928) Electro-surgery as and aid to the removal of intracranial tumors. Surg Gynecol Obstet 47: 751.
13. Davis MJE, Murdock CJ, Cope GD, Kallas IJ, Lovett MD (1988) Radiofrequency catheter ablation for refractory arrhythmias. Pace 11: 918. (abstr).
14. Evans GT, Scheinman MM (1988) The percutaneous cardiac mapping and ablation registry: final summary of results. Pace 11: 1621–1626.
15. Farin G (1987) Möglichkeiten und Probleme der Standardisierung der Hochfrequenzleistung, in: Lux G, Senn K, (eds), Hochfrequenzdiathermie in der Endoskopie pp. 34–46. Berlin, Heidelberg, New York: Springer Verlag.

16. Fisher JD, Kim SG, Matos JA, Waspe LE, Brodman R, Merav AM (1985) Complications of catheter ablation of tachyarrhythmias: occurrence, protection, prevention. *Clin Prog Electrophysiol and Pacing* 3: 292–298.
17. Fisher JD, Brodman R, Kim SG, Mercando AD (1987) Nonsurgical ablation of accessory pathways: physical, anatomical, and clinical considerations. *J Electrophysiol* 1: 47–57.
18. Gallagher JJ, Svenson H, Kasell JH, Lerman LD, Bardy GH, Broughton A, Critelli G (1982) Catheter technique for ablation of the atrioventricular conduction system. *N Engl J Med* 306: 194–200.
19. Goy JJ, Kappenberger L (1988) Different techniques for catheter ablation. *Pace* 11: 910 (abstr).
20. Haines DE (1989) Impedance rise during radiofrequency ablation is due to sudden boiling at the catheter tip and is prevented by tip temperature monitoring. *Circulation* 78 (Suppl II): II-156 (abstr).
21. Haverkamp W, Hindricks G, Gülker H, Rissel U, Pfennings W, Borggrefe M, Breithardt G (1989) Coagulation of ventricular myocardium using radiofrequency energy: bio-physical aspects and experimental findings. *Pace* 12: 187–195.
22. Haverkamp W, Hindricks G, Rissel U, Budde T, Pfennings W, Gülker H, Breithardt G (1989) Temperature-guided radiofrequency coagulation of myocardial tissue. *J Am Coll Cardiol* 13: 169A (abstr).
23. Hindricks G, Haverkamp W, Rissel U, Richter KD, Gülker H (1988) Experimental observations on the use of radiofrequency energy for ablation of ventricular tissue. *New trends Arrhyt* IV (1–2): 337–342.
24. Hindricks G, Haverkamp W, Dute U, Richter KD, Gülker H (1988) Inzidenz ventrikulärer Arhythmien nach Gleichstromablation, Hochfrequenzstromablation und Laser-Photo-ablation. *Z Kardiol* 77: 696–703.
25. Hindricks G, Haverkamp W, Gülker H, Rissel U, Budde T, Richter KD, Borggrefe M, Breithardt G (1989) Radiofrequency coagulation of ventricular myocardium: improved prediction of lesions size by monitoring catheter tip temperature. *Europ Heart J* 10: 972–984.
26. Hindricks G, Haverkamp W, Pfennigs W, Rissel U, Gülker H, Breithardt G (1989) Hochfrequenzablation mit automatischer Leistungsanpassung—akute und subakute Gewebeeffekte. *Z Kardiol* 78 (suppl 1): 35 (abstr).
27. Hoyt RH, Huang SK, Markus FI (1987) Factors influencing transcatheter radiofrequency ablation of the myocardium. *J Appl Cardiol* 1: 469–486.
28. Huang SK, Lee MA, Bazgan ID, Chang MS (1988) Radiofrequency catheter ablation of the atrioventricular junction for refractory supraventricular tachyarrhythmias. *Circulation* 78 (suppl II): II-156 (abstr).
29. Huang SK, Bharati S, Graham AR, Lev M, Marcus FI, Odell RC (1987) Closed chest catheter desiccation of the atrioventricular junction using radiofrequency energy—a new method of catheter ablation. *J Am Coll Cardiol* 9: 349–358.
30. Huang SK, Garham AR, Hoyt RH, Odell RC (1987) Transcatheter desiccation of the left ventricle using radiofrequency energy: a pilot study. *Am Heart J* 114: 42–48.
31. Jackman WM, Kuck KH, Naccareli GV, Carmen L, Pitha J (1988) Radiofrequency current directed across the mitral anulus with a bipolar epicardial–endocardial catheter electrode configuration in dogs. *Circulation* 78: 1288–1298.
32. Kottkamp H, Hindricks G, Haverkamp W, Krater L, Rissel U, Borggrefe M, Gülker H, Breithardt G (1989) Significance of electrode configuration and temperature monitoring during transcatheter radiofrequency application for ablation of left-sided accessory pathways. *Europ Heart J* 10: 221 (abstr).
33. Kuck KH, Kunze KP, Geiger M, Schlüter M (1989) Attempted ablation of left-sided accessory pathways by radiofrequency current. *J Am Coll Cardiol* 13: 168A (abstr).
34. Kuck KH, Kunze KP, Schlüter M, Geiger M, Jackman WM, Naccarelli V (1988) Modification of left-sided accessory pathway by radiofrequency current using bipolar epicardial-endocardial electrode configuration. *Europ Heart J* 9: 927–933.

35. Kunze KP, Schlüter M, Kuck KH (1988) Modulation of AV nodal conduction: definitive treatment for AV nodal tachycardia? *Circulation* 78: II–304 (abstr).
36. Langberg J, Griffin JC, Herrer JM, Chin MC, Lev M, Bharati S, Scheinman MM (1989) Catheter ablation of accessory pathways using radiofrequency energy in the canine coronary sinus. *J Am Coll Cardiol* 13: 491–196.
37. Langberg JJ, Chin MC, Herre JM, Griffin, Dullet N, Scheinman MM (1989) Catheter ablation of the atrioventricular junction using radiofrequency energy. *J Am Coll Cardiol* 13: 169A (abstr).
38. Lavergne TL, Sebag CI, Guize LJ, Blanc JJ, le Heuzey JY, Mottè GA, Bèrad TJ, Ourbak PA (1988) Transcatheter radiofrequency modification of atrioventricular conduction for refractory supraventricular tachycardia. *Circulation* 78 (Suppl II): II–305 (abstr).
39. Lavergne T, Prunier L, Cuize L, Bruneval P, van Euw D, le Herzey JY, Peronneau P (1989) Transcatheter radiofrequency ablation of atrial tissue using a suction catheter. *Pace* 12: 177–186.
40. Marcus FI, Blouin LT, Bharati S, Lev M, Wharton K (1988) Production of first degree atrioventricular block in dogs, using closed chest electrode catheter with radiofrequency. *J Electrophysiol* 2: 315–326.
41. Naccarelli GV, Rinkenberger L, Dougherty AH, Fitzgerald DM, Zinner A, Kuck KH, Jackman WM (1989) Successful radiofrequency catheter ablation of right anteroseptal accessory atrioventricular connections. *J Am Coll Cardiol* 13: 176A (abstr.)
42. Reidenbach HD (1983) *Hochfrequenz- und Lasertechnik in der Medizin.* Berlin, Heidelberg, New York: Springer Verlag.
43. Saksena S, Marcantuono D, Janssen M, Osypka P (1988) Pulsed radiofrequency ablation with conventional electrode catheters: experimental studies and early clinical observations. *Pace* 11: 489.
44. Warin JF, Haissaguerre M (1989) Fulguration of accessory pathways in any location: report of seventy cases. *Pace* 12: 215–219.

29. The role of the surgeon in the management of supraventricular arrhythmias

C. J. MURDOCK, G. M. GUIRAUDON, G. J. KLEIN, R. W. YEE, and A. D. SHARMA

Introduction

In order for surgery to provide a reasonable, effective therapeutic alternative to drug therapy in patients with supraventricular arrhythmias, the following criteria must be fulfilled:

1. The mechanism of the arrhythmia responsible for the patients symptoms must be identified.
2. The site of origin of the tachycardia, or the pathway responsible for its maintenance must be located.
3. The area in question must be accessible to surgical ablation.
4. Surgical ablation must be achieved with an acceptable mortality and morbidity.

Indications for surgery in patients with supraventricular tachycardia may include the following from strongest to most weak: patients with out of hospital cardiac arrest; potentially life threatening arrhythmia; drug resistant arrhythmia; tachycardia induced cardiomyopathy; pregnancy; drug intolerance; failure or contraindications to alternative therapies; commitment to life-long drug therapies; lifestyle/occupation limitations (e.g., pilots, athletes, etc.); asymptomatic patients with Wolff-Parkinson-White (WPW) syndrome and a short RR interval during atrial fibrillation.

Surgical ablation of accessory pathways in patients with symptomatic WPW syndrome and modification of atrioventricular (AV) nodal conduction in patients with AV node reentrant tachycardia (AVNRT) is a reasonable therapeutic alternative. Operations can be performed with a high success rate and with minimal morbidity at institutions performing a large volume of arrhythmia surgery. Less commonly, the operative approach may be used in patients with drug refractory and highly symptomatic atrial tachycardia, flutter and fibrillation.

V. Hombach et al. (eds), Interventional Techniques in Cardiovascular Medicine, 245–248.
© 1991 *Kluwer Academic Publishers*.

Wolff-Parkinson-White syndrome

All patients with WPW syndrome are potential surgical candidates. The reentry circuit is large and can be located using electrophysiologic techniques. The accessory pathway is almost invariably accessible to surgical ablation and if the pathway participates in the tachycardia, cure can be achieved.

The first successful surgical approach to the WPW syndrome was by W. C. Sealy et al. in 1968 [1]. Since then Sealy, J. J. Gallagher et al. [2] and J. L. Cox [3] have perfected the technique using an endocardial approach. With cardiac arrest and bypass, an endocardial atrial incision is made in the region of the accessory pathway, and the epicardial fat pad dissected.

The epicardial approach [4–6] is based on pathological observations that most accessory pathways course within the coronary sulcus. This approach combines 2 steps: (1) dissection of structures within the AV sulcus; and (2) cryoablation of the AV junction. After medium sternotomy is performed, an intraoperative electrophysiologic study is performed to confirm the location of the accessory pathway. Seventeen sites are mapped around the AV ring anterogradely during sinus rhythm or atrial pacing and retrogradely during reciprocating tachycardia or ventricular pacing. After identifying the location of the accessory pathway, the coronary sulcus is dissected either using a direct approach or by en bloc mobilization of the epicardial fat pad. Because the operation is carried out on the normothermic beating heart, the exact location of the accessory pathway is identified by loss of preexcitation with the blunt dissection. Once loss of preexcitation is confirmed by further electrophysiologic testing, cryotherapy is performed. Epicardial cryoablation is performed using a 0.5 cm and/or a 1.5 cm diameter cryoprobe, cooled to –60 degrees C, for 2 minutes. Multiple lesions are made in the dissected area. The cryoprobe is applied onto the atrial wall, impinging onto the AV junction, and in contact with the ventricular myocardium. When accessory pathway conduction is present after dissection, the pathway is assumed to be subendocardial in location. A 0.5 cm probe is placed inside the atrium and the AV junction is cryoablated in the region of interest.

This operation has been performed in 316 patients [7], aged 7 months to 74 years (mean 33 years). Associated heart disease was present in 23 patients. All patients had paroxysmal tachycardia, 55 had syncope and 80 had spontaneous atrial fibrillation. There were no perioperative deaths and no long term complications. One patient had a pacemaker inserted for postoperative complete heart block but normal conduction has returned. Intraoperative complications occurred in 9 patients (hemorrhage from an atrial tear in 4 patients, hemorrhage from coronary sinus injury in 3 patients, coagulopathy in 1 patient and noncardiogenic pulmonary edema in 1 patient). Postoperative complications occurred in 8 patients (re-sternotomy for bleeding in 5 patients, low cardiac output state in 1 patient, stroke in 1 patient and chylopericardium in 1 patient). Accessory pathway ablation required a second operation in 7 patients. An undetected second pathway became manifest in 3 patients and was surgically ablated. Overall 336 pathways were ablated and 3 obtunded in 316 patients.

The epicardial approach is thus successful and associated with low morbidity. It has the advantages of continuous monitoring of the ECG to detect potential damage to the AV node in critically located pathways, provides immediate assessment of accessory pathway ablation without delay for rewarming the heart, allows ablation of multiple pathways in sequence and usually avoids the need for cardiopulmonary bypass.

Atrioventricular nodal reentrant tachycardia

Until recently, surgical treatment of AVNRT was limited to the production of complete heart block. Successful AV nodal modification surgery has subsequently been described by Johnson and Ross [8, 9], who reported the results of surgical dissection in the region of the AV node for modifying the substrate for AVNRT, reporting a cure rate of 96%.

Similarly, we developed a technique of skeletinization of the AV node [10]. In this series, a primary success rate of 92% in 32 patients was achieved. Three patients have had recurrence of tachycardia 11, 11 and 7 months after the initial operation. All 3 patients have been arrhythmia-free since their secon operation. No patients have had permanent complete heart block and there have been no complications (mean follow up 17 months). Post-operative electrophysiological correlates of a successful outcome were complete ventriculo-atrial conduction block or a retrograde Wenckebach cycle length of > 400 ms.

Atrial fibrillation, atrial flutter and ectopic atrial tachycardia

Cases of ectopic atrial tachycardia are rare, accounting for < 10% of cases of supraventricular tachycardia. Where this arrhythmia is refractory to drug therapy and highly symptomatic, surgical excision of the atrial focus may be considered. Similarly, on rare occasions classical atrial flutter may be mapped and surgically ablated [11].

Atrial fibrillation unresponsive to drug therapy may be treated by ablation of the AV junction either by catheter or direct surgical techniques. We have designed an operation in which a corridor of atrial tissue is preserved between the sinus and AV nodes and the rest of the atria electrically isolated from this corridor, and hence the AV node [12]. The corridor of tissue cannot fibrillate because of the reduced critical mass and the sinus pacemaker function and AV nodal conduction are preserved. The operation has been performed successfully on 8 patients.

Conclusion

All patients with WPW syndrome or AV node reentrant tachycardia are potential candidates for surgical ablation. Surgery for these conditions is curative in a high percentage of patients and is associated with very low morbidity and mortality. The indication for surgery depends on the risk of life of the arrhythmia, the severity of patients symptoms, the availability of successful alternative therapy with lower mortality and morbidity, the surgical expertise of the referral centre and patients preference.

References

1. Sealy WC, Hattler BG, Blumenschein SD et al.(1969) Surgical treatment of the Wolff-Parkinson-White syndrome. *Ann Thorac Surg* 8: 1–11.
2. Sealy WC, Gallagher JJ, Pritchett ELC (1978) The surgical anatomy of Kent bundles based on electrophysiological mapping and surgical exploration. *J Thorac Cardiovasc Surg* 76: 804–815.
3. Cox JL, Gallagher JJ, Caine ME (1985) Experience with 118 consecutive patients undergoing operation for the Wolff-Parkinson-White syndrome. *J Thorac Cardiovasc Surg* 90: 490–501.
4. Guiraudon GM, Klein GJ, Gulamhusein S et al. (1984) Surgical repair of the Wolff-Parkinson-White syndrome: A new closed-heart technique. *Ann Thorac Surg* 37: 67–71.
5. Guiraudon GM, Klein GJ, Sharma AD et al. (1986) Closed heart technique for Wolff-Parkinson-White syndrome: Further experience and potential limitations. *Ann Thorac Surg* 42: 651–657.
6. Klein GJ, Guiraudon GM, Perkins DG et al. (1984) Surgical correction of the Wolff-Parkinson-White syndrome in the closed heart using cryosurgery: a simplified approach. *J Am Coll Cardiol* 3: 405–409.
7. Guiraudon GM, Klein GJ, Sharma AD, Yee RW, McClellan DG (1989) Surgery for the Wolff-Parkinson-White syndrome: the epicardial approach. *Sem Thorac Cardiovasc Surg* 1: 21–33.
8. Johnson DC, Nunn GR, Richards DA, Uther JB, Ross DL (1987) Surgical therapy for supraventricular tachycardia, a potentially curable disorder. *J Thorac Cardiovasc Surg* 93: 913–918.
9. Ross DL, Johnson DC, Denniss AR, Cooper MJ, Richards DA, Uther JB (1985) Curative surgery for atrioventricular junctional (AV nodal) reentrant tachycardia. *J Am Coll Cardiol* 6: 1383–1392.
10. Guiraudon GM, Klein GJ, Sharma AD, Yee RW, McClellan DG (1986) Surgical treatment of supraventricular tachycardia: a 5 year experience. *Pace* 9: 1376–1380.
11. Klein GJ, Guiraudon GM, Sharma AD (1986) Demonstration of macroreentry and feasibility of operative therapy in the common type of atrial flutter. *Am J Cardiol* 57: 587–591.
12. Guiraudon GM, Campbell CS, Jones DL (1985) Combined sinoatrial node — atrioventricular isolation: a surgical alternative to His bundle ablation in patients with atrial fibrillation. *Circulation* 72: 211–220.

30. Catheter mapping of ventricular tachycardia

K.-H. KUCK, M. SCHLÜTER, K.-P. KUNZE and M. GEIGER

Introduction

The electrophysiologic mechanism underlying ventricular tachycardia after myocardial infarction is generally thought to be reentry [1, 2], with one limb of the reentrant circuit exhibiting normal conduction properties, the other representing an (abnormal) area of slow conduction (Figure 1). This concept has been proven in several animal studies, and recently evidence has also been given in intraoperative studies in humans.

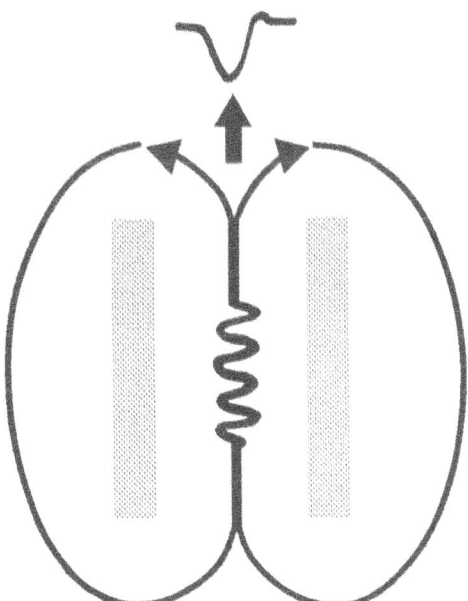

Figure 1   Sketch of the 'Figure of eight' model of reentry The shaded bars represent regions of conduction block, the undulated line represents the area of slow conduction, and the solid lines represent paths of normal conduction Electrical activity exciting the reentrant circuit (thick arrow) gives rise to the sketched QRS complex while at the same time re-activating the circuit (two curved arrows)

V Hombach et al (eds), Interventional Techniques in Cardiovascular Medicine, 249–261
© 1991 *Kluwer Academic Publishers*

In 1977, Josephson et al. [3] introduced catheter mapping of the right and left ventricle in patients with ventricular tachycardia. The technique consisted of recording the local electrical activity, via electrode catheters, at 7 different sites in the right ventricle and 12 sites in the left ventricle during ventricular tachycardia induced in the electrophysiologic laboratory. Potentials obtained from each site were analyzed for their timing with respect to a reference point (e.g., the onset of the QRS complex) as well as for their width, amplitude and morphology. Such an activation map enabled the identification of the site of earliest endocardial activation. This site was considered to represent the origin of ventricular tachycardia [4].

This technique became the 'gold' standard for ventricular tachycardia mapping. Determination of the 'origin' of ventricular tachycardia by this method allowed surgical exclusion or resection of such an area [5]. In patients in whom ventricular tachycardia could not be induced in the operating room, the surgical procedure was based upon the results of preoperative catheter mapping. Intraoperative maps from patients in whom the clinical tachycardia was inducible in the operating room confirmed the

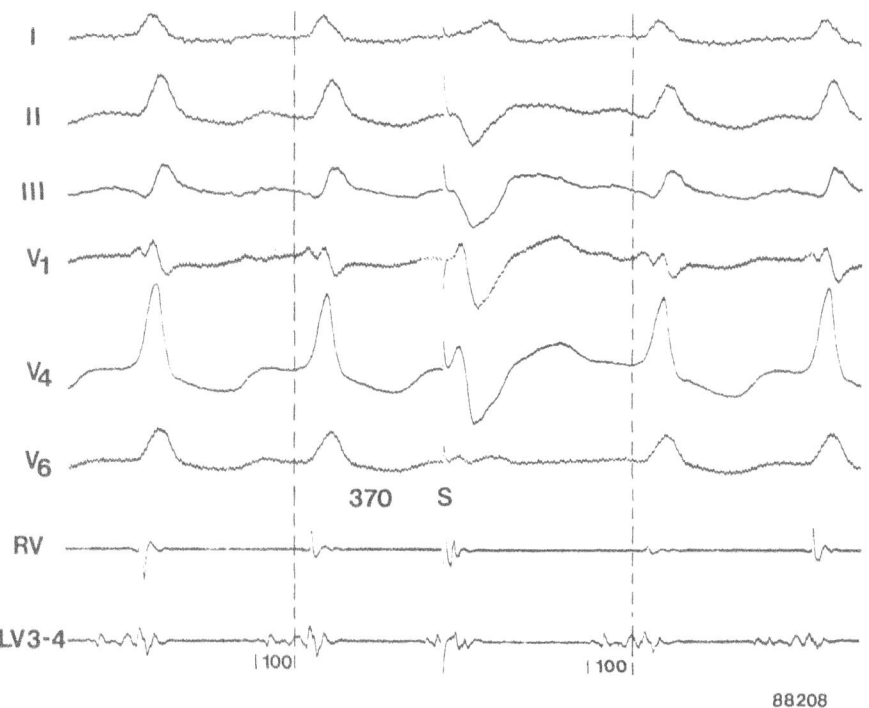

88208

Figure 2.   Right ventricular stimulation (coupling interval 370 ms) during ventricular tachycardia. Note in the tachycardia beats preceding and following the extrastimulus identical morphology and timing (100 ms prior to QRS onset) of isolated diastolic potential recorded at left ventricular site LV 3–4 (Josephson nomenclature). This feature constitutes an 'early' potential. Six surface ECG leads are shown in addition to the two endocardial leads.

preoperative catheter findings in almost all patients, thereby underlining the accuracy and reproducibility of catheter mapping data [6].

Activation mapping

Since the concept of tachycardia activation mapping is based on the assumption that an earliest potential can be recognized, extreme care must be taken in the interpretation of such a tachycardia map with regard to whether the 'earliest' potential is indeed early, i.e., preceding the next QRS complex, rather than late, i.e., following the previous QRS complex. An easy and elegant way to differentiate between these possibilities is to introduce a premature beat during ventricular tachycardia. An early potential will then exhibit a fixed coupling interval with the first ventricular tachycardia beat following the premature beat (Figure 2). In contrast, a potential that represents late activation during ventricular tachycardia will either change its temporal relation, according to the prematurity of the extrastimulus, with respect to the preceding tachycardia beat or it will disappear completely. This is evidence that a late potential is not part of the reentrant circuit necessary to maintain the tachycardia (Figure 3), but represents activation of a 'bystander' area.

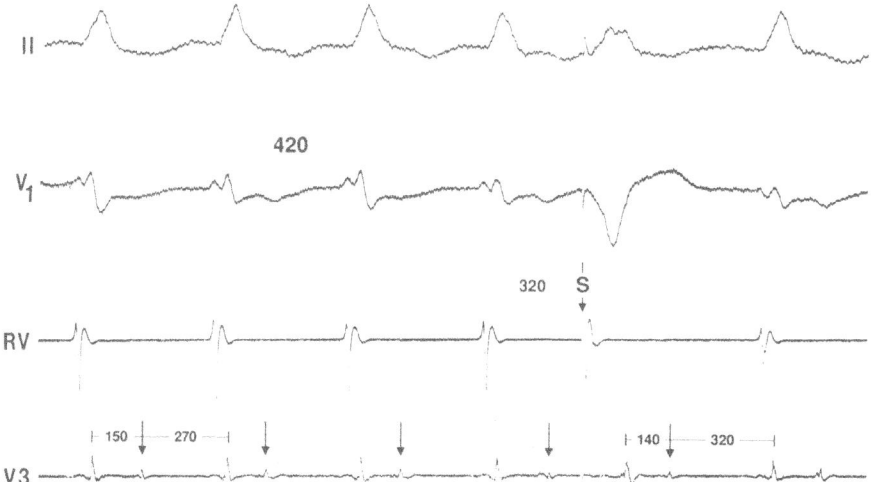

Figure 3. Right ventricular stimulation (coupling interval 320 ms) during ventricular tachycardia of 420 ms cycle length. Note in the tachycardia beats preceding and following the extrastimulus timing of the isolated diastolic potentials recorded at left ventricular site LV 3 is not identical. During spontaneous tachycardia the isolated potential (arrow) follows the local left ventricular potential by 150 ms and precedes the next ventricular potential by 270 ms. In contrast, after the extrastimulus (S), the isolated potential follows local left ventricular activity by 140 ms and precedes the next one by 320 ms. This feature constitutes a 'late' potential, representing activation of a 'bystander' area. Two surface ECG leads are shown in addition to the two endocardial leads.

As long as surgical resection or isolation of myocardial tissue was the only approach to ventricular tachycardia ablation, the catheter mapping technique aiming at identification of the site of earliest endocardial activation appeared accurate enough to produce excellent clinical results. More than 80% of patients who underwent mapping-guided arrhythmia surgery remained free of tachycardia recurrences [7].

When catheter ablation was introduced as a therapeutic alternative for ventricular tachycardia control, results were poor in comparison with the excellent surgical results [8, 9]. An explanation for the different outcome of both procedures may be found in the amount of tissue ablated by either technique. Whereas surgical techniques ablate several square centimeters, catheter ablation injury is limited to volumes of 0.5 to 4 cc [10].

The limited success of mapping-guided catheter ablation raised questions as to the value of activation mapping during ventricular tachycardia which aimed at the determination of the site of earliest endocardial activation as an indirect parameter for the site of 'origin' of ventricular tachycardia. Theoretically, several aspects are not taken into account in the 'earliest site of activation' tachycardia map hypothesis. If reentry is considered the underlying mechanism, one should be able to demonstrate electrical activity in the ventricular tachycardia reentrant circuit throughout the whole of systole and diastole (Figure 4). This, however, is often limited by the inability to map percutaneously all endocardial sites in detail and by the fact that parts of the reentrant circuit may lie intramurally or epicardially and can therefore not be accessed by an endocardial mapping technique. Furthermore, the earliest site of endocardial activation may represent only the exit or one of several exits from the reentrant circuit, with the circuit itself or a critical part of it embedded in deeper myocardial layers, e.g., in an intraseptal location of the reentrant circuit. If the exit is destroyed by application of electrical current, the reentrant circuit may remain functionally intact and continue to give rise to ventricular tachycardia after the ablation procedure.

Recent investigations have demonstrated that results of catheter ablation are markedly improved if electrical current is delivered to the area of slow conduction within the reentrant circuit [11–17]. The existence of such an area has been confirmed in many animal experiments [18, 19]. Identification of this area and subsequent current delivery should eliminate ventricular tachycardia effectively, because the area of slow conduction is an essential part of the reentrant circuit. Identification of, and stimulation at, this area has led to alternative catheter mapping techniques.

Pace mapping

The area of slow conduction is characterized on the intracardiac electrogram by a low-amplitude potential which may be recorded either as an isolated diastolic potential or as a split potential. Its onset in relation to the onset of

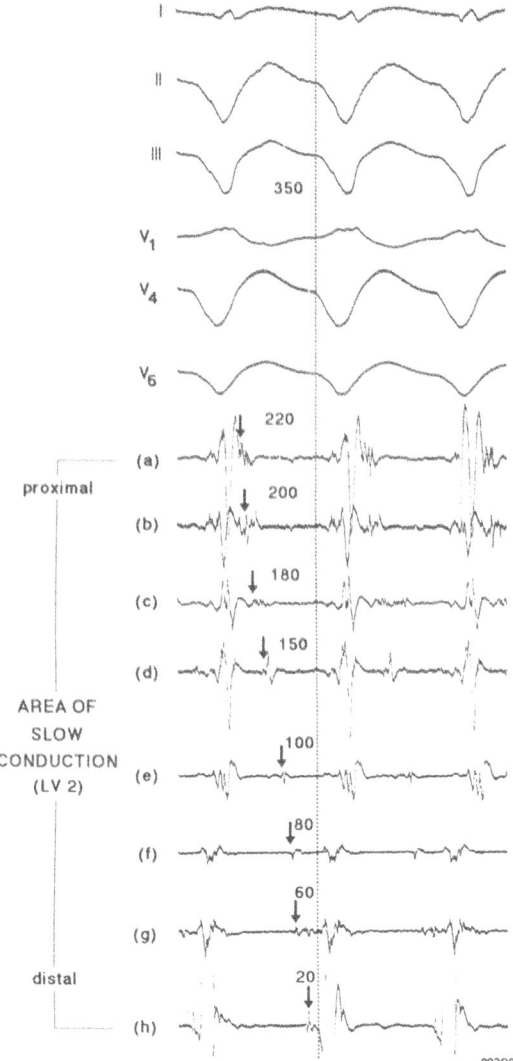

Figure 4. Complete endocardial map of the area of slow conduction. The area was located at the apical left ventricular septum (site LV 2) and extended for about 2 cm in caudo-cranial direction. Moving the mapping catheter along this area, isolated diastolic low-amplitude potentials (arrows) were recorded from eight sites (labeled (a) through (h), with (a) representing the most proximal and (h) the most distal part of the area of slow conduction). Note that the onset of the isolated potential could be recorded throughout the whole of diastole. It occurred initially right after the QRS complex when the mapping catheter was located at the proximal area of slow conduction (site LV 2) (a)), i.e., at the entrance of the reentrant circuit, and was shifted towards the onset of the next QRS complex when the mapping catheter was moved from the proximal to the distal end of the area of slow conduction (site LV 2 (h)), i.e., to the exit from the reentrant circuit.

the ventricular tachycardia QRS complex varies and depends on the location of the catheter within the area of slow conduction and the ability to record electrical activity from it. As for activation maps, it must be proven that such an area of slow conduction is indeed a necessary part of the reentrant circuit and not just a 'bystander' area.

Pacing the area of slow conduction during ventricular tachycardia at a cycle length slightly shorter than the intrinsic ventricular tachycardia cycle length should elicit the same QRS morphology as during spontaneous ventricular tachycardia, provided that the activation sequence during pacing is the same as during ventricular tachycardia (Figure 5). This will be the case if the orthodromic wave front of the intrinsic ventricular tachycardia collides with the pacing-induced antidromic wave front and the paced orthodromic wavefront itself activates the heart in a similar fasion as the intrinsic wave front ('entrainment').

However, it must be taken into consideration that the paced QRS complex can match the intrinsic ventricular tachycardia QRS complex over an area of paced sites that may extend to several square centimeters. Since pacing occurs at an area of slow conduction the stimulated QRS complex matching the intrinsic QRS complex will follow the stimulus artifact with a certain latency. This interval (stimulus artifact to the onset of the QRS complex (SA-QRS)) varies according to the catheter position within the area of slow conduction. When pacing is performed at this area, the SA-QRS interval should match the timing in relation to the QRS onset of spontaneous intrinsic electrical activity at any site within the area of slow

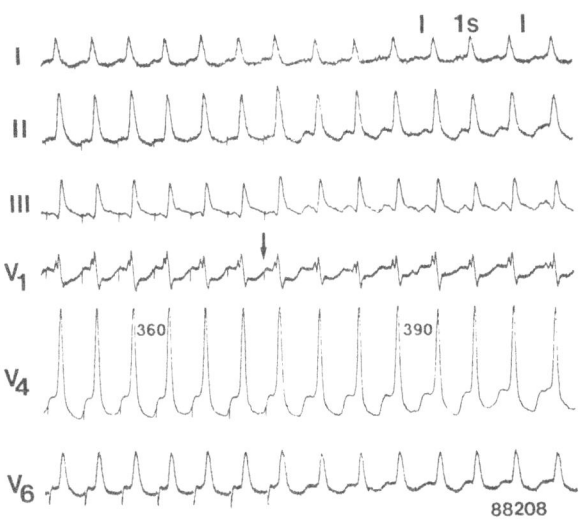

Figure 5. Entrainment of ventricular tachycardia. Note identical QRS morphology during pacing at 360 ms (left hand side of panel; last drive stimulus marked by arrow) and during intrinsic ventricular tachycardia of 390 ms cycle length (right hand side of panel).

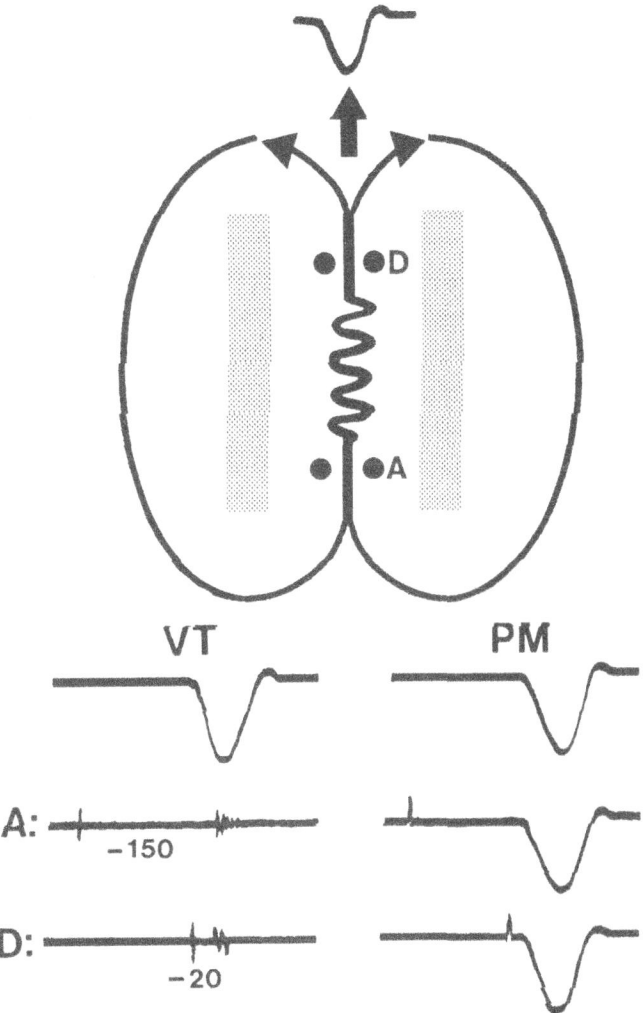

Figure 6. Schematic diagram showing temporal relations during intrinsic ventricular tachycardia (VT; left lower panel) und during pace mapping (PM; right lower panel) of the area of
slow conduction at its proximal (site A) and distal ends (site D). For both sites the interval
between stimulus artifact and QRS onset during PM is identical to the interval between the
local diastolic low-amplitude potential and QRS onset during VT. Sketch of reentrant circuit is
explained in Figure 1.

conduction (Figure 6). Changes in the SA-QRS interval maintaining the
same QRS morphology allow the identification of different regions within
the area of slow conduction, e.g., an area close to the entrance to, or an
area close to the exit from, the reentrant circuit.

The described technique of pace mapping may allow to identify precisely
the anatomical locations of the entrance and exit sites of the reentrant

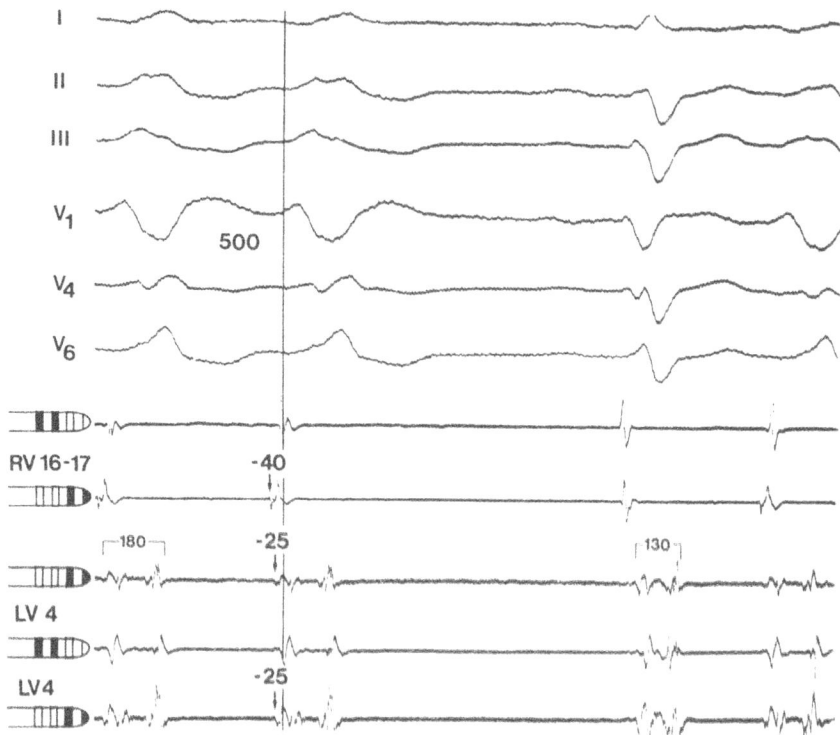

Figure 7.   Surface electrocardiograms (I-III, V_1, V_4, V_6) and endocardial map of ventricular tachycardia interrupted by a sinus beat. Earliest ventricular activation is recorded, during tachycardia (−40 ms) as well as during sinus rhythm, at the proximal right ventricular septum (RV 16–17). Earliest left ventricular activation during tachycardia (−25 ms) is recorded at the opposite septal site, i.e. the proximal left ventricular septum (LV 4). At this site, a fractionated low-amplitude potential of 180 ms duration is recorded during tachycardia and a split potential of 130 ms duration during sinus rhythm. This suggests an area of slow conduction embedded subendocardially in the ventricular septum. The vertical line represents the onset of the ventricular tachycardia QRS complex. Top and bottom electrograms from site LV 4 were recorded through the same electrode pair, but at different amplifications.

circuit and the area of slow conduction. Pacing at the exit site and at the area of slow conduction should elicit the intrinsic ventricular tachycardia QRS morphology, but without a latency between stimulus artifact and QRS onset in the former pacing mode and a marked latency in the latter.

In a septal origin of ventricular tachycardia the exit from the reentrant circuit may be located at the right ventricular septum leading to early right ventricular activation and left bundle branch block QRS morphology of the tachycardia, whereas the area of slow conduction may be located subendo-cardially within the ventricular septum [14, 20] (Figure 7). This implies that in a 'septal' ventricular tachycardia right ventricular mapping is mandatory.

The area of slow conduction may be identified during sinus rhythm by the

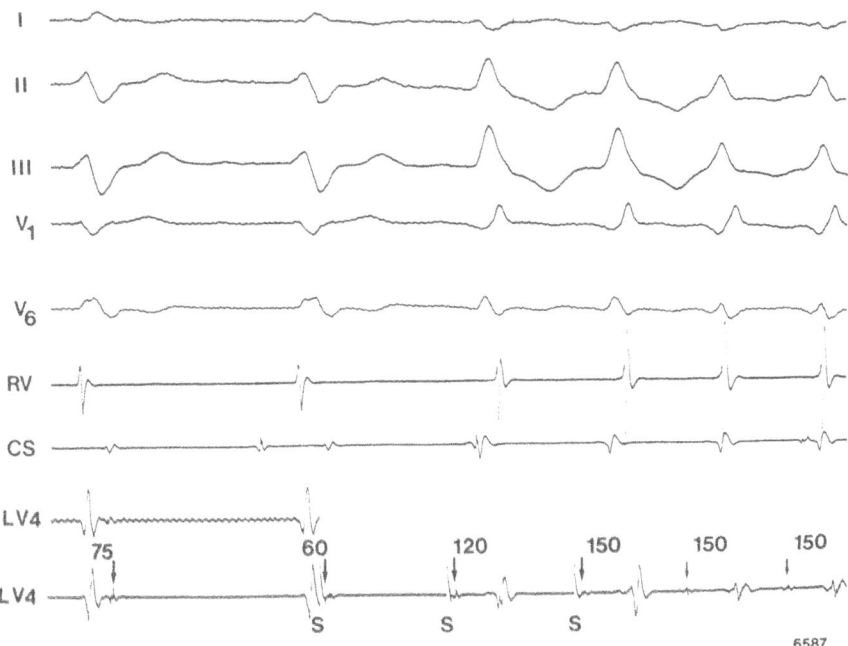

Figure 8.   Left ventricular pacing at the area of slow conduction (located at site LV 4), initiated during sinus rhythm (left two beats) such that the isolated potential (arrow) which follows the local ventricular potential by 75 ms (first beat) is advanced by 15 ms to follow the local ventricular potential by 60 ms (second beat). Continued pacing activates the isolated potential 120 ms (third beat) and 150 ms (fourth beat) prior to the local ventricular potential. This pacing sequence initiates ventricular tachycardia during which the 150 ms interval remains constant. Note that the morphology of the two stimulated QRS complexes is almost identical to the tachycardia QRS complexes. Abbreviations: RV = right ventricle; CS = coronary sinus.

recording of a distinct late potential. Pacing at this site during sinus rhythm may lead to selective activation of the area of slow conduction earlier than expected by the intrinsic sinus impulse (Figure 8). Continued pacing may lead to ventricular activation from this site and initiation of a sustained ventricular tachycardia without a premature beat. Again, the SA-QRS interval should be identical to the interval between the onset of spontaneous electrical activity at this site and the onset of the QRS complex during intrinsic ventricular tachycardia.

Pacing the area of slow conduction should not only elicit the same QRS morphology as during intrinsic ventricular tachycardia, but should also lead to the same endocardial activation sequence of the surrounding tissue. This implies that the morphologies and timing of potentials recorded from all areas mapped during intrinsic ventricular tachycardia should not change during pacing at the area of slow conduction (Figure 9).

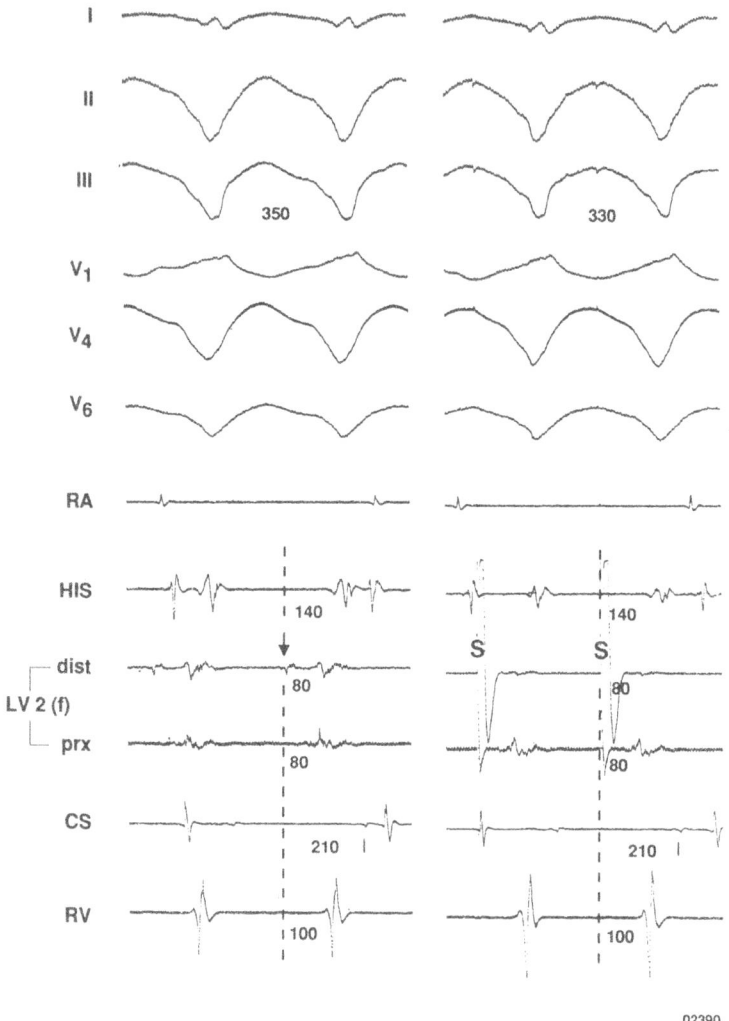

Figure 9. Ventricular tachycardia of 350 ms cycle length (left panel) and pace mapping at 330 ms during tachycardia (right panel). Note identical QRS complexes in both panels. Furthermore, note that morphologies and timing of local potentials recorded from four endocardial sites (HIS, LV 2, CS, RV) remain identical, since pacing is performed from the distal electrode pair located at the area of slow conduction (site LV 2 (f); see Figure 4). Abbreviations: dist = distal electrode pair; prx = proximal electrode pair.

Decremental conduction

Pacing the area of slow conduction at a rate higher than that of the intrinsic ventricular tachycardia leads to a progressive increase of latency between the stimulus and the QRS complex (Figure 10). This phenomenon can be

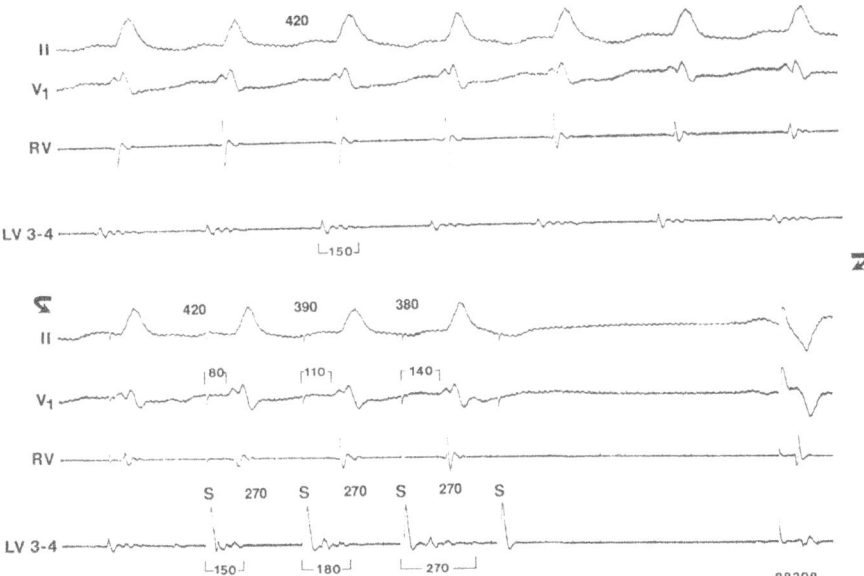

Figure 10. Left ventricular pacing at 270 ms of the area of slow conduction (located at site LV 3–4) initiated during ventricular tachycardia (cycle length 420 ms). The duration of the fractionated potential recorded from the area of slow conduction is 150 ms. The first paced beat captures the area of slow conduction without changing the fractionated potential. The next two paced beats prolong the potential to 180 and 270 ms, respectively, before the fourth drive beat fails to capture the area of slow conduction but terminates the tachycardia. Note unchanged tachycardia QRS morphology and decreasing cycle length (from 420 to 380 ms), but increasing latency between stimulus artifact and QRS onset (from 80 to 140 ms). Two surface ECG leads are shown in addition to the two endocardial leads.

explained by decremental conduction properties of the area of slow conduction. Continued pacing may cause conduction block within the area of slow conduction without ventricular capture.

Conclusion

Since the experimental demonstration of reentry as the underlying mechanism of post-myocardial infarction ventricular tachycardia it has been postulated that a reentrant circuit is the anatomical substrate in the majority of patients with ventricular tachycardia. Intraoperative mapping techniques have provided evidence in favor of this hypothesis. Catheter ablation techniques, however, frequently failed to control the arrhythmia if current was delivered to the site of earliest endocardial activation. Newer mapping techniques aimed at the identification of an area of slow conduction appear to improve catheter ablation results, provided that proof could be obtained prior to current delivery that the area of slow conduction was critical to the maintenance of ventricular tachycardia. To this end, multiple pacing interventions are required.

References

1. El-Sherif N, Smith RA, Evans K (1981) Canine ventricular arrhythmias in the late myocardial infarction period. 8. Epicardial mapping of reentrant circuits. *Circ Res* 49: 255–265.
2. Hope RR, Sherlag BJ, El-Sherif N, Lazzara R (1978) Ventricular arrhythmias in healing myocardial infarction. Role of rhythm versus rate in re-entrant activation. *J Thorac Cardiovac Surg* 75: 458–466.
3. Josephson ME, Horowitz LN, Farshadi A (1978) Continuous local electrical activity. A mechanism of recurrent ventricular tachycardia. *Circulation* 57: 659–665.
4. Josephson ME, Horowitz LN, Spielman SR, Waxman HL, Greenspan AM (1982) Role of catheter mapping in the preoperative evaluation of ventricular tachycardia. *Am J Cardiol* 49: 207–220.
5. Horowitz LN, Harken AH, Kastor JA, Josephson ME (1980) Ventricular resection guided by epicardial and endocardial mapping for treatment of recurrent ventricular tachycardia. *N Engl J Med* 302: 589–593.
6. Josephson ME, Horowitz LN, Spielman SR, Greenspan AM, VandePol C, Harken AH (1980) Comparison of endocardial catheter mapping with intraoperative mapping of ventricular tachycardia. *Circulation* 61: 365–404.
7. Borggrefe M, Podczeck A, Ostermeyer J, Breithardt G, and the Surgical Ablation Registry (1987) Long-term results of electrophysiologically guided antitachycardia surgery in ventricular tachyarrhythmias: a collaborative report on 665 patients, in: Breithardt G, Borggrefe M, Zipes DP (eds), *Nonpharmacological Therapy of Tachyarrhythmias*, pp. 109–132. Mount Kisco; Futura Publishing.
8. Hartzler GO (1983) Electrode catheter ablation of refractory focal ventricular tachycardia. *J Am Coll Cardiol* 6: 1107–1113.
9. Evans GT jr, Scheinman MM, Zipes DP et al. (1988) The Percutaneous Cardiac Mapping and Ablation Registry: final summary of results. *Pace* 11: 1621–1626.
10. Hauer RNW, Straks W, Borst C, Robles de Medina EO (1986) Electrical catheter ablation in the left and right ventricular wall in dogs: Relation between delivered energy and histopathologic changes. *J Am Coll Cardiol* 8: 637–643.
11. Morady F, Scheinman WM, Griffin JC, Herre JM, Kou WH (1989) Results of catheter ablation of ventricular tachycardia using direct current shocks. *Pace* 12: 252–257.
12. Morady F, Frank R, Kou WH et al. (1988) Identification and catheter ablation of a zone of slow conduction in the reentrant circuit of ventricular tachycardia in humans. *J Am Coll Cardiol* 11: 772–782.
13. Fontaine G, Tonet JL, Frank R, Rougier I (1989) Clinical experience with fulguration and antiarrhythmic therapy for the treatment of ventricular tachycardia. Follow-up of 43 patients. *Chest* 95: 785–797.
14. Kuck KH, Schlüter M, Kunze KP, Geiger M (1989) Pleomorphic ventricular tachycardia: demonstration of conduction reversal within the reentry circuit. *Pace* 12: 1055–1064.
15. Fitzgerald DM, Friday KJ, Yeung Lai Wah JA, Lazzara R, Jackman WM (1988) Electrogram patterns predicting successful catheter ablation of ventricular tachycardia. *Circulation* 77: 806–814.
16. Breithardt G, Borggrefe M, Karbenn U, Schwarzmaier J, Laucevicius A. (1986) Therapie refraktärer ventrikulärer Tachykardien durch transvenöse, elektrische Ablation. *Z Kardiol* 75: 80–90.

17. Stevenson WG, Weiss J, Wiener I, Wohlgelernter D, Yeatman L (1987) Localization of slow conduction in a ventricular tachycardia circuit: implications for catheter ablation. *Am Heart J* 114: 1253–1258.
18. Brachmann J, Kabell G, Scherlag B, Harrison L, Lazzara R (1983) Analysis of interectopic activation patterns during sustained ventricular tachycardia. *Circulation* 67: 449–456.
19. Hope RR, Scherlag BJ, Lazzara R (1980) Excitation of ischemic myocardium: altered properties of conduction, refractoriness, and excitability. *Am Heart J* 99: 753–765.
20. Josephson ME, Horowitz LN, Farshadi A, Spielman SR, Michelson EL, Greenspan AM (1979) Recurrent sustained ventricular tachycardia. 4. Pleomorphism. *Circulation* 59: 459–468.

31. Catheter ablation of ventricular tachycardia by direct current

H. KLEIN, H. J. TRAPPE, J. TRÖSTER and A. AURICCHIO

Introduction

Non-pharmacological treatment of ventricular tachycardia has become increasingly important in recent years. This has mainly been due to disappointing results of conventional antiarrhythmic drug therapy as well as to undesirable pro-arrhythmic effects being revealed even of the newer drugs and, on the other hand, to the technical improvement of implantable devices.

Electrophysiologically-guided surgery has long been accepted for patients with monomorphic sustained ventricular tachycardia proving refractory to antiarrhythmic drug therapy. This approach is restricted to patients showing sufficient ventricular function, however, and this, in turn, is a condition hardly ever met in this group of patients.

These are the aspects supporting the desire for a curative approach enabling the arrhythmogenic focus to be destroyed without requiring open-heart surgery.

Growing experience has been reported by many centers using electrode catheters positioned at the atrio-ventricular junction or at the insertion site of an accessory pathway for ablation by direct current [18, 19]. However, catheter ablation at the site of ventricular tachycardia origin has not been accepted as a routine procedure yet [9, 14].

There are various physical effects of the ablation procedure that are being discussed to be responsible for the alteration of myocardial tissue generating or sustaining a re-entrant circuit [2, 5]. For instance, there is an immense barotraumatic effect caused by gas bubble collapse that may lead to disruption of myofibrils and cause a conduction block [3]. In addition, there are thermal effects brought about by high temperatures developing at the tip of the electrode catheter which may produce local endocardial and subendocardial necrosis.

There are also electrical effects caused in the critical area by high current density that are responsible for circumscribed electrophysiological changes, such as an alteration in the duration of action potential, heterogeneity of

263

V. Hombach et al. (eds), Interventional Techniques in Cardiovascular Medicine, 263–278.

refractoriness, and impairment of impulse conduction. The actual mechanism of 'fulguration' has not been fully understood yet and is thus requiring further experimental and clinical investigation.

Where should ablation be performed?

In the early days of our ablation experience it had been our belief that energy application should be important at the area of earliest endocardial activation recorded during activation mapping of ventricular tachycardia. This always had to be effected prior to the onset of the tachycardia QRS complex. From experimental studies [20] we learned, however, that it would be more appropriate to detect the critical isthmus of the re-entrant circuits i.e., the area of maximum slowing of impulse conduction. If our understanding of the re-entry mechanism should be correct, this area ought to be locatable immediately prior to the 'onset' of the re-entrant circuit as this would represent the earliest activation preceding the QRS complex.

In case the assumed mechanism of tachycardia is not re-entrant but focal (abnormal automaticity), earliest endocardial activation must be traced by activation mapping.

In patients whose clinical tachycardia cannot reproducibly be induced, pace-mapping is the only method for identifying the area of energy application. However, even in those cases permitting identification of the arrhythmogenic area during ventricular tachycardia, additional pace-mapping should be performed. Identical QRS complex morphology of paced and inherent tachycardia beat is most likely to confirm the area of tachycardia origin.

Characteristics of the area of slow conduction

By activation mapping during ventricular tachycardia there may be electrograms found to be preceding the QRS complex, whereas others are detected very late after the onset of the tachycardia QRS complex. The sites of both these recordings are located very close to each other. With some experience, however, we are able to record mid-diastolic potentials or mid-diastolic fractionated activity indicating that we are recording signals from the area of maximum slowing in conduction (Figures 1, 2). Pacing from this site of recording produces the same QRS complex as ventricular tachycardia does (pace-mapping). There must be the same long interval between the stimulus artifact and the onset of QRS complex, and a further delay between stimulus and QRS complex should be produced as stimulation is increased. Rapid pacing at this critical isthmus of tachycardia should result in entrainment without producing fusion beats (pseudo-entrainment), and premature stimuli in this area may cause local capture, but no propagated wave front to

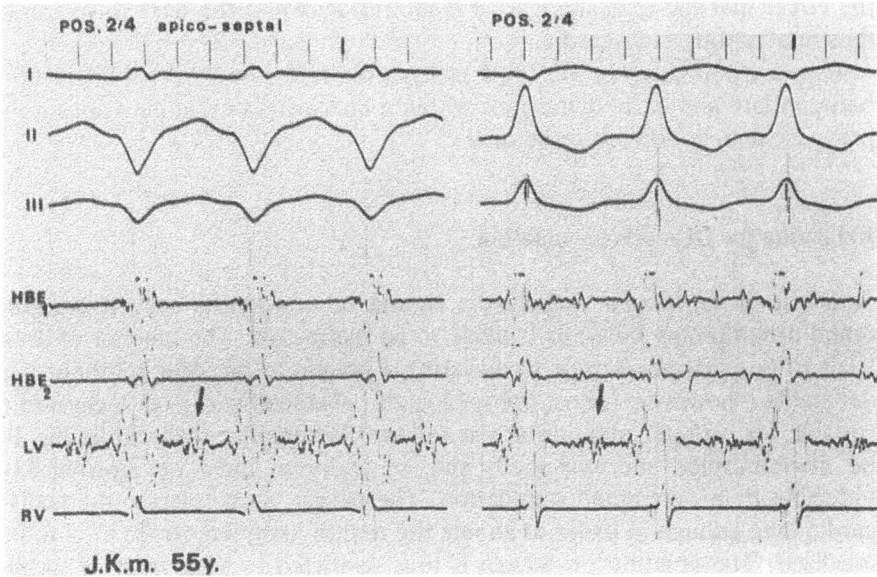

Figure 1. Electrogram recordings from the area of slow conduction. Arrows indicate mid-diastolic potentials. Activation mapping at the apico-septal site during two different tachycardia morphologies. Note that the area of slow conduction is recorded at the same position in both tachycardia morphologies. HBE 1 and 2 = His bundle recordings; LV = left ventricular recording; RV = right ventricular recording.

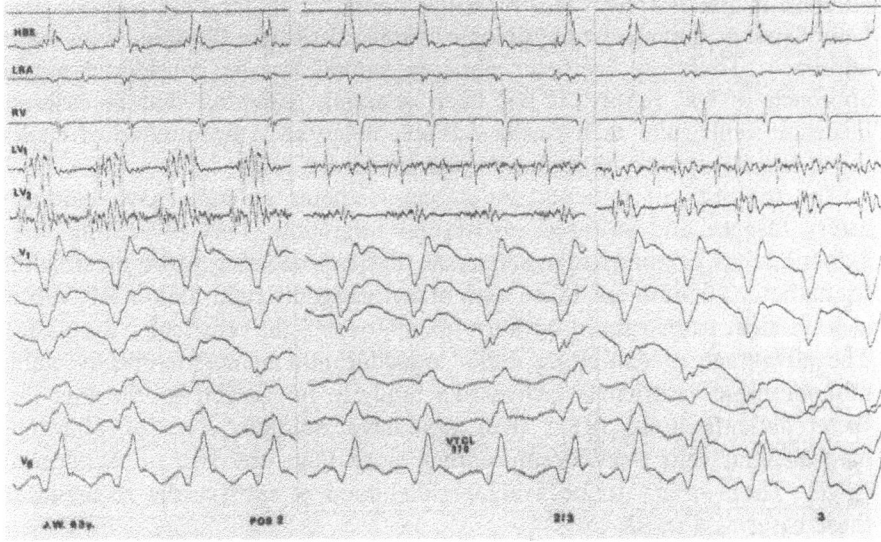

Figure 2. Activation mapping during ventricular tachycardia. Note the mid-diastolic potentials in LV-1 at position 3, early and fractionate activity in LV-1 and 2 at position 2. Recordings at HBE = His bundle; LRA = low right atrium; RV = right ventricle; LV_1 and LV_2 = left ventricle; V_1 to V_6 = chest leads of ECG; VTCL = ventricular tachycardia cycle length.

the effect that the excitable gap is made refractory to the next wave front, thus interrupting tachycardia.

Especially in cases of very fast tachycardia rates, however, a distinction between late and early deflections within a tachycardia cycle may not rarely prove extremely difficult to be made.

Indication for DC-catheter ablation

Ablation of ventricular tachycardia should be considered only if conventional drug therapy failed or is likely to be ineffective. The number of drug trials to be performed prior to declaring a patient to be 'drug-refractory' is debatable, however. Electrophysiological characteristics of tachycardia suitable for catheter ablation are as follows: Ventricular tachycardia has to be monomorphic and sustained, and, in addition, must be reproducibly inducible by programmed stimulation. The patient must tolerate the tachycardia long enough in order to enable the critical arrhythmogenic area to be localized. The ablation procedure is thus restricted to such rates of tachycardia that are slow enough not to cause hemodynamic instability or intolerable ischemia.

Since we are still in the process of learning, it is not believed that ablation should be attempted only in patients who are not candidates for electrophysiologically-guided surgery. On the contrary, we prefer to attempt ablation in patients who still have the option of undergoing surgery since hemodynamic and electrophysiologic characteristics are the same with either approach. Therefore, catheter ablation should not be considered as the approach of last report. It has been generally accepted that in cases of incessant ventricular tachycardia catheter ablation is the method of choice for at least temporary termination of tachycardia.

The majority of patients undergoing catheter ablation have coronary artery disease and suffered myocardial infarction, thus presenting large akinetic areas or ventricular aneurysm. Patients seeming to be most suited for catheter ablation are those with arrhythmogenic right and/or left ventricles, in most cases caused by fibro-lipomatosis (right ventricular dysplasia). The advantage of exhibiting easily inducible and hemodynamically stable monomorphic ventricular tachycardia tends to be waived by the fact that these patients more often than not have multiple sites of abnormal myocardium, thus possibly presenting more than one site of tachycardia origin. There seems to be a higher likelihood of tachycardia recurring in these cases as a result.

The worst type of underlying disease in patients undergoing catheter ablation is dilative cardiomyopathy. These patients often show poor ventricular function, and the barotraumatic effect of fulguration may cause further impairment of ventricular function. In addition to the undesirable hemodynamic effect, ventricular tachycardia often proves to be not inducible during ablation.

Ablation procedure

Catheter ablation is performed under general anesthesia. We place quadripolar catheters in the left and right ventricle, a tripolar one at the bundle of His and a bipolar catheter in the right atrium. Sustained monomorphic ventricular tachycardia is induced by programmed stimulation, and thorough endocardial activation mapping is performed in both ventricles with careful hemodynamic monitoring being guaranteed.

After assessment of the area of slow conduction as identified by mid-diastolic potentials, pacing from this area is mandatory in order to verify 'pseudo-entrainment', stimulus latency and termination of tachycardia. Pace-mapping during sinus rhythm is then performed.

The first DC-shock amounting to 360–400 J of stored energy is delivered at the area of maximum slowing of conduction after ventricular tachycardia being re-induced. Cathodal shocks are applied using a conventional R-wave-synchronized defibrillator. The anode electrode is placed at the left lateral chest wall, using commercially available adhesive patch electrodes.

Re-induction of ventricular tachycardia is attempted 10–15 mins after the initial DC-shock. In case of re-inducibility further detailed activation mapping will be required.

The number of shocks applied depends upon both the electrophysiologic and hemodynamic situation of the individual patient. We never deliver more than three shocks via one 6 or 7 F catheter, and a maximum of 10 shocks may be applied to a patient during a single ablation session even though ventricular tachycardia may remain inducible.

Upon completion of ablation careful monitoring must be performed in the CCU measuring pulmonary wedge pressure and MB-CK enzyme levels for another 3 to 4 days.

Control stimulation is done 4 to 6 weeks after ablation in our unit; some investigators prefer re-studying their patients earlier after the procedure.

Inducing a previously clinically undocumented tachycardia during or after catheter ablation is yet a matter of debate. It certainly indicates the presence of arrhythmogenic tissue (possibly remaining after incomplete ablation) that may sustain another re-entrant circuit, thus leaving the patient at risk of further tachycardia episodes. Re-mapping during tachycardia and a second ablation session may then be reasonable; this is dependent on the clinical and hemodynamic state of the patient, however. Unless there had been two or more distinct arrhythmogenoc areas that could be traced during activation mapping, in many cases the arrhythmogenic area was found to be identical in both forms of tachycardia, with the direction of the propagating wave front emerging from the area of slow conduction being different according to tachycardia morphologies.

Experience in catheter ablation of ventricular tachycardia

Our own experience in catheter ablation of ventricular tachycardia todate includes 49 patients. In six cases a second ablation session was performed because of initial failure. Patients undergoing ablation were 48 men and one woman. The mean age was 49 years, ranging from 36 to 71 years. 33 patients suffered from coronary artery disease with a history of myocardial infarction, while there was no coronary artery disease in 16 cases. Of these 12 showed arrhythmogenic right and 4 left ventricular disease. Hemodynamic and angiographic studies of left and/or right ventricles were performed in all 49 patients.

Of all patients, the mean left ventricular ejection fraction was 31%, ranging from 15 to 70%. In patients with coronary artery disease, LV-EF

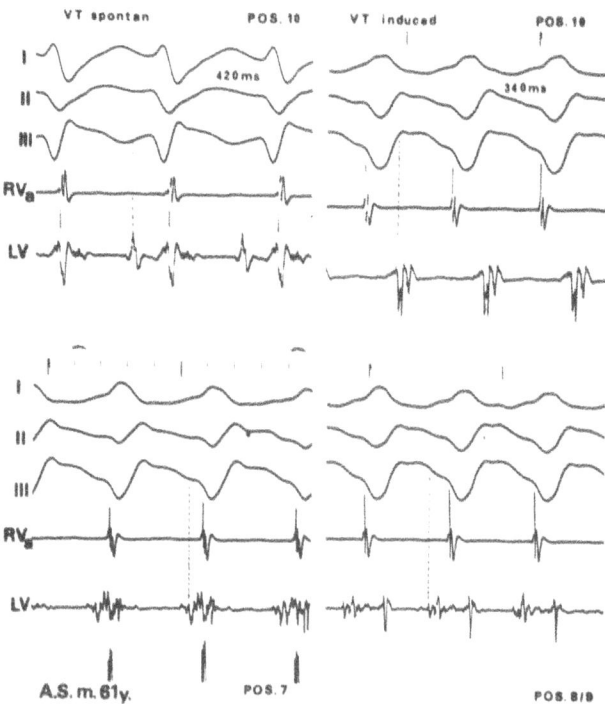

Figure 3.   Activation mapping during spontaneous ventricular tachycardia (upper left pannel) and at various sites (positions 10, 7, 8/9) during induced tachycardia. Note the earliest recording at position 10 during spontaneous VT becoming a very late recording during induced VT. I, II, III = limb leads of ECG; RV$_a$ = right ventricular apex recording; LV = left ventricular recording.

was significantly lower (24%) than in the group of non-coronary artery disease (48%, ranging from 41–70%).

Electrophysiologic characteristics of ventricular tachycardia assessed during pre-ablation EP studies showed a mean tachycardia rate of 178 bmp (125–195 bmp) for the 33 coronary artery disease patients, and of 198 bmp (175–230 bpm) for the 16 non-coronary artery disease patients. Of the group of coronary artery disease patients, 10 patients showed an incessant type of tachycardia. In the group of patients with coronary disease 26 of 33 (79%) showed one morphology of clinically documented tachycardia as against two in 7 cases (21%). During ablation single-type or monomorphic ventricular tachycardia was induced in no more than 17 patients (51%), however, whereas 16 patients (49%) exhibited multiple morphologies with up to four different types of tachycardia (Figure 3).

The difference between the clinically documented type of tachycardia and those induced during catheter ablation was even more impressive in the group of non-coronary patients. Ten of 16 patients showed only one morphology of the clinical type, whereas in 9 patients (56%) two to three different morphologies were inducible during ablation (Figure 4).

Results of catheter ablation

In 31 patients of our initial series, ablation was attempted at the site of earliest endocardial activation during ventricular tachycardia, whereas DC energy was delivered at the area of slow conduction in the last 18 patients.

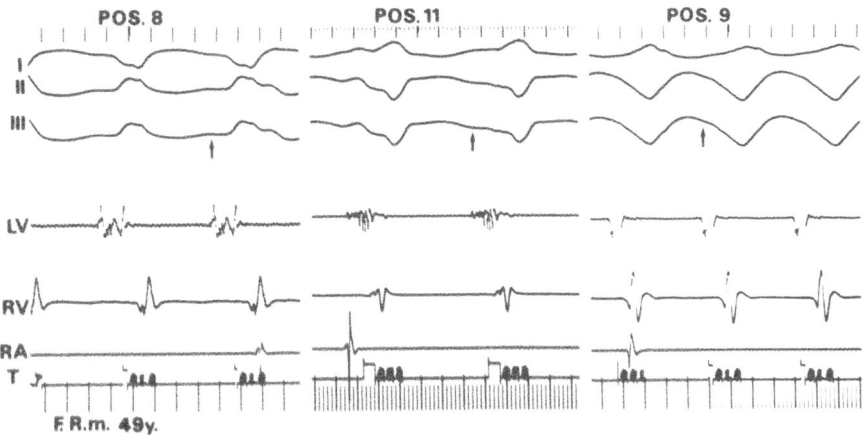

Figure 4. Activation mapping during ablation procedure. Note that three different VT morphologies have their earliest activity at different sites (positions 8, 11 and 9). I, II, III = limb leads of ECG. Recordings at LV = left ventricle, RV = right ventricle; RA = right atrial bipolar recording; T = time line.

The mean interval between earliest activation recorded and the onset of QRS complex during tachycardia was 74 msec (40–130 msec) in 17 coronary patients, and 35 msec (10–70 msec), respectively, in 14 non-coronary patients. Ablation at the site of slow conduction was performed in 16 coronary patients and no more than two patients with arrhythmogenic right ventricular disease.

Ablation at the site of earliest activation

Patients suffering from coronary artery disease (CAD) received a mean of 4.3 shocks/patient during an ablation session as against a mean of 5.9 shocks/patient in cases of non-CAD. At the end of the ablation procedure ventricular tachycardia was no longer inducible in 8 patients with CAD (47%) and in 6 without CAD (43%), respectively.

Control stimulation after 4–6 weeks revealed that only 7 CAD-patients (41%) and 5 without CAD (36%) remained non-inducible. Mean follow-up was 37 months for both groups, with ventricular tachycardia spontaneously recurring in 9 patients with CAD (53%) and in 11 without CAD (78%), respectively, thus totalling 20 cases (64%). At the time of control stimulation performed 4–6 weeks after ablation ventricular tachycardia was not inducible in 5 of these patients (25%). Of 11 patients (36%) without tachycardia recurring spontaneously during the follow-up period, four suffering from CAD still proved to be inducible at the time of control stimulation (Table 1).

Table 1. Ablation at the site of earliest activation

	CAD 17				NON-CAD 14			
	NI		I		NI		I	
Inducibility after ablation	8		9		6		8	
Inducibility after 4 weeks	NI	I	I	NI	NI	I	I	NI
	5	3	7	2	3	3	6	2
	NI		I		NI		I	
Follow-up 37 months	7		10		5	9		
	VT	NO	VT	VT	VT	NO	VT	VT
	3	4	4	6	2	3	–	9

CAD = coronary artery disease; NON-CAD = patients without coronary artery disease; NI = non-inducible; I = inducible; VT = spontaneously occurring ventricular tachycardia; NO VT = no recurrence of ventricular tachycardia.

Ablation at the area of slow conduction

16 CAD patients were applied a mean of 3.2 DC shocks/patient as against 5.8 in two cases of non-CAD. In 12 CAD patients (74%) ventricular

tachycardia was not inducible upon termination of ablation. Of these, tachycardia remained non-inducible in 10 cases (62%) during control stimulation performed after 4–6 weeks. Two patients continued to show inducibility upon termination of ablation. In the two non-CAD patients ventricular tachycardia was inducible both upon termination of ablation and during control stimulation. Mean follow-up time in this group has been 25 months. Ventricular tachycardia recurred in 5 patients with CAD (31%) and in one case without. Of these, two had not been inducible by control stimulation performed after four weeks. Of the 11 patients with spontaneous tachycardia not relapsing, three showed inducibility at control after four weeks (Table 2).

Table 2. Ablation at the area of slow conduction

	CAD 16				NON-CAD 2		
	NI		I		NI		I
Inducibility after ablation	12		4		–		2
	NI	I	I	NI	I	NI	
Inducibility after 4 weeks	8	4	2	2	2	–	
	NI		I		NI		I
Follow-up 25 months	10		6		–		2
	VT	NO	VT	VT	VT	NO	VT
	2	8	3	3	1	1	

see Table 1.

Catheter ablation in patients with incessant ventricular tachycardia

Among 33 CAD patients, ten showed an incessant type of tachycardia lasting a mean of 4.1 days (range 1–26). Of these, 8 had been under antiarrhythmic drug therapy at the time of referral. Tachycardia rate was slower (ranging from 120 to 193 bpm with a mean of 156) than in the group of patients showing non-incessant tachycardia. In 8 of these 10 patients ventricular tachycardia showed right bundle branch block morphology.

In all patients ablation was attempted as an emergency measure with endocardial mapping being performed in general anesthesia. In seven cases we were able to trace the area of slow conduction, and in three patients energy was applied at the site of earliest activation.

In all patients ventricular tachycardia could be terminated by the very first DC shock delivered at the critical area of tachycardia 'origin'. Upon termination of ablation, ventricular tachycardia was not re-inducible in 8 out of ten patients concerned. Antiarrhythmic drugs were discontinued in all patients until control stimulation was performed. In five patients ventricular tachycardia was inducible upon control study; 7 patients, however, did not experience a recurrence of tachycardia for a follow-up period of at least 12 months. During long-term follow-up six patients required additional non-pharmacological approaches because of recurrent tachycardia (three cases) and aortocoronary bypass grafting (three cases). Two of these patients received an implantable defibrillator, and four underwent electrophysiologically-guided endocardial resection.

Overall result after DC catheter ablation

Catheter ablation is considered 'successful' if there is no recurrence of spontaneous ventricular tachycardia during follow-up, irrespective of the fact that ventricular tachycardia was inducible upon termination of the procedure or at control stimulation. Inducibility of ventricular tachycardia at control study that may give rise to antiarrhythmic drug therapy being initiated is not regarded as an 'unsuccessful' result.

In our series comprising 49 patients, 23 (47%) underwent successful catheter ablation; of these 19 suffered from CAD and four did not. 15 patients (65%) continued on antiarrhythmic drug therapy after control stimulation; There was no Class I drug given, six patients received amiodarone, and nine sotalol. There were only 8 patients not receiving any antiarrhythmic drug therapy and not experiencing recurrent ventricular tachycardia.

A 'moderate' result of ablation was achieved by patients experiencing a single episode of spontaneous tachycardia recurring after control stimulation, with a history of more frequent occurrences of tachycardia prior to ablation and irrespective of antiarrhythmic drug therapy after control stimulation. This applies to 7 patients (14%) of our patient population.

A complete 'failure' of ablation in controlling ventricular tachycardia episodes was encountered in 19 patients (39%) with multiple episodes of ventricular tachycardia or ventricular fibrillation continuing to occur.

Six patients were subjected to ablation a second time after first relapse of spontaneous tachycardia (Figure 5). In four of these repeated catheter ablation again was unsuccessful with ventricular tachycardia remaining inducible even after second control stimulation, and spontaneous ventricular tachycardia episodes occurring. There were only two patients with CAD in whom ventricular tachycardia was not inducible any more and no spontaneous recurrence was noted.

Myocardial damage after catheter ablation

Determinations of creatinine kinase enzymes within 3 to 4 days after DC catheter ablation revealed a significant difference between CAD and Non-CAD patients. In CAD patients the mean maximum creatinine kinase level was 270 ($\pm$ 330) U/l as against 490 ($\pm$ 370) U/l in non-CAD patients. Measurement of isoenzyme levels of MB-CK yielded the same effect. In the

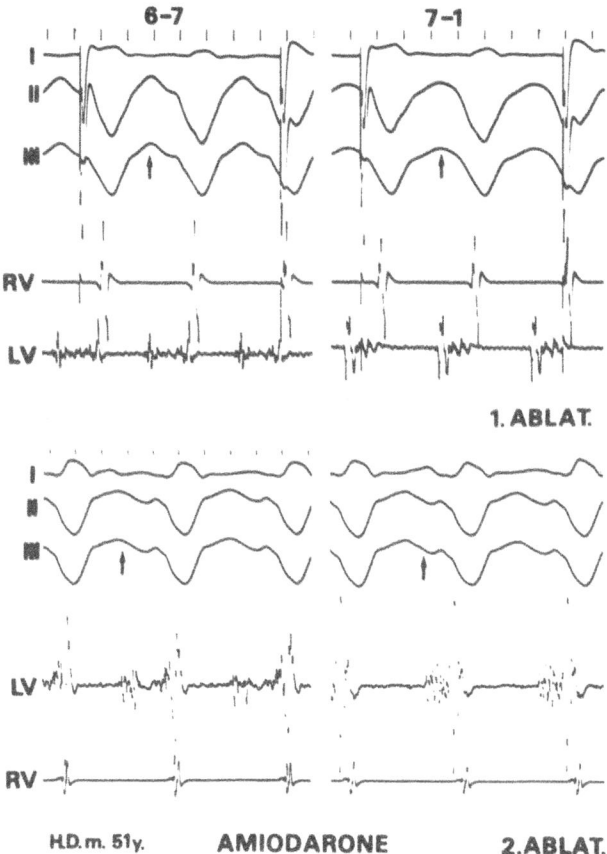

Figure 5. Activation mapping during two ablation sessions. During the second ablation procedure the patient was treated with amiodarone. Note that the earliest activity is recorded at the same site during both ablation sessions (arrows). I, II, III = limb leads of ECG. Recordings at LV = left ventricle; RV = right ventricle.

group of Non-CAD patients MB-CK enzyme levels were significantly higher (64 ± 43 U/l) than with CAD-patients (47 ± 31 U/l). This finding clearly indicates that there is a likelihood of impairment of ventricular function caused by the actual technique. A rise in enzyme levels may mainly result from the barotraumatic effect and can be critical in patients whose ventricular function has been poor already prior to catheter ablation.

Cardiac events and other treatment modalities after catheter ablation

In the course of follow-up after catheter ablation four cardiac events were recorded in our patient population. Two patients died suddenly, 6 and 9 months, respectively, after ablation. Most likely sudden death was caused by a sudden arrhythmic event. Two patients died of cardiac failure or low cardiac output, three weeks and 10 months after ablation, respectively. Two patients developed heart failure thus necessitating heart transplantation.

17 patients required other non-pharmacological measures. In 10 CAD patients electrophysiologically-guided endocardial resection was performed, 7 patients were implanted an automatic defibrillator after catheter ablation had turned out to be unsuccessful and with ventricular function not permitting endocardial resection.

Complications of DC catheter ablation

Death related to ablation occurred in two (3–4%) of ablation sessions totalling 55. One was a patient who had received 10 DC discharges during the procedure, and developed acute cardiac failure three weeks later; he died of low cardiac output. The second patient developed an electro-mechanical dissociation immediately after the first discharge; he was put in the operating theater under permanent cardiac massage and survived an emergency endocardial resection, but died three weeks after the intervention due to pump failure.

Immediately after ablation severe pulmonary edema was developed by two patients who gradually recovered. In both these cases ventricular tachycardia ablation had been successful. Complex ventricular arrhythmia pertaining for six days occurred in two patients after the procedure, with polymorphic tachycardia episodes looking quite different from the inherent type of ventricular tachycardia.

Less severe problems related to ablation included three patients developing arterial vessel problems, and two cases of arterial hemorrhage occurring two days after the procedure. In one patient temporary neurologic problems with reversible paralysis of the left upper limb were noted for two days. Perforation of the ventricular wall or cardiac tamponade never occurred in our series; in two patients minor pericardial effusion was found after ablation at the site of the right ventricular outflow tract.

Discussion

Although catheter ablation has already been listed as an armament of non-pharmacological therapy of ventricular tachycardia we must accept that we are dealing yet with an experimental approach requiring further investigation and additional experience. Results reported so far [4, 6, 7, 12, 15, 19] are less than satisfying, with the number of experienced centers remaining rather small. The patient population undergoing catheter ablation for ventricular tachycardia in each of the centers hardly exceeds 50 cases so far, and it has even been concluded by some authors already that fulguration represents a promising therapeutic approach in most cases of tachycardia failing to respond to antiarrhythmic drug therapy [11].

As our own results would indicate, effective or successful ablation may be achieved in no more than 50% of cases, which is in accordance with results reported by other authors [7, 12] comparing effectiveness of single ablation sessions. As reported by Borggrefe [7], of his series comprising 53 cases, 16 patients required a second and 5 a third ablation session. In 74% of his patient population there has been no recurrence of spontaneous tachycardia; in no less than 50% of cases, however, ventricular tachycardia remained to be inducible, and (similar to our results) 61% of patients are continuing on an antiarrhythmic drug regimen.

Haissaguerre [13] reported on 31 patients with a success rate approaching 85% of patients that have been either with or without antiarrhythmic drug therapy. In a series of 43 patients reported on by Fontaine [12] the initial ablation session failed in 43% and included two procedure-related deaths; in 20 patients undergoing a second session the failure rate was 25%, including another two deaths. Of this study population some patients had to tolerate no less than four ablation sessions. The overall success rate after three months of follow-up was stated by Fontaine to be a complete success in 49% and a 'partial' success in 43%, thus adding up to 92% of clinical efficacy of catheter ablation.

Procedure-related death rate has been 4% in our patient population, thus confirming other reports; according to Fontaine [12] the death rate in his series has been 8.5%, and as stated by Borggrefe [6, 7] three patients died within the first week after ablation.

Comparison of results of different authors and arrival at final conclusions is proving rather difficult in view of considerable variations existing between the reports available in respect of indication, underlying disease, ventricular function and definition of 'success' and 'failure' of catheter ablation.

Physical effects of DC catheter ablation are poorly understood; there has been some concern, however, about the barotrauma involved in the technique [1, 3, 5]. Although we do not know whether the barotraumatic effect may to some degree be responsible for the long-term effectiveness of DC catheter ablation, we are reluctant about repeating ablation in a group of patients whose LV ejection fraction is below 40%. Myofibril rupture to an unknown degree is certainly a matter of concern in patients in bad need of unaffected myocardial tissue. This is emphysized by a fairly high rise in MB-CK enzymes observed in particular in the group of patients not suffering from coronary artery disease. Investigation of various defibrillator characteristics with the object of reducing the barotraumatic effect [1, 8] and experimental work on other forms of energy such as radiofrequency and laser energy, will contribute to better results to be achieved with catheter ablation.

The extent of tissue lesion or of local necrosis produced by the direct electrical or thermal effect of catheter ablation is of great importance. Probably the circumscribed myocardial damage produced at the tip of the catheter placed into the critical region for permanent interruption of reentrant circuits is too small to guarantee higher success rates. This aspect is supported by the size of endocardial and subendocardial tissue resected by electrophysiologically-guided surgery for ventricular tachycardia. However, we understand, too, that the extent of the lesion inversely correlates with the hemodynamic effects of catheter ablation.

There has been general consent about the optimum site for energy application. In the early days of ablation, we all looked for earliest endocardial activation during ventricular tachycardia activation mapping. It may well have been for this reason that we failed to destroy the most critical part of the renentrant circuit, i.e., the area of slow conduction. With improving our mapping techniques by tracing the area of slow conduction [10, 11, 17] and adding pace-mapping and stimulation from the site of slow conduction, the success rate of catheter ablation has since been increasing significantly. This has been shown by our study comparing results achieved by ablation at both the site of earliest activation and the area of slow conduction, respectively.

We learned, however, that it may sometimes be difficult — if not impossible — to detect the critical area of slow conduction; this is the case particularly in those patients who are not suffering from coronary artery disease. In addition, the characteristic features of the area of slow conduction are still a matter of debate.

The majority of patients undergoing catheter ablation will be those suffering from coronary artery disease with a history of myocardial infarction. Most investigators (including ourselves) report on better results in patients with CAD than in those suffering from cardiomyopathy or arrhythmogenic right ventricular disease.

There has been one report [16], however, showing fairly good results (60–70%) of catheter ablation achieved in patients with arrhythmogenic right ventricular disease.

It is hardly debatable that incessant ventricular tachycardia represents an indication for catheter ablation. Fortunately enough, however, this type of tachycardia is not encountered very often, as currently there does not seem to be any better approach than catheter ablation for at least temporary termination of the incessant character of ventricular tachycardia. Our best results have been achieved in patients with the incessant type of ventricular tachycardia.

From our study we would conclude that it will not be until DC catheter ablation for ventricular tachycardia will have been further improved and will have to be able to produce better results that it may be accepted as a routine procedure [15]. This approach will continue to be restricted to centers offering a sophisticated electrophysiologic equipment and command of other possibilities of non-pharmacological treatment modalities such as cardiac surgery in particular. Mapping techniques, hardware equipment and electro-physiological as well as physical understanding will certainly soon be improving; but we are also in need of generally accepted criteria in respect of both optimum indication and hemodynamic state as well as the most appropriate method of procedure.

Before we may claim catheter ablation to be a promising measure of therapy in ventricular tachycardia and compare this approach with other treatment modalities, we shall have to define and agree on criteria as to what is considered a successful ablation and what has to be regarded as a failure. We shall have to shed light on the significance of inducibility of tachycardia persisting even if there is no spontaneous recurrence of arrhythmia episodes; we also shall have to discuss the interpretation of continuous antiarrhythmic drug therapy, and what must be accepted as procedure-related death. We all agree that currently there are a large number of questions remaining in respect of catheter ablation for ventricular tachycardia that are going to be solved in the near future.

References

1. Ahsan AJ, Cunningham D, Rowland E, Rickards AF (1989) Catheter ablation without fulguration: design and performance of a new system. *Pace* 12 (II): 131–135.
2. Bardy GH, Coltori F, Ivey TD, Yerkovich D, Green LH (1985) Effect of damped sine-wave shocks on catheter dielectric strength. *Am J Cardiol* 56: 769–772.
3. Bardy GH, Coltori F, Ivey TD, Alferness C, Rackson M, Hansen K, Stewart R, Green LH (1986) Some factors affecting bubble formation with catheter-mediated defibrillator pulses. *Circulation* 73: 525–538.
4. Belhassen B, Miller HJ, Geller E, Laniado S (1986) Transcatheter electrical shock ablation of ventricular tachycardia. *J Am Coll Cardiol* 7: 1347–1355.
5. Boyd EGCA, Holt PM (1985) An investigation into the electrical ablation technique and a method of electrode assessment. *Pace* 8: 815–824.
6. Borggrefe M, Breithardt G, Podczek A, Rohner D, Martinez-Rubio A (1989) Catheter ablation of ventricular tachycardia using defibrillator pulses: electrophysiological findings and long-term results. *Europ Heart J* 10: 591–601.
7. Borggrefe M, Hindrichs H, Haferkamp W, Karbenn U, Budde Th, Martinez-Rubio A, Breithardt G (1990) Katheterablation bei ventrikulären Tachykardien. *Herz* 15: 103–110.
8. Cunningham D, Rowland E, Rickards AF (1986) A new low enery power source for catheter ablation. *Pace* 9 (II): 1384–1390.
9. Evans GT, Scheinman MM (1986) Catheter ablation for control of ventricular tachycardia: a report of the percutaneous cardiac mapping and ablation registry. *Pace* 9 (II): 1391–1395.
10. Fitzgerald DM, Friday KJ, Yeung Lai-Wah JA, Lazzara R, Jackman WM (1988) Electrogram patterns predicting successful catheter ablation of ventricular tachycardia. *Circulation* 77: 806–814.
11. Fontaine G, Cansell A, Tonet JL, Frank R, Gallais Y, Rougier J, Grosgogeat Y (1988) Techniques and methods for catheter endocardial fulguration. *Pace* 11: 592–602.
12. Fontaine G, Tonet JL, Frank R, Rougier J (1989) Clinical experience with fulguration and antiarrhythmic therapy for the treatment of ventricular tachycardia: longterm follow-up of 43 patients. *Chest* 95: 785–797.
13. Haissaguerre M, Warin JF, Lemétayer Ph, Guillem JP, Blanchot P (1989) Fulguration of

ventricular tachycardia using high cumulative energy: results in thirty-one patients with a mean follow-up of twenty-seven months. *Pace* 12 (II): 245–251.

14. Hartzler GO (1983) Electrode catheter ablation of refractory focal ventricular tachycardia. *J Am Coll Cardiol* 2: 1107–1113.

15. Klein H, Trappe HJ, Hartwig CA, Kuehn E (1986) Problems and pitfalls with catheter ablation of ventricular tachycardia. *New Trends Arrhythm* 21: 257–263.

16. Leclercq JF, Chouty F, Cauchemez B, Leenhardt A, Coumel P, Slama R (1988) Results of electrical fulguration in arrhythmogenic right ventricular disease. *Am J Cardiol* 62: 220–224.

17. Morady F, Frank R, Kou WH, Tonet JL, Nelson SD, Kounde S, de Buitleir M, Fontaine G (1988) Identification and catheter ablation of a zone of slow conduction in the reentrant circuit of ventricular tachycardia in humans. *J Am Coll Cardiol* 11: 772–782.

18. Scheinman MM, Evans-Bell T (1984) The executive committee of the percutaneous cardiac mapping and ablation registry: catheter ablation of the atrioventricular junction: a report of the percutaneous mapping and ablation registry. *Circulation* 70: 1024–1029.

19. Scheinman MM, Davis JC (1986) Catheter ablation for treatment of tachyarrhythmias: present role and potential promise. *Circulation* 73: 10–13.

20. Waldo AL, Henthorn RW (1989) Use of transient entrainment during ventricular tachycardia to localize a critical area of re-entry circuit for ablation. *Pace* 12: 231–244.

32. Catheter ablation of ventricular tachycardia using radiofrequency current

G. BREITHARDT, G. HINDRICKS, W. HAVERKAMP,
M. BORGGREFE, A. MARTINEZ-RUBIO and TH. BUDDE

Introduction

Catheter ablation has evolved as an alternative to antitachycardia surgery and has proven effective in the disruption of either atrio-ventricular (AV) conduction [1–3] or accessory AV-connections [4, 5] as well as in the treatment of selected patients with ventricular tachycardia [6–9]. The Percutaneous Cardiac Mapping and Ablation Registry [10] has shown that direct-current (DC) catheter ablation is effective, resulting in tachycardia control in about 50 to 70% of cases. However, despite these encouraging results, there are several disadvantages associated with the use of high-energy pulses. These disadvantages have stimulated our interest in the search for other ablative energy sources suitable for catheter ablation. As early as in 1983, we became interested in the application of radio-frequency (RF) current. However, our early results were discouraging since no coagulation of the myocardium but instead generation of deep holes resulted from unipolar or bipolar radio-frequency current application (A. Laucevicius, G. Breithardt, M. Borggrefe: Personal communication). These discouraging results were obviously due to the fact that an energy source with a too high output was used. Subsequent studies resulted in the use of devices with lower outputs [11]. These studies as well as other studies have shown that radio-frequency current is obviously a save and an effective energy source for inducing heart block as well as areas of discrete coagulation necrosis in ventricular tissue in experimental animals [11–53].

Direct-current catheter ablation ('fulguration')

Methodology

The method most widely used for catheter ablation has been the application of high-energy direct-current to the myocardium. After identification of the region of earliest activity during tachycardia (the so-called 'site of origin') or

279

V. Hombach et al. (eds), Interventional Techniques in Cardiovascular Medicine, 279–297.
© 1991 *Kluwer Academic Publishers.*

the specific structures of the HIS-bundle by intracardiac mapping techniques, a shock between 50 to 400 Joules is delivered via the ablation catheter synchronously with the QRS-complex. The shock is generated by a defibrillator unit, the catheter usually serving as cathode and a plate electrode placed at the back of the patient used as anode. However, some groups including ours have initially used the opposite polarity. Although the mapping procedure for identification of the arrhythmogenic structures can be performed without anaesthesia, the shock has to be applied in general anaesthesia because of the painful effects of high-energy direct-current pulses. This implies that immediate electrophysiological testing of the efficacy of the shock applied will always take place under the effects of narcotic agents.

Mechanisms of direct-current ablation

Experimental studies and a few clinical observations suggest that barotrauma and/or thermal effects mediated by the application of direct-current may play a role in the therapeutic effects of catheter ablation [54–63]. Some of the consequences of high-energy direct-current application is the formation of gas bubbles [64–66] as well as the potential for thrombus formation [67, 68]. Anodal catheter discharges, higher energies, and smaller electrode surfaces seem to be the determining factors for an increased probability of gas bubble formation. Another limitation of direct-current catheter ablation is the limited stability of electrode catheters in terms of their ability to tolerate more than one consecutive high-energy shock [69]. Furthermore, there is the potential for induction of ventricular tachyarrhythmias which was mainly observed in the experimental setting [70–72]. Surprisingly, the arrhythmogenic potential of catheter ablation in man seems to be small [7, 8, 73–79].

Own experience

Our earlier results in the first group of 24 consecutive patients have recently been published [8, 9]. In the meanwhile, a total of 53 patients have been studied using high-energy direct-current ablation [80]. 35 of these patients had coronary artery disease whereas the remaining patients had dilative cardiomyopathy (n = 9), arrhythmogenic right centricular disease (n = 5), valvular heart disease (n = 3) or no structural heart disease (n = 1). Twelve of the patients with coronary heart disease had previously undergone cardiac surgery. Mean ejection fraction in the patients with coronary heart disease was 34 ± 7%. In 16 patients, two and in another 5 patients, three ablation sessions were necessary. The site of ablation was in the left ventricle in 43 patients. There were three deaths (5.7%) in conjunction with the procedure. One patient died despite immediate surgical intervention from perforation of an electrode catheter that was distant from the site of ablation. Another patient developed an inferior wall myocardial infarction (in the presence of a left ventricular anterior wall aneurysm) due to thrombotic occlusion of the right coronary artery (most probably not due to embolization) which caused immediate cardiogenic shock. The third death occurred in a patient who was brought to the catheterization laboratory in cardiogenic shock due to incessant ventricular tachycardia. After hospital discharge, another 6 patients died during a mean follow-up period of 18 ± 13 months: two patients died suddenly, one of them after progression of heart failure; two patients died non-suddenly from heart failure; one patient died from acute respiratory distress syndrome (ARDS) and one patient died perioperatively after heart transplantation. Spontaneous recurrences of sustained ventricular tachycardia occurred in 8 cases within the first month and in one patient later. In those with spontaneous recurrences, antitachycardia surgery was performed in three, implantation of an AICD (automatic implantable cardioverter-defibrillator; CPI) in four, and of an automatic cardioveter (Medtronic) in another patient. Post-ablation electrophysiological studies after about one week later revealed that ventricular tachycardia had been rendered non-inducible in 47% of patients, and made more difficult to induce in another 17%.

One of the most compelling findings was that ventricular tachycardia was non-inducible in almost all patients at the end of the ablation session whereas it became inducible again in about one third of patients.

Transient nature of the ablative effects

Besides the above-mentioned limitations, one of the major problems that we have encountered during our ongoing experience with direct-current ablation has been the transient nature of tissue effects. The 'regeneration' of arrhythmogenic myocardial structures may lead to recurrences of tachycardias after initially successful catheter ablation. Several mechanisms may be responsible for this effect.

Histological studies have demonstrated a three-layered pattern of necrosis immediately around the site of ablation [81]. On the surface of the myocardium, there was a crater of necrotic debris. The tissue below the crater was composed of a halo of myocytes with pycnotic nuclei of contraction bands. The third layer of tissue injury was composed of myocytes with typical contraction bands and foci of fiber disruption and haemorrhage. The area of myocardium exhibiting abnormal electrophysiological variables was greater than that in which contraction bands of necrosis were found. This suggests that a border zone of abnormal but viable cells may be present after high-energy ablation. This border zone of abnormal but viable cells may be responsible for the final recovery of the electrical properties of the tissue. This is an obvious limitation of the technique of direct-current catheter ablation. As soon as ventricular tachycardia can no longer be induced during an ablation procedure, there is no way to predict whether the arrhythmogenic tissue is going to remain unresponsive or whether it is going to recover its electrical properties. Our still limited experience suggests that frequently the ablated area recovers its electrophysiological properties. Therefore, improved techniques that result in more predictable and permanent tissue damage need to be developed in order to avoid these obvious limitations of the delivery of high-energy shocks. This may be accomplished by either improving the characteristics of high-energy direct-current or by exploring other energy sources. In our recent in-vitro studies using radio-frequency current via conventional electrode catheters, zones of coagulation and also tissue defects could be induced. The dimensions of these defects were dependent on energy dose and duration [11]. Probably, radio-frequency energy causes more permanent tissue damage.

Radio-frequency alternating-current catheter ablation

Application of radio-frequency current in surgery

Radio-frequency alternating-current has been used for cutting and coagulation during surgery since more than 20 years [82–85]. In contrast to the surgical knife, the use of radio-frequency current simultaneously provides for precise cutting and coagulation effects depending on various technical parameters (Table 1). With recent technical improvements, the method has also been applied during endoscopic interventions, such as the resection of small tumors or the treatment of ulcer bleeding in gastroenterology.

Tissue effects of alternating-current application

Three main effects of radio-frequency current application to biological tissues have to be considered [55]:

Table 1. Factors which determine the influence of radiofrequency alternating current on biological tissue (modified from Haverkamp et al., *Pace* 12: 187, 1989)

Mode of power output (monopolar vs. bipolar)
Delivered waveform (modulated vs. unmodulated)
Current frequency
Phase displacement
Current density
Tissue temperature
Tissue impedance
Internal resistance of the generator ('power characteristic')
Heat transfer properties of the tissue
Convective heat loss
Contact of the electrode to tissue
Shape and size of the electrode
Contact pressure of the ablation catheter

1. *The thermal effect* causes a warming up and heating of the tissue during current application. Temperature changes in the tissue are related to tissue impedance, current density, and duration of application. Thermal coagulation of the tissue is achieved by slow heating of the tissue and by vaporization of water of intra- and extra-cellular fluids. The velocity of this heating process is related to the amount of energy applied. If the heating of the tissue is slow, the intra-cellular vaporizing pressure will be low, and the non-fluid structures (e.g., proteins) of muscle, connective and other tissues will be thermally coagulated without disruption or blowing-up of the wall components. If, however, higher electrical energies are applied over a short period of time, the temperature of the cellular fluids will arise rapidly. Hereby, the increase in intra-cellular vaporizing pressure is going to blow-up cellular wall structures instead of resulting in coagulation, thereby producing disconnection of the tissue components. This 'blow-up' effect, in microscopical dimension, is used in electrical cutting procedures. Basically, cutting as well as coagulation effects can be achieved with either direct or alternating current application.

2. *The faradic effect* means that electrically excitable cells will be excited by current application. Using alternating current, maximal excitatory effects in human tissue are observed at frequencies between 50 to 1000 Hz. If current frequency is increased to more than 300,000 Hz, the faradic effect is abolished. Therefore, radio-frequency current application does not induce unwanted faradic effects if sufficiently high-frequencies are used.

3. A third phenomenon observed with current application to biological tissue is *the electrolytic effect*. With direct-current application, ionized components of cellular fluids will be mobilized between cathode and anode in a direction corresponding to their electrical polarity. Application of radio-frequency alternating current, however, will only result in a kind of 'oscillation' of ionized components since the high-frequency changes of polarity will not create a permanent direction of the electrical field.

In conclusion, the major mechanism of radio-frequency current is tissue coagulation. The energy applied should be sufficiently low to avoid the effects of rapid increases in intra-cellular pressure.

Radio-frequency generator and electrode catheters

Different radio-frequency generators have been used for transcatheter intra-cardiac ablation. Most devices generate radio-frequency currents in the range between 300 KHz and 2 MHz. Before using a specific device for intracardiac ablation, some important data on the power characteristics of the generator have to be obtained. In our experimental and clinical studies, we have been using the HAT 100 RF-generator (Dr. Osypka GmbH,

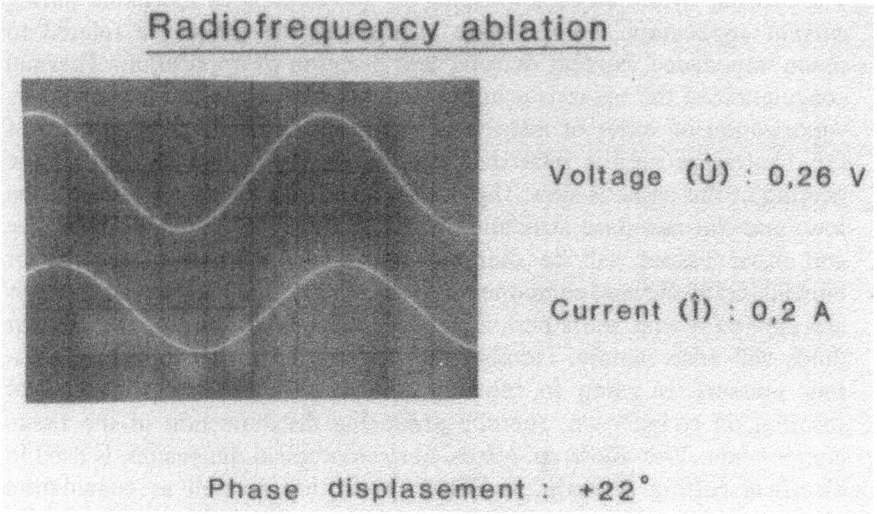

Figure 1.   Oscilloscopic recordings of voltage (upper curve) and current (lower curve) waveforms of unmodulated 750 kHz radiofrequency current. Peaks of current and voltage slightly out of phase.

Grenzach-Whylen, Germany, F.R.). The power output of this device has ten different settings ranging between 2.5 and 50 W at a tissue resistance of 480 ohms. However, the power actually applied to tissue varies as a function of the tissue impedance: according to the power characteristics of the HAT 100 measured via carbon resistors, maximal power is delivered at a resistance of 480 ohms whereas at higher or lower resistances, delivered power markedly decreases [50]. Thus, depending on the tissue characteristics, the delivered power may vary markedly. Therefore, direct measurements of current and voltage should be performed during each application to calculate delivered power. However, data obtained from current and voltage measurements can only be considered accurate if no significant phase displacement during current delivery occurs (Figure 1) [14]. This is due to fact that the delivered power is calculated as the product of phase angle (cosinus alpha), voltage and current [86]. However, as long as current and voltage are constant without a sudden rise in impedance, the phase shift of the HAT 100 RF-generator is usually below 10 degrees and therefore seems to be of negligible importance.

Since most of the tissue injury caused by radio-frequency current is mainly due to thermal mechanisms, a temperature-guided radio-frequency generator has recently been introduced (HAT 200, Dr. Osypka GmbH, Grenzach-Wyhlen, Germany, F.R.) [13, 51]. This microprocessor-controlled device delivers energy as a function of a preselected catheter tip temperature which is measured with a built-in catheter-tip thermistor. Hereby, current delivery is limited by temperature development, thus avoiding overheating and arching of the coagulating electrode. The efficacy of a specific coagulation process to induce tissue injury can be estimated from the ratio of delivered power and developed temperature: slow temperature development at the catheter tip even at a high power output suggests an insufficient electrode-tissue contact and an ineffective coagulation. On the contrary, fast temperature rise followed by down-regulation of delivered power indicates a good tissue-electrode contact by detecting the heat that is reflected from the tissue. Initial experimental experience with the new device is encouraging [13, 51]. However, the clinical usefulness of temperature-guided radio-frequency ablation remains to be established.

A variety of catheters have been used for radio-frequency ablation. Besides standard electrode catheters, different catheters have been designed to improve the feasibility of radio-frequency ablation including needle- or screw-in electrodes, rectangular electrodes with large surfaces, suction electrodes, steerable catheters, and catheters with built-in thermo-elements for temperature monitoring [12, 22, 35, 37–39, 44, 45, 47]. Most approaches, in fact, have improved the feasibility of transcatheter radio-frequency current delivery with respect to a certain aspect of the procedure. However, needle- or screw-in electrodes ensure good tissue contact but may induce unwanted traumatic tissue damage. In-vitro experiments have shown that electrodes with large surfaces produce large lesions but they may be more difficult to position than smaller electrodes when applied percutaneously. Thermo-sensitive electrodes improve the monitoring of current delivery and tissue effects but are lacking the advantages mentioned above. By taking the biophysical aspects of the technique into consideration, an ideal electrode for radio-frequency ablation is presently not available.

Delivered power, energy and catheter tip temperature

A good correlation between delivered power or total applied radio-frequency energy and lesion size has been observed in several 'in vitro' experimental studies [11, 12, 15]. However, these findings cannot be extended to the percutaneous transcatheter application to the beating heart [12, 19]. The differences between 'in-vitro' and 'in-vivo' findings can be explained because major variables that govern the effects of radio-frequency currents (such as tissue-electrode contact, constant heat loss due to convection, etc.) can presently only be controlled and standardized 'in-vitro'.

A major problem is the preselection of an adequate power setting before a specific coagulation. Power should be high enough to result in a smooth coagulation of the target tissue but not too high to avoid overheating of the active electrode which may lead to arching. The so-called 'arching-phenomenon' occurs when catheter tip temperature exceeds approximately 140°C. At this point, tissue proteins or blood proteins first start to coagulate followed by carbonization at the catheter tip [12, 27, 48]. The formation of a thin layer of carbonized tissue results in partial block of heat transfer to the tissue followed by excessive heating of the catheter tip and the risk of vaporization. The flow of current is interrupted by a sudden increase in voltage, a drop of current and an increase in resistance. In addition, a significant phase displacement of current and voltage occurs, resulting in a decreasse of actual current efficacy [14]. When arching occurs, radio-frequency currents are 'out-of-control' and the discharge should be immediately interrupted. Some generators prevent these adverse effects by automatic discontinuation of current flow when impedance rise occurs. However, as mentioned above, multiple variables affect the flow of current to tissue. Since some variables can only be partially controlled, the choice of an adequate power setting is difficult. Application of the same current over 10 sec may result in a constant flow of current at one time but may lead to arching after a few seconds during another discharge.

Even when a constant flow of current is obtained, it remains unclear whether tissue effects are actually achieved or whether the energy is simply delivered to blood due to insufficient contact of the active electrode to the myocardium [50]. Therefore, additional measurements are necessary to control the coagulation process. As the effects of radio-frequency current are mainly based on thermal mechanisms, monitoring catheter tip temperature, a concept first introduced by Hindricks and Haverkamp in 1987 [47–49], provides additional and significant informations about tissue effects. Monitoring temperature at the catheter tip has been shown to make the procedure more controllable [47, 48]. Monitoring of the catheter tip temperature provides information on the electrode-tissue contact and helps to control for lesion size [12, 47]. Furthermore, the temperature signals can be used for the early detection of arching and overheating of the electrode with the subsequent risk of crater formation and myocardial perforation [12].

Macroscopic and microscopic findings

The macroscopic appearance of ventricular lesions induced by coagulation temperatures below 120°C consists of spherically shaped and well delineated areas of necrosis surrounded by a haemorrhagic zone (Figure 2). In the centre of the lesion, a discrete pit due to maximal cell dessication can often be observed. Acute histological changes show dessication and shrinking of the contractile elements with a relative increase in intercellular space and extravasation of red blood cells. The endocardium is often not disrupted. However, long coagulation times, overheating of the electrode or high-contact pressure can affect the integrity of the endocardium [12]. Long-term observations on the histological changes induced by radio-frequency energy in the region of the AV-node showed distinct fibrotic areas with inflammatory cell infiltrations and cartilage formation of tissue [87].

In a previous study (Figure 3), depth and diameter of the coagulation zones were measured for three levels of applied energies (level I: 2.5 W, level V: 25 W, level X: 50 W) and three different coagulation periods (10,

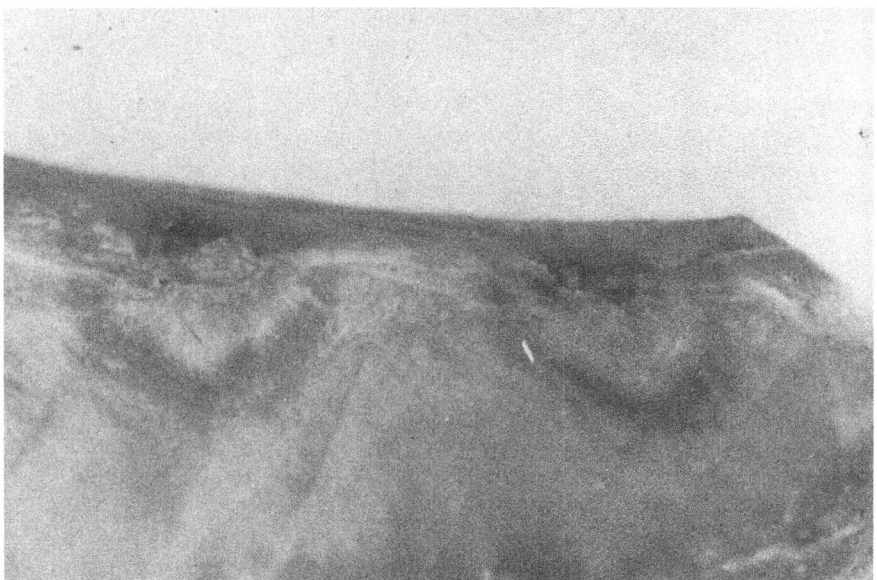

Figure 2.   Cross section of radiofrequency-induced ventricular lesion showing discrete central pit and coagulation necrosis surrounded by a haemorrhagic margin.

30 and 60 sec) [11]. A total of 216 coagulations was performed in left lateral, left septal, and right ventricular myocardium. The diameters of the coagulation zones ranged between 1.8 to 3.7 mm (at 2.5 W, 10 sec) and 6.2 to 8.9 mm (at 50 W, 60 sec). The depth of the coagulation zones was 0.7 to 1.6 mm at 2.5 W and 10 sec, and increased to 3.5 to 4.8 mm at 50 W and 60 sec. In general, using a catheter with a higher internal resistance (e.g., 65 ohm) resulted in smaller coagulation zones than using a catheter with a lower internal impedance (e.g., 5 ohm). The depth and diameter of the coagulation zones was in proportion to the energies applied, the pulse duration, and the catheters used.

Similar results were obtained for bipolar radio-frequency ablation of postmortal myocardium. Using the distal two electrodes of a quadripolar USCI catheter for current delivery in bovine left ventricular myocardium under in vitro conditions, Hoyt et al. [15] found a power of 5 W and a pulse duration of 5 sec to be the minimum threshold for induction for myocardial damage. They concluded the pulse duration and power level were the most significant determinants of the extent of myocardial damage in radiofrequency ablation.

Clot formation

To evaluate the risk of blood clotting, the distal electrode of a USCI quadripolar catheter was placed in heparinized blood without myocardial

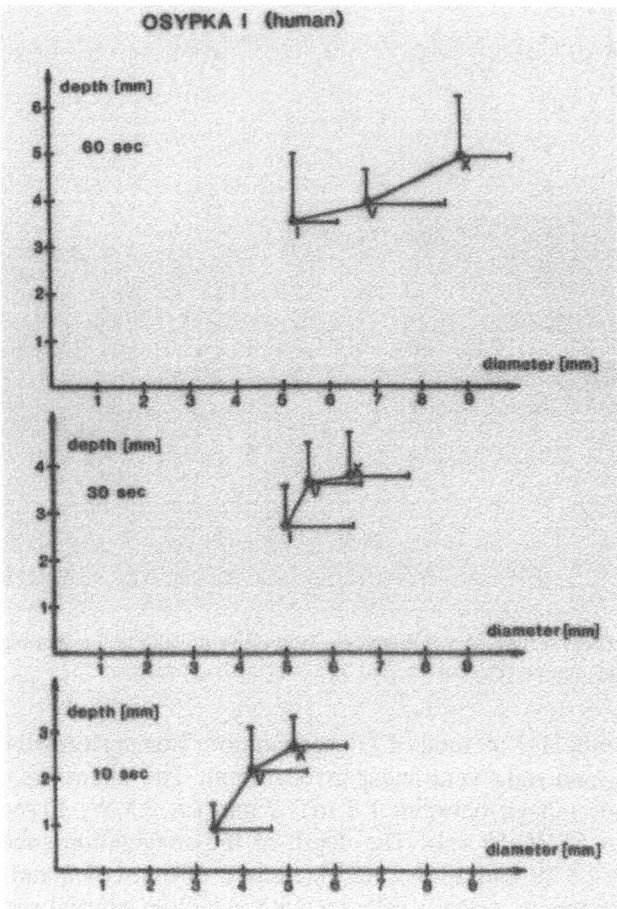

Figure 3.   Depths and diameters of coagulation zones in human myocardium. Power settings: I (2.5 W), V (25 W), and X (50 W); coagulation times: 10, 30 and 60 sec, respectively. (From: ref. 11).

tissue [11]. If there was no movement of the blood, multiple clots of up to 2 mm in diameter were found after filtration of the blood. The blood around the distal electrode was darkened and some of the clots were attached to the catheter electrode. If the catheter was placed on myocardium (5 g weight) in a bath of non-mobilized human blood, there was clot and gas bubble formation with power settings of 25 W and a pulse duration of 3 to 4 sec or more using the HAT 100 device by Dr. Osypka.

During the second part of the study, the influence of blood movement or catheter flushing on clot formation was studied in heparinized blood using electrode catheters with a central lumen ending at three 1 mm outlets at the distal electrode. If, by using a magnetic agitator, the blood was moved with streaming velocities of up to 0.8 m/sec without flushing through the catheter,

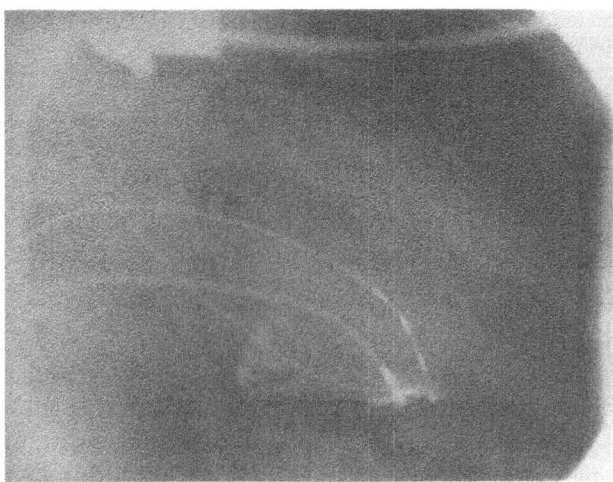

Figure 4. Injection of a mixture of saline and contrast medium (1: 1) through the central lumen of an electrode catheter (having one end hole and side-holes) during RF-coagulation in the right ventricle. Hereby, the exact position of the catheter tip in relation to the ventricular wall can be visualized.

no clots were detectable after filtration of the blood. With immobilized blood, again clots of up to 2 mm in diameter were found in the filtered blood. With higher streaming velocities, a line of coagulation material at the border between the distal electrode and the insulation material of the interelectrode catheter segment was a consistent finding. If, however, in addition to using the agitator during current application, the catheter was flushed with saline solution at a flow rate of 50 ml/min, with streaming velocities of the blood of 0.3 m/sec or higher, there were no clots either in the filtered blood or at the catheter itself. If flushing was performed during catheter coagulation of human postmortal myocardium, even in immobilized heparinized blood, there was no clot formation either in filtered blood or at the catheter.

From these data, it might be concluded that the risk of gross blood coagulation will be limited by the physiological blood movement and additionally suppressed by flushing the distal electrode of the catheter with a saline solution. Another option is to use a mixture of saline with a contrast agent (1 : 1) which gives the same effects but also helps to early detect the penetration of the catheter tip into the ventricular wall (Figure 4).

Radio-frequency catheter ablation of ventricular tachycardia

Present experience with the use of radio-frequency alternating current for the treatment of drug-refractory ventricular tachycardia is mainly based on

Table 2. Clinical results of attempted radiofrequency ablation for drug-refractory ventricular tachyarrhythmias (x = personal communication)

	No of pts.	Success	Failure
Goy	1	–	1
Davies	1	1	–
Kunze and Kuck	7	–	4
Gonska	6	4	2
Klein (x)	3	1	2
Borggrefe	7	4	3

experimental findings. Several investigators have shown that radio-frequency energy is able to induce coagulation necrosis in ventricular myocardium [12, 45, 88, 94]. However, most studies in the beating heart were done in structurally non-diseased myocardium. The fact obviously limits the applicability of these experimental data to the clinical setting.

Only a few preliminary reports on the clinical efficacy of radio-frequency catheter ablation for the treatment of ventricular tachyarrhythmias in man exist (Table 2). Based on this currently available information and our own experience, the efficacy of radio-frequency current in patients with underlying structural heart disease is far from being established. There is strong evidence that the structural changes of diseased myocardium (e.g, fibrotic tissue and scars) affect the response of tissue to radio-frequency currents. This may explain the low success rate in patients treated up to now with radio-frequency energy for ventricular tachycardia [27, 43, 46, 80, 89–91]. Further experimental and clinical studies are necessary to improve the feasibility of radio-frequency currents as a means of non-pharmacological treatment of ventricular tachyarrhythmias.

Kunze et al. [27] studied 7 patients with sustained ventricular tachycardia which was incessant in 4 patients. Six patients had coronary artery disease whereas one patient had ventricular tachycardia of right ventricular origin. The localization procedure included the search for mid-diastolic potentials as well as the detection of sites at which pacing caused a marked delay between the stimulus and the complexes of ventricular tachycardia. Radio-frequency pulses of 30 to 40 W for 10 to 30 sec were applied. In 5 patients, electrical current was applied between a catheter in the left ventricle and a back paddle whereas in 2 patients the current was applied transseptally. In all 4 patients with incessant ventricular tachycardia, there was no termination and no change in cycle length of ventricular tachycardia. In those 3 patients with paroxsysmal ventricular tachycardia, it was still inducible. A subsequent attempt with direct-current catheter ablation led to termination and non-inducibility in all patients.

Gonska and co-workers [90] assessed the effect of radio-frequency current in 6 patients with recurrent monomorphic sustained ventricular tachycardia, all due to coronary artery disease and previous myocardial infarction. Four patients had an anterior wall aneurysm. Ventricular tachycardia originated from the septum in 3, from the anterior-medial aspects of the left ventricle in 2 and from the postero-medial aspects in one patient. The duration of fragmented activity during sinus rhythm was 155 ± 50 msec. The time from earliest endocardial activity to the onset of QRS during ventricular tachycardia was 73 ± 10 msec. The morphology of QRS during pace-mapping was identical to the morphology of ventricular tachycardia at the site where catheter ablation was finally attempted. Radio-frequency impulses of 50 Ws were applied. During a follow up of up to 4 months, one patient had a spontaneous recurrence of non-sustained ventricular tachycardia and one patient died suddenly.

Another study was done by Davies et al. [43] who used 750 KHz radio-frequency pulses of up to 70 W output for up to 50 sec. One patient had recurrent sustained ventricular tachycardia. Ventricular tachycardia was no longer inducible immediately after and 5 days after ablation. During follow-up of 5 months, this patient had no recurrences of ventricular tachycardia. Another case was reported by Goy et al. [89] in whom radio-frequency catheter ablation had no effect on ventricular tachycardia.

We have studied a total of 7 patients at a mean age of 51 ± 16 years (6 male and one female patient). Four patients had coronary artery disease, one patient dilated cardiomyopathy, and one patient had primary electrical disease. Six patients presented with chronic recurrent sustained ventricular tachycardia whereas one patient had 'automatic' ventricular tachycardia (i.e., ventricular tachycardia was not inducible but occurred spontaneously as frequent bouts). The site of ablation was in the left ventricle in 5 cases and in the right ventricle in the remaining two patients. The median number of radio-frequency pulses was 8 (range 6 to 9 pulses/patient). At the end of the ablation procedure, the clinical ventricular tachycardia was no longer inducible in 4 patients whereas it was still inducible in two cases. In the remaining patient with 'automatic' ventricular tachycardia, there were only short episodes of non-sustained tachycardias. At a second electrophysiological study one week later, clinical tachycardia was still inducible in two cases whereas non-clinical ventricular tachycardia was induced in three patients. There were two patients with spontaneous recurrences of ventricular tachycardia which included the patient with 'automatic' ventricular tachycardia. The three patients in whom only non-clinical ventricular tachycardia was inducible, were discharged. During a follow-up of 31, 35, and 36 months, respectively, there were no spontaneous recurrences of ventricular tachycardia. In the remaining 4 patients in whom clinical ventricular tachycardia was still inducible or there were spontaneous recurrences during the first week, a second procedure using direct-current was performed. This was effective in only two of these cases.

Complications of radio-frequency catheter ablation

Compared to the well-known complications of high-voltage direct-current catheter ablation, radio-frequency current application seems to carry a lower risk of procedure-related complications. In our own clinical series, there were no severe complications (no arrhythmias, no hemodynamic complications or ischaemia, no thrombotic or embolic complications). All patients were treated with low-dose heparin followed by either aspirin or coumarin derivatives for at least 3 months after the procedure. This very low incidence of severe complications has been confirmed by other groups [14, 25–27, 30]. The only significant complication in man was reported by Steinbach et al. [92]. After repeated unipolar energy discharges for ablation of the AV-junction, the distal ('active') catheter electrode broke off the catheter and remained in the heart when the catheter was removed. This fracture of the electrode was presumably due to overheating of the catheter tip. Temperature monitoring might have prevented this severe complication.

In our series of ablation of various types of arrhythmias (see also Borggrefe et al. in this book), mild chest pain or discomfort occurred during energy discharge in about 40% of patients. In 2 patients (not belonging to those with ventricular tachycardia), general anaesthesia was necessary because of intense chest pain during radio-frequency application.

Arrhythmogenic potential

In animal studies, we and others have rarely observed the induction of severe ventricular tachyarrhythmias [44, 53]. During delivery of radio-frequency current to ventricular myocardium using a unipolar electrode configuration, ventricular fibrillation was induced in two animals when the impulse was not synchronised to the QRS complex. Other data showed that the arrhythmias preferentially occurred immediately after the onset of energy discharge, and that they can be prevented by QRS-synchronized current delivery [93]. For still unknown reasons, severe ventricular arrhythmias seem to occur more often during bipolar as compared to unipolar radio-frequency current application [44].

Risk of perforation

Perforation of the left ventricular wall has been observed in the experimental animal [52]. This complication was seen during radio-frequency ablation at high-power settings and a high-contact pressure. Perforation of ventricular myocardium might have been related to overheating of the coagulating electrode resulting in arching. Perforation may thus be prevented by automatic discontinuation of current flow as soon as a sudden increase in the impedance occurs or, again, by a tip temperature feed-back control mechanism of the power output.

Future perspectives

The use of radio-frequency currents seems to be feasible and relatively save for the management of ventricular tachyarrhythmias. This technique seems to have both potential theoretical and practical advantages particularly with respect to unwanted side effects and procedure-related complications. Our clinical experience with the use of radio-frequency energy for the treatment of drug-refractory ventricular tachyarrhythmias is still limited. Larger studies are obviously needed using improved techniques such as catheter tip temperature monitoring before more definite conclusions on the clinical usefulness of this technique can be drawn.

In the future, a better design of the electrode catheters with the possibility of monitoring the effects on the tissue are mandatory. Furthermore, a stable electrode-tissue contact is necessary to allow the induction of more extended lesions. In addition, more precise localization techniques such as the delineation of the area of slow conduction within the reentrant circuit might help to improve the feasibility of radio-frequency catheter ablation. With regard to the radio-frequency generators, power-regulated or temperature-guided devices seem to have advantages over the currently available designs. Thus, this presently still experimental technique seems to be promising for the future.

References

1. Gallagher JJ, Svenson H, Kasell JH, Lerman LD, Bardy GH, Broughton A, Critelli G (1982) Catheter technique for ablation of the atrioventricular conduction system. *N Engl J Med* 306: 194–200.
2. Scheinman MM, Morady F, Hess DS, Gonzales R (1982) Catheter-induced ablation of the atrioventricular junction to control refractory supraventricular arrhythmias. *JAMA* 248: 851–855.
3. Scheinman MM, Evans-Bell T and the Executive Committee of the Percutaneous Cardiac Mapping and Ablation Registry. (1984) Catheter ablation of the atrioventricular junction: a report of the percutaneous mapping and ablation registry. *Circulation* 70: 1024–1029.
4. Morady F, Scheinman MM (1984) Transvenous catheter ablation of a posteroseptal accessory pathway in a patient with the Wolff-Parkinson-White syndrome. *N Engl J Med* 310: 705–707.
5. Fisher JJ, Brodman R, Kim SG et al. (1984) Attempted nonsurgical electrical ablation of accessory pathways via the coronary sinus in the Wolff-Parkinson-White syndrome. *J Am Coll Cardiol* 4: 685–694.
6. Fontaine G, Frank R, Tonet JL, Cansell A, Grosgogeat Y (1984) Catheter ablation of ventricular tachycardia (abstr). *Eur Heart J* 5 (abstr suppl 1): 127.
7. Hartzler GO (1983) Electrode catheter ablation of refractory focal ventricular tachycardia. *J Am Coll Cardiol* 2: 1107–1113.
8. Breithardt G, Borggrefe M, Karbenn U, Scharzmaier J, Laucevicius A (1986) Therapie refraktärer ventrikulärer Tachykardien durch transvenöse, elektrische Ablation. *Z Kardiol* 75: 80–90.
9. Borggrefe M, Breithardt G, Podczeck A, Rohner D, Budde Th, Martinez-Rubio A (1989)

Catheter ablation of ventricular tachycardia using defibrillator pulses: electrophysiological findings and long-term results. *Eur Heart J* 10: 591–601.

10. Evans GT, Scheinman MM (1988) The percutaneous cardiac mapping and ablation registry: final summary of results. *Pace* 11: 1621–1626.

11. Budde Th, Borggrefe M, Podczeck A, Jacob B, Langwasser J, Frenzel H, Breithardt G (1987) Radiofrequency ablation: an improvement of ablation techniques in comparison to direct-current delivery? In: Breithardt G, Borggrefe M, Zipes DP (eds), *Non-Pharmacological Therapy of Tachyarrhythmias*, pp. 221–241. Mount Kisco: Futura Publishing Company.

12. Hindricks G, Haverkamp W, Gülker H, Rissel U, Budde T, Richter KD, Borggrefe M, Breithardt G (1989) Radiofrequency coagulation of ventricular myocardium: improved prediction of lesions size by monitoring catheter tip temperature. *Europ Heart J* 10: 972–984.

13. Hindricks G, Haverkamp W, Pfennigs W, Rissel U, Gülker H, Breithardt G (1989) Hochfrequenzablation mit automatischer Leistungsanpassung—akute and subakute Geweebeeffekte. *Kardiol* 78 (suppl 1): 35 (abstr).

14. Hoffmann E, Haberl R, Pulter R, Dainat C (1987) Phase displacement between voltage and current during radiofrequency catheter ablation. *Circulation* 76 (suppl V): IV–278 (abstr).

15. Hoyt RH, Huang SK, Markus FI (1987) Factors influencing trans-catheter radiofrequency ablation of the myocardium. *J Appl Cardiol* 1: 469–486.

16. Huang SK, Lee MA, Bazgan ID, Chang MS (1988) Radiofrequency catheter ablation of the atrioventricular junction for refractory supraventricular tachyarrhythmias. *Circulation* 78 (suppl II): II–156 (abstr).

17. Huang SK, Bharati S, Graham AR, Lev M, Marcus FI, Odell RC (1987) Closed chest catheter desiccation of the atrioventricular junction using radiofrequency energy—a new method of catheter ablation. *J Am Coll Cardiol* 9: 349–358.

18. Huang SK, Bharati S, Lev M, Marcus FI (1987) Electrophysiologic and histologic observations of chronic atrioventricular block induced by closed-chest catheter desiccation with radiofrequency energy. *Pace* 10: 805–816.

19. Huang SK, Garham AR, Hoyt RH, Odell RC (1987) Transcatheter desiccation of the left ventricle using radiofrequency energy: a pilot study. *Am Heart J* 114: 42–48.

20. Huang SK, Graham AR, Bharati S, Lee M, Gorman G, Lev M (1988) Short and long-term effects of transcatheter ablation of the coronary sinus by radiofrequency energy. *Circulation* 78: 416–427.

21. Hunalin A, Saksena S (1989) Comparative effects of radiofrequency and laser ablation in normal and diseased ventricular myocardium. *Am Coll Cardiol* 13: 175A (abstr).

22. Jackman WM, Kuck KH, Naccareli GV, Carmen L, Pitha J (1988) Radiofrequency current directed across the mitral anulus with a bipolar epicardial-endocardial catheter electrode configuration in dogs. *Circulation* 78: 1288–1298.

23. Kottkamp H, Hindricks G, Haverkamp W, Krater L, Rissel U, Borggrefe M, Gülker H, Breithardt G (1989) Significance of electrode configuration and temperature monitoring during transcatheter radiofrequency application for ablation of left-sided accessory pathways. *Europ Heart J* 10: 221 (abstr).

24. Kuck KH, Kunze KP, Müller HJ, Antz M (1987) Physical concepts for the application of radiofrequency current at the left atrioventricular ring. *Pace* 10: 426 (abstr).

25. Kuck KH, Kunze KP, Geiger M, Schlüter M (1989) Attempted ablation of left-sided accessory pathways by radiofrequency current. *J Am Coll Cardiol* 13: 168A (abstr).

26. Kuck KH, Kunze KP, Schlüter M, Geiger M, Jackman WM, Naccarelli V (1988) Modification of left-sided accessory pathway by radiofrequency current using bipolar epicardial-endocardial electrode configuration. *Europ Heart J* 9: 927–933.

27. Kunze KP, Kuck KH, Schlüter M (1989) Radiofrequency or direct current for ablation of ventricular tachycardia. *J Am Coll Cardiol* 13: 176A (abstr).

28. Kunze KP, Schlüter M, Kuck KH (1988) Modulation of AV nodal conduction: definitive treatment for AV nodal tachycardia? *Circulation* 78: II 304 (abstr).

29. Langberg J, Griffin JC, Herre JM, Chin MC, Lev M, Bharati S, Scheinman MM (1989) Catheter ablation of accessory pathways using radiofrequency energy in the canine coronary sinus. *J Am Coll Cardiol* 13: 491–496.
30. Langberg JJ, Chin MC, Herre JM, Griffin, Dullet N, Scheinman MM (1989) Catheter ablation of the atrioventricular junction using radiofrequency energy. *J Am Coll Cardiol* 13: 169A (abstr).
31. Lavergne TL, Sebag CI, Guize LJ, Blanc JJ, le Heuzey JY, Mottè GA, Bèrad TJ, Ourbak PA (1988) Transcatheter radiofrequency modification of atrioventricular conduction for refractory supraventricular tachycardia. *Circulation* 78 (suppl II): II-305 (abstr).
32. Lavergne T, Prunier L, Cuize L, Bruneval P, van Euw D, le Herzey JY, Peronneau P (1989) Transcatheter radiofrequency ablation of atrial tissue using a suction catheter. *Pace* 12: 177–186.
33. Marcus FI, Blouin LT, Bharati S, Lev M, Wharton K (1988) Production of first degree atrioventricular block in dogs, using closed chest electrode catheter with radiofrequency. *J Electrophysiol* 2: 315–326.
34. Naccarelli GV, Rinkenberger L, Dougherty AH, Fitzgerald DM, Zinner A, Kuck KH, Jackman WM (1989) Successful radiofrequency catheter ablation of right anteroseptal accessory atrioventricular connections. *J Am Coll Cardiol* 13: 176A (abstr.)
35. Blouin LT, Marcus FI (1989) The effect of electrode design on the efficacy of delivery of radiofrequency energy to cardiac tissue in vitro. *Pace* 12: 136–143.
36. Borggrefe M, Budde T, Podczeck A, Breithardt G (1987) High frequency alternating current ablation of accessory pathway in humans. *J Am Coll Cardiol* 10: 576–582.
37. Borggrefe M, Karbenn U, Haverkamp W, Hindricks G, Breithardt G (1989) Radiofrequency ablation of accessory pathways. *Pace* 12: 644 (abstr).
38. Borggrefe M, Budde Th, Podczeck A, Breithardt G (1987) Hochfrequenzablation der atrioventrikulären Überleitung und akzessorischer Leitungsbahnen—Erste klinische Erfahrungen. *Z Kardiol* 76 (suppl 1): 59 (abstr).
39. Borggrefe M, Budde Th, Podczeck A, Breithardt G (1987) Application of transvenous radiofrequency alternating current ablation in humans. *Circulation* 76 (suppl IV): IV–406 (abstr).
40. Budde Th, Breithardt G, Borggrefe M, Podczeck A, Langwasser J (1987) Erste Erfahrungen mit der Hochfrequenzstromablation des AV-Leitungssystems beim Menschen. *Z Kardiol* 76: 204–211.
41. Budde Th, Borggrefe M, Martinez-Rubio, Karbenn U, Haverkamp W, Hindricks G, Breithardt G (1989) Ergebnisse der Hochfrequenz-Katheterablation des AV-Überleitungssystems beim Menschen. *Z Kardiol* 78 (suppl 1): 18 (abstr).
42. Budde Th, Borggrefe M, Martinez-Rubio A, Karbenn U, Breithardt G (1989) Late occurrence of total AV-block after initially only partial destruction of the AV-conduction system with catheter ablation. 4th European Symposium on Cardiac Pacing, Stockholm, May 28th–31st 1989, Abstract Book: 138.
43. Davis MJE, Murdock CJ, Cope GD, Kallas IJ, Lovett MD (1988) Radiofrequency catheter ablation for refractory arrhythmias. *Pace* 11: 918 (abstr).
44. Franklin JO, Oeff M, Langberg JJ, Herre JM, Griffin JC, Chin MC, Scheinman MM (1988) Arrhythmias during unipolar and bipolar radiofrequency catheter ablation in the canine ventricle. *Pace* 11: 489 (abstr).
45. Franklin JO, Langberg JJ, Oeff M, Finkbeiner WE, Herre JM, Griffin JC, Scheinman MM (1989) Catheter ablation of canine myocardium with radiofrequency energy. *Pace* 12: 170–176.
46. Furman R, Gadhoke A, Osypka P, Saksena S (1987) Feasibility of radiofrequency ablation of supraventricular and ventricular tachyarrhythmias. *Pace* 10: 414 (abstr).
47. Haines DE, Watson DD, Cidio H (1987) Monitoring electrode tip temperature during radiofrequency fulguration of ventricular myocardium is strongly predictive of lesions size. *Circulation* 76: IV–406 (abstr).
48. Haines DE (1988) Impedance rise during radiofrequency ablation is due to sudden boiling

at the catheter tip and is prevented by tip temperature monitoring. *Circulation* 78 (suppl II): II–156 (abstr).

49. Haverkamp W, Hindricks G, Rissel U, Behrenbeck Th, Gülker H (1987) Determinanten der endokardialen Hochfrequenz-Katheterablation. *Herzschrittmacher* 7: 63 (abstr).

50. Haverkamp W, Hindricks G, Gülker H, Rissel U, Pfennings W, Borggrefe M, Breithardt G (1989) Coagulation of ventricular myocardium using radiofrequency energy: Bio-physical aspects and experimental findings. *Pace* 12: 187–195.

51. Haverkamp W, Hindricks G, Rissel U, Budde T, Pfennings W, Gülker H, Breithardt G (1989) Temperature-guided radiofrequency coagulation of myocardial tissue. *J Am Coll Cardiol* 13: 169A (abstr).

52. Hindricks G, Haverkamp W, Rissel U, Richter KD, Gülker H (1988) Experimental observations on the use of radiofrequency energy for ablation of ventricular tissue. *New Trends Arrhyt* IV: 337–342.

53. Hindricks G, Haverkamp W, Dute U, Richter KD, Gülker H (1988) Inzidenz ventrikulärer Arhythmien nach Gleichstromablation, Hochfrequenzstromablation und Laser-Photo-ablation. *Z Kardiol* 77: 696–703.

54. Gonzalez R, Scheinman M, Margaretten W, Rubinstein M (1981) Closed-chest electrode-catheter technique for His bundle ablation in dogs. *Am J Physiol* 241: H283–H287.

55. Coltorti F, Bardy G, Reichenbach D, Greene HL, Thomas R, Breazale DG, Alferness C, Ivey TD (1985) Catheter-mediated electrical ablation of the posterior septum via the coronary sinus: electrophysiologic and histologic observations in dogs. *Circulation* 72: 612–622.

56. Bardy GH, Ideker RE, Kasell J, Worley SJ, Smith WM, German LD, Gallagher JJ (1983) Transvenous ablation of the atrio-ventricular conduction system in dogs: electrophysiologic and histologic observations. *Am J Card* 51: 1775–1782.

57. Kempf FC jr, Falcone RA, Marchlinski FE, Josephson ME (1984) The electrophysiologic effects of high energy electrical discharges in the ventricle. *J Am Coll Cardiol* 3: 554 (abstr).

58. Lerman BB, Weiss JL, Bulkley BH, Becker LC, Weisfeldt ML (1984) Myocardial injury and induction of arrhythmia by direct current shock delivered via endocardial catheters in dogs. *Circulation* 69: 1006–1012.

59. Doherty PW, McLaughlin PR, Billingham M, Kernoff R, Goris ML, Harrison DC (1979) Cardiac damage produced by direct current countershock applied to the heart. *Am J Cardiol* 43: 225–232.

60. Anderson HN, Reichenbach D, Steinmetz GP, Merendino KA (1964) An evaluation and comparison of effects of alternating and direct current electrical discharges on canine hearts. *Ann Surg* 160: 251.

61. Van Vleet JF, Tacker WA jr, Geddes LA, Ferrans VJ (1978) Sequential cardiac morpho-logic alterations induced in dogs by single transthoracic damped sinusoidal waveform defibrillator shocks. *Am J Vet Res* 39: 271–278.

62. Van Vleet JF, Tacker WA jr, Geddes LA, Ferrans VJ (1978) Sequential ultrastructural alterations in ventricular myocardium of dogs given large single transthoracic damped sinusoidal waveform defibrillator shocks. *Am J Vet Res* 41: 493–501.

63. Ward DE, Davies M (1984) Transvenous high energy shock for ablating atrioventricular conduction in man — Observations on the histological effects. *Br Heart J* 51: 175–178.

64. Boyd EG, Holt PM (1985) Advantages of using cathodal impulses for electrical ablation in the left ventricle. *Circulation* 72, suppl III: 390 (abstr).

65. Nathan AW, Bennet DH, Ward DE, Bexton RS, Camm AJ (1984) Catheter ablation of atrioventricular conduction. *Lancet* 1: 1280–1287.

66. Bardy GH, Coltorti F, Ivey TD, Alferness C, Rackson M, Hansen K, Stewart R, Greene L (1986) Some factors affecting bubble formation with catheter-mediated defibrillator pulses. *Circulation* 73: 525–538.

67. Kunze KP, Schlüter M, Costard A, Nienhaber CA, Kuck KH (1985) Right atrial thrombus formation after transvenous catheter ablation of the atrioventricular node. *J Am Coll Cardiol* 6: 1428–1430.

68. Fisher JD, Kim SG, Matos JA, Waspe LE, Brodman R, Merav A (1985) Complications of catheter ablation of tachyarrhythmias: occurrence, protection, prevention. *Clin Prog Electrophys and Pacing* 4: 292–298.
69. Uebis R, Recker S, Diederich KJ, Effert S (1985) Belastbarkeit verschiedener Katheter für die elektrische Unterbrechung der AV-Überleitung. *Z Kardiol* 74: 714–717.
70. Lerman BB, Weiss JL, Bulkley BH, Becker LC, Weisfeldt ML (1984) Myocardial injury and induction of arrhythmia by direct current shock delivered via endocardial catheter in dogs. *Circulation* 69: 1006.
71. Westveer DC, Nelson T, Stewart JR, Thornton EP, Gordon S, Timmis GC (1985) Sequelae of left ventricular electrical endocardial ablation. *JACC* 5: 956–960.
72. Kempf FC, Falcone RA, Iozzo RV, Josephson ME (1985) Anatomic and hemodynamic effects of catheter-delivered ablation energies in the ventricle. *Am J Cardiol* 56: 373–377.
73. Fontaine G, Frank R, Tonet JL, Cansell A, Grosgogeat Y (1984) Catheter ablation of ventricular tachycardia. *Eur Heart J* 5: (suppl): I–127 (abstr).
74. Huang SK, Marcus FI, Ewy GA (1985) Clinical experience with endocardial catheter ablation for refractory ventricular tachycardia. *JACC* 5: 473 (abstr).
75. Klein H, Werner PC, Kühn E, Frank G, Lichtlen PR (1985) Behandlung von Kammer-tachykardien durch Ablation über Elektrokatheter. *Z Kardiol* 74: (suppl) III–97 (abstr).
76. Puech P, Gallay P, Grolleau R, Koliopoulus N (1984) Traitement par électrofulguration endocvitaire d'une tachycardie ventriculaire droite. *Arch Mal Coeur* 77: 826–834.
77. Ruffy R, Kim SS, Lal R (1985) Paroxysmal fascicular tachycardia: electrophysiologic characteristics and treatment by catheter ablation. *JACC* 5: 1008–1014.
78. Scheinman MM (1985) Electrical ventricular endocardial ablation: a tomato ripe or rotted? *JACC* 5: 961–962.
79. Borggrefe M, Breithardt G (1986) Ectopic atrial tachycardia after transvenous catheter ablation of a posteroseptal accessory pathway. *J Am Coll Cardiol* 8: 441–445.
80. Borggrefe M, Martinez-Rubio A, Budde Th, Karbenn U, Block M, Chen X, Breithardt G (1989) Ablation of ventricular tachycardia foci. *Eur Heart J* 10 (abstr suppl): 222.
81. Levine JH, Spear JF, Weisman HF, Kadish AH, Prood C, Siu CO, Moore EN (1986) The cellular electrophysiologic changes induced by high-energy electrical ablation in canine myocardium. *Circulation* 73: 818–829.
82. Bellmann G, Börner G, Kirsch E (1962) Elektrochirurgie. In: Handbuch medizinischer Elektronik I, VEB Verlag Technik, Berlin.
83. Kirsch E, Koenig G (1965) Das Elektrochirurgiegerät. *Medizintechnik* 5: H.3.
84. Oringer MJ (1969) Evaluation of dental electro-surgical devices. *J Amer Dent Ass* 78: 799–802.
85. Seemen v. H (1965) Die praktische Bedeutung der Elektrochirurgie. *Dtsch Z Chir* 284: 536.
86. Reidenbach HD (1983) *Hochfrequenz- und Lasertechnik in der Medizin*. Springer Verlag, Berlin, Heidelberg, New York.
87. Bharati S, Lev M (1989) Histopathologic changes in the heart including the conduction system after catheter ablation. *Pace* 12: 159–169.
88. Ring ME, Huang SK, Graham AR, Gorman G, Bharati S, Lev M (1987) Trans-septal catheter ablation with radiofrequency. *Circulation* 76 (suppl IV): IV–279 (abstr).
89. Goy JJ, Kappenberger L (1988) Different techniques for catheter ablation. *Pace* 11: 910 (abstr).
90. Gonska BD, Brune S, Bathge KP, Kreuzer H (1988) Catheter ablation of ventricular tachycardia with high frequency current. *Europ Heart J* 9 (suppl 1): 263 (abstr).
91. Klein H., personal communication.
92. Frohner G, Podczeck A, Steinbach K. Submitted for publication.
93. Rissel U, Hindricks G, Haverkamp W, Gülker H (1989) Arrhythmieinduktion unter EKG-getriggerter Hochfrequenzablation. *Z Kardiol* 78 (suppl I): 40 (abstr).
94. Saksena S, Marcantuono D, Janssen M, Osypka P (1988) Pulsed radiofrequency ablation with conventional electrode catheters: experimental studies and early clinical observations. *Pace* 11: 489 (abstr).

33. Catheter ablation for arrhythmias using lasers

A. W. NATHAN

Introduction

At St Bartholomew's Hospital in London over 60 patients have been treated for supraventricular tachycardias with catheter ablation techniques. In addition a small number have been treated for ventricular tachycardia. In each case capacitive direct current shocks have been used. Many different sorts of energy sources can be used for catheter ablation. These include conventional capacitive direct current shocks and their derivatives, with a short time constant in order to try and avoid arcing, radiofrequency, ultrasound, and cryothermy, as well as lasers. However almost no experience has been gained using this latter mode of therapy, despite much interest using the laser elsewhere in the heart, for example, in the coronary arteries.

The objectives of catheter ablation are to create an effective lesion in order to destroy or modify an arrhythmia focus, circuit or conduction pathway. In doing this the very minimum damage should be caused to adjacent tissues which do not form a critical part of the arrythmia substrate. The type of energy used or its amount is quite unimportant providing that these objectives are adhered to.

When considering how to create an effective lesion for ablation many factors must be considered. Indeed it is not possible to define a single kind of lesion that would be suitable for all different arrhythmia types as different types of lesion are required for different arrhythmia substrates. Defining a lesion to destroy an accessory pathway is fairly straightforward and to cause complete ablation of AV conduction is not difficult, although the sort of lesion that should be created in patients with duality of AH conduction and AV nodal reentrant tachycardia is more difficult to define. More difficult still to define are lesions that are necessary for the treatment of ventricular tachycardia. As will be discussed elsewhere in this volume, patients with ventricular tachycardia have substrates of varying types and sizes with an area of slow conduction thought to be critical. Methods of identifying and mapping this area are still in their infancy.

If one considers classical, arcing capacitive of DC shock ablation there

V. Hombach et al. (eds), Interventional Techniques in Cardiovascular Medicine, 299–301.
© 1991 *Kluwer Academic Publishers.*

are a number of, by now well known, characteristics. Usually simple 'pacing' catheters are used and almost no special equipment is necessary. The injury is relatively uncontrolled and diffuse and barotrauma is produced which is probably unnecessary for its success. Except in patients in whom AV block is necessary the overall safety and efficacy is disappointing.

There has been some interest in using lasers as energy sources for catheter ablation. This is because lasers have been used to ablate arrhythmia substrates during open heart procedures and the experience is encouraging. Lasers can produce well defined lesions with little collateral damage and experience during open heart procedures has shown them to be potentially less proarrhythmic than other energy sources.

When considering lasers there are of many different types. The waveform may be continuous or pulsed. There are a number of different laser sources, including argon, Nd-Yag, excimer and flashlight excited dye. The different forms of lasers have different powers with different tissue specificities and cause different lesion profiles in terms of depth, surface area, collateral damage and so on. The time period required for ablation varies, as does the ease of coupling the laser fibres to the various different lasers. Continuous wave lasers with sources such as argon tend to produce ragged lesions with considerable collateral damage, whereas pulsed lasers, particularly dye and excimer lasers produce extremely discrete lesions with almost no collateral damage what so ever.

Whatever sort of laser is used a special catheter is required capable of both mapping and ablation. Exceptionally careful mapping will be necessary and fibres should be as flexible as possible to aid manoeuvrability although this is always difficult with optical fibres. Pressure on the catheter tip is essential and tissue contact is usually necessary as blood can form a barrier between the tissue to be lased and the laser fibre, some method of catheter fixation will be necessary as suggested by Weber et al. [1].

However, it must be remembered that operative experience has shown that in some cases very large lesions are necessary and intra-operative experience has shown, that a mean lesion size for successful therapy is 9 ± 6 cm$_2$.

At the time of writing the author is not aware of any human experience with catheter based laser ablation techniques for arrhythmias. Experimental work is also limited but Curtis et al. [2] have shown the feasibility of inducing AV block in the experimental situation using drugs, although perforation certainly occurred during their experience. Examining their results and also Weber's it is clear that the lesions caused are deep and narrow and would not be ideal for treating arrhythmias other than those dependent on the AV node and possibly AV accessory pathways. Of course it is certainly conceivable that with careful and limited lasing shallower lesions could be created.

At present lasers do not seem to be ideal energy sources for most forms of catheter ablation although it seems certain that different groups will continue with research, and that some experience will be gained in the human before too long. However it is very important that the lure of available technologies must be withstood by all those investigating this field and a systematic approach to ablation must define the necessary technology, rather than the other way around. Although this technology may turn out to be some form of laser, much development will be necessary before it becomes a realistic option.

References

1. Weber H, Enders S, Keiditsch E (1989) Percutaneous Nd: YAG laser coagulation of ventricular myocardium in dogs using a special electrode laser catheter. *Pace* 12: 899–910.
2. Curtis AB, Abela GS, Griffin JC, Hill JA, Normann SJ (1989) Transvascular argon laser ablation of atrioventricular conduction in dogs: feasibility and morphological results. *Pace* 12: 347–357.

34. Chemical ablation in the pig heart by subendocardial injection of ethanol via catheter

P. WEISMÜLLER, U. MAYER, P. RICHTER, F. HEIECK, M. KOCHS, M. HÖHER, B. KUHNT and V. HOMBACH

Introduction

There are different methods of interventional treatment for control of ventricular tachycardia, namely surgical ablation of the arrhythmogenic area, application of direct current (DC) or high frequency energy via catheter, and the implantation of an automatic cardioverter defibrillator. All these routinely used methods have their disadvantages: DC catheter ablation only succeeds in 33% of patients without further medication and in another 38% taking antiarrhythmic agents. Furthermore, this method has the burden of a high number of serious complications [1]. Operative resection of arrhythmogenic foci is effective, but perioperative mortality has to be taken into account. The number of implantations of a cardioverter defibrillator is increasing. But, these devices do not cure the patients, but rescue them in malignant arrhythmia. The patients are highly dependent on permanent control of the devices. These have to be exchanged frequently.

Therefore, there still is the need to find a safe and easily applicable method for ablation of arrhythmogenic areas in ventricular myocardium of patients faced with the risk of sudden cardiac death.

Local application of chemicals is able to damage arrhythmogenic myocardium. Already in 1964 complete heart block was induced in dogs by injection of formaldehyde in the region of His [2]. Damiano et al. [3] could lower ventricular fibrillation threshold in dogs by applying Lugol's solution on ventricular endocardium intraoperatively. Chilson et al. [4] were able to ablate an experimentally induced ventricular tachycardia in dogs in 60% by endocardial Phenol application at the focus of tachycardias intraoperatively. Inoue et al. [5] ablated Aconitine-induced ventricular tachycardia in dogs by intracoronary injection of alcohol. Brugada et al. [6] treated ventricular tachycardia in man by intracoronary ethanol injection after identification of the artery supplying the arrhythmogenic area with blood. Ayisi et al. [7] were able to damage the focus of tachycardias in 5 patients by direct subendocardial injection of ethanol during surgery.

V. Hombach et al. (eds), Interventional Techniques in Cardiovascular Medicine, 303–306.

It was the purpose of this study to characterize the effect of subendocardial application of ethanol via catheter in an experimental setting.

Methods

In 6 landrace pigs a 7 F bipolar catheter with lumen was placed in the left ventricle via sectio of the right A. carotis communis under general anesthesia with halothane. A 3 F catheter with an apical 2 mm needle was inserted through the lumen. Subendocardial injection was performed under fluoroscopic control. Different quantities and concentrations of ethanol and iopamidol (Solutrast[R]) were injected at the apex, lateral wall and septum of the heart (a) 2 ml ethanol 48% + iopamidol 50%; (b) 1 ml: ethanol 48% + iopamidol 50%; (c) 2 ml ethanol 72% − iopamidol 25%. In each animal 3 injections with the different solutions were performed during the procedure.

All animals were sacrificed 25 days later, the hearts were removed and a pathological (macroscopic and histologic) assessment for characterisation of lesions was performed: the Formalin-fixed hearts (175–220 gr) — cut in transverse sections (5–7 mm) from apex to base — were embedded in paraffine and stained H & E and v.Gieson-Elastica.

Dimensions of lesions were calculated as follows:

Area: Apicobasal diameter × circumferential diameter × $\pi/4$.
Volume: Area × depth /1.5

In two animals Holter monitoring was performed for 20 hours after the procedure.

Results

All pigs survived without further complications. Myocardial perforation with pericardial injection of the solution occurred twice without further problems. Ventricular tachycardias were seen only during the procedure of ethanol injection, partly induced mechanically. In two pigs Holter monitoring revealed only some single ventricular ectopic beats.

During pathological assessment most of the lesions were seen macro-

Table 1. Characteristics of lesions

Solution:	(a) n = 8	(b) n = 5	(c) n = 5
Maximum diameter (mm)	10.6 (± 3.1)	11.4 (± 3.4)	10.8 (± 3.4)
Area (mm^2)	49 (± 32)	47 (±29)	42 (± 18)
Volume (mm^3)	61 (± 41)	92 (± 92)	56 (± 19)

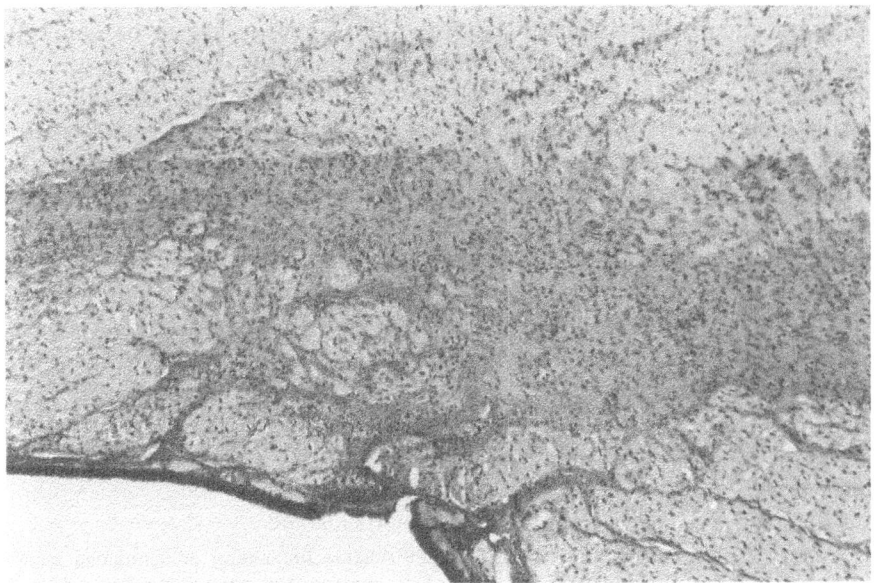

Figure 1. Subendocardial scar; Pig 3, lateral wall, magnification 200x, 0.5 ml ethanol + 0.5 ml iopamidol, v.Gieson Elastica.

scopically already. The scars were not configured like a ball: Figure 1 shows a typical scar. The lesion is oriented in the direction of the myocardial fibers. Scars were also seen along the vessels.

Table 1 shows the dimensions of the lesions.

Dimensions of lesions were not found to be highly dependent on quantity and concentration of ethanol in the used solutions, but on fibre orientation and presence of vessels at the site of injection. Mostly, the shape of the lesions resembled a disc in the subendocardium.

Discussion

To our knowledge the procedure of direct endocardial injection of chemicals via catheter without operation has not been studied, yet; in this experimental work dimensions of lesions were evaluated.

In the used model it is shown in 18 different ethanol injections that controlled myocardial damage can be achieved without major complications. More than one lesion can be induced during one procedure. Dimensions of myocardial damage are about 1/10 the volume of those seen during direct current application [8]. The lesions extend subendocardially. This is important, because it is known, that ventricular arrhythmias mostly originate from the endocardium [9].

In man DC ablation is performed in a zone of slow conduction in the reentrant circuit, the common pathway. This pathway has to be carefully identified by mapping techniques before ablation [10]. So, our results are preliminary, because arrhythmogenic areas did not have to be found before. Furthermore, in the used model ethanol was injected into normal myocardium. In humans the myocardium of arrhythmia origin is located in the borderzone of a scar. The pattern of distribution of ethanol may be different. These problems may be solved in a chronic infarction animal model before subendocardial ethanol application in man.

But we may conclude that percutaneous direct subendocardial application of ethanol causes controlled local necrosis and subsequent scarring of the lesion, which we suggest may be a promising new approach to ablate ventricular tachycardia.

References

1. Evans GT, Scheinmann MM (1986) Catheter ablation for control of ventricular tachycardia: a report of the percutaneous cardiac mapping and ablation registry. *Pace* 8 (II): 1391–1395.
2. Williams JCP, Lambert EH (1964) Production of heart block in dogs without thoracotomy. *Federation Proc* 23: 413 (abstr).
3. Damiano RJ, Smith PK, Fripp HF, Asano Tetsuo, Small KW, Lowe JE, Ideker RE, Cox JL (1986) The effect of chemical ablation of the endocardium on ventricular fibrillation threshold. *Circulation* 74 (3): 645–652.
4. Chilson DA, Peigh PS, Mahomed Y, Waller BF, Zipes DP (1986) Chemical ablation of ventricular tachycardia in the dog. *Am Heart J* 111: 1113–1118.
5. Inoue H, Waller BF, Zipes DP (1987) Intracoronary Ethyl alcohol or Phenol injection ablates Aconitine-induced ventricular tachycardia in dogs. *J Am Coll Cardiol* 10, 6 1342–1349.
6. Brugada P, de Swart H, Smeets JLRM, Wellens HJJ (1989) Transcoronary chemical ablation of ventricular tachycardia. *Circulation* 79: 475–482.
7. Ayisi K, Darup J, Drebber HJ, Rodewald G, Kuck KH (1989) Alcohol-induced Coagulation necrosis in cardia tissue: A new concept in the surgical management of recurrent ventricular arrhythmias. *Thorac cardiovasc surgeon* 37: 76–79.
8. Hauer RNW, Straks W, Borst C, Robles de Medina EO (1986) Electrical ablation in the left and right ventricular wall in dogs: relation between delivered energy and histopathologic changes. *J Am Coll Cardiol* 8: 637–643.
9. Harris L, Downar E, Mickleborough L, Parson I (1987) Activation sequence of ventricular tachycardia: endocardial and epicardial mapping studies in the human ventricle. *J Am Coll Cardiol* 10: 1040–1047.
10. Morady F, Frank R, Kou WH, Tonet CL, Nelson SD, Kounde S, Buitleir M, Fontaine G (1988) Identification and catheter ablation of a zone of slow conduction in the reentrant circuit of ventricular tachycardia in humans. *J Am Coll Cardiol* 11: 775–782.

35. Long-term results of antitachycardia electrotherapy in ventricular tachyarrhythmia

M. MANZ and B. LÜDERITZ

Introduction

The development of the implantable defibrillator (AICD) is considered a major advancement in the therapy of the sudden death syndrome, since for the first time recurrent ventricular fibrillation could be treated by this device [1–4]. In most patients with recurrent circulatory arrest, ventricular tachycardia is the primary arrhythmia, which can be interrupted by antitachycardia pacing. Though antitachycardia pacing may initiate ventricular fibrillation, it has several advantages as primary electrical therapy in patients with recurrent ventricular tachycardia: (a) availability without delay; (b) no relevant depletion of batteries; (c) painlessness [5, 6]. In addition, antibradycardia pacing is possible. Since antitachycardia pacing systems with back up defibrillation have not been readily available, two separate units had to be implanted in selected patients with recurrent ventricular tachycardia [7]. The longterm results of these patients are reviewed.

Patients and methods

Patients with recurrent ventricular tachycardia, which could be repeatedly terminated by overdrive pacing, were considered candidates for this type of treatment. Criteria for the combined use of the implantable defibrillator and antitachycardia pacemaker were (1) drug refractory, symptomatic, persistent monomorphic VT, which was sustained but did not deteriorate into ventricular fibrillation within 30s. (2) Termination of ventricular tachycardia had to be possible by a maximum of 6 synchronized ventricular premature beats (minimal interval 240 ms) from the apex of the right ventricle.

As automatic defibrillator, the AICD pulse generator was used in all patients together with two sensing electrodes and a pair of energy-discharging electrodes. As antitachycardia pacemaker, the 'Tachylog' antitachycardia device was implanted in all patients. Overdrive stimulation was selected. During operation, the signals of the sensing electrodes, the patch electrodes

V. Hombach et al. (eds), Interventional Techniques in Cardiovascular Medicine, 307–310.

and the bipolar electrode in the right ventricular apex were recorded. Defibrillation thresholds were determined. In addition, the possible interactions of the two electrical devices were assessed. After surgery, Holter monitoring was performed for 10 days. Thereafter, patients were followed on an outpatient basis at intervals of two months. By telemetry of the automatic implantable defibrillator, the charging time and the patients' pulse rate were determined. In addition, the number of tachycardia episodes, the rate of the last tachycardia and the rate increase of the last tachycardia could be counted [7].

Results

The antitachycardia devices (Tachylog and AICD) were implanted in 6 patients with a mean age of 60 +/−8 years. Five patients had coronary artery disease and one dilative cardiomyopathy. The rate of ventricular tachycardia at baseline in the electrophysiologic study was 209+/−10/min. Under antiarrhythmic drug treatment, the rate of VT decreased to 177+/−15/min. Since one patient died after 1 1/4 months due to heart failure and pneumonia, long-term results of five patients were available.

Follow-up

During the mean follow-up period of 56+/−7 months, five patients had one and three patients two AICD replacements; the Tachylog system had to be replaced in two cases due to battery depletion.

During a period of 2.5 years, patient I had 50 successful terminations of VT episodes at the same time, the AICD was activated 11 times. Thereafter reinfarction deteriorated the hemodynamic status of the patient, overdrive pacing became ineffective, and the antitachycardia pacing mode was switched off. The patient in congestive heart failures died 56 months after AICD implantation.

In patient II numerous VT episodes occurred, which were interrupted 448 times by overdrive pacing and 91 times by discharges of the AICD. Three periods of numerous interventions of the electrical device within a short period of time were observed in this patient. Therefore, activation of the system due to atrial tachyarrhythmias cannot be excluded. Another cause might have been the interaction of the two systems which is unlikely however, since one of these episodes occurred before the implantation of the Tachylog system. Overdrive pacing remained effective, and the length of the burst could be reduced from 4 to 2 stimuli.

In patient III, IV and V the vast majority of VT episodes could be stopped by the antitachycardia pacemaker, whereas the AICD was discharged only in few instances. Throughout the period of antitachycardia pacing, the VT could be reliably interrupted by burst pacing in these cases.

In this small group of patients, the successful use of antitachycardia pacing together with back-up defibrillation could be demonstrated during a follow-up period of 4 to 5 years. Except for one patient in which antitachycardia pacing became ineffective after 2.5 years, termination of the tachycardia episodes by burst pacing remained possible throughout that time. No sudden death occurred in the patient group.

A comparable high number of interventions of the antitachycardia pacemaker as well as AICD discharges were observed. There were several explanations for this observation: (1) The high number of spontaneous VT's was one of the reasons to select these patients for antitachycardia pacing. (2) The pacemaker identified ventricular tachycardia after four sensed intervals, therefore non-sustained ventricular tachycardia has triggered the termination mode of the Tachylog. (3) Since tachycardia detection and termination of the pacemaker had to be completed before the AICD was charged, only 1 to 2 pacemaker interventions were possible. (4) The antitachycardia pacemaker has activated the defibrillator in some instances, in case the burst was followed by some ventricular premature beats.

In advanced antitachycardia devices, programmability of the detection mode and detection time will avoid most of these limitations. It can be expected, that the combination of antitachycardia overdrive pacing together with back-up defibrillation will become a successful therapy in patients with recurrent ventricular tachycardia [8].

Table 1

Pat. no.	Age (yrs) and sex	VT rate (min^{-1})	AICD cut-off rate	Tachylog	Follow-up AICD	months
I	66 m	171	156	50	57	46
II	53 m	160	156	448	91	65
III	70 m	162	156	326	20	51
IV	59 m	188	156	505	19	59
V	63 m	182	173	428	33	61
VI	50 m	200	156	∅	8	11/4

References

1. Mirowski M, Reid PR, Watkins L, Weisfeldt ML, Mower MM (1981) Clinical treatment of life-threatening ventricular tachyarrhythmias with the automatic implantable defibrillator. *Am Heart J* 102: 265.
2. Mirowski M, Reid PR, Winkle RA, Mower MM, Watkins L, Stinson EB, Griffith LSC, Kallman CH, Weisfeldt ML (1983) Mortality in patients with implantable automatic defibrillators. *Ann Intern Med* 98: 585.
3. Echt DS, Armstrong K, Schmidt P, Oyer PE, Stinson EB, Winkle RA (1985) Clinical experience, complications, and survival in 70 patients with the automatic implantable cardioverter/defibrillator. *Circulation* 71: 289.

4. Winkle RA, Mead RH, Ruder MA, Gaudiani VA, Smith NA, Buch WS, Schmidt P, Shipman T (1989) Long-term outcome with the automatic implantable cardioverter-defibrillator. *J Am Coll Cardiol* 13: 1353.
5. Fisher JD, Mehra R, Furman S (1978) Termination of ventricular tachycardia with burst of rapid ventricular pacing. *Am J Cardiol* 41: 94.
6. Lüderitz B, Naumann d'Alnoncourt C, Steinbeck G, Beyer J (1982) Therapeutic pacing in tachyarrhythmias by implanted pacemakers. *Pace* 5: 366.
7. Manz M, Gerckens U, Funke HD, Kirchhoff PG (1986) Combination of antitachycardia pacemaker and automatic implantable cardioverter/defibrillator for ventricular tachycardia. *Pace* 9: 676.
8. Newman DM, Lee MA, Heere JM, Langberg JJ, Scheinman MM, Griffin JC (1989) Permanent antitachycardia pacemaker therapy for ventricular tachycardia. *Pace* 12: 1387.

36. Implantable cardioverter-defibrillators: patient selection, devices and results

A. J. CAMM, M. A. de BELDER and G. A. HAYWOOD

Introduction

Over 8000 patients have received implantable cardioverter-defibrillators (ICDs) over the last 10 years and the rate of implantation continues to increase. ICDs are now an accepted therapeutic modality in the management of patients with recurrent ventricular arrhythmias and are uniquely suited to certain patient groups [4]. There are however problems associated with their use in terms of cost, patient acceptability and the need for device renewal which mean that the devices are far from a panacea for sudden cardiac death.

Patient selection

ICDs must be considered within the context of the overall management strategy for patients with recurrent ventricular arrhythmias. The goals of management are to prevent sudden death or the recurrence of symptomatic arrhythmias. The techniques used to achieve this should minimise the need for invasive investigation and therapy and result in as few long term side effects for the patient as possible [1]. In addition, the large number of patients involved, means that the economic impact of different therapies must be considered.

The therapeutic options can be summarised as:

1. No treatment.
2. Drug therapy with single or multiple agents.
3. Surgery—Aneurysmectomy, subendocardial resection, encircling procedures, cryotherapy.
4. Catheter ablation techniques.
5. Implantable cardioverter-defibrillators.

There is no universally accepted protocol for selection of therapy in recurrent ventricular arrhythmias. One approach has been to use exhaustive

311

V. Hombach et al. (eds), Interventional Techniques in Cardiovascular Medicine, 311–317.

serial testing with different drug treatments chosen on a trial and error basis with evaluation of efficacy by ambulatory monitoring or programmed electrical stimulation. Only when the patient remains inducible after therapeutic trials of several drugs are other modalities considered. This is a prolonged, traumatic process for the patient and places major demands on acute cardiology units in terms of bed occupancy and physician and catheter laboratory time. Alternatively a more 'pragmatic' approach can be used.

The pragmatic approach

This can be summarised thus:
Select ideal candidates for definitive therapy:

a) ICD implantation.
b) Surgery.
c) Transplantation.
etc.

For the rest: Test inducibility after class 1 anti-arrhythmic agent — if non-inducible, select an antiarrhythmic drug according to clinical and electrophysiological parameters.
For the rest: Select best end strategy:

a) Amiodarone.
b) Surgery.
c) ICD.
d) Transplantation.

The indications for ICD implantation are generally taken as the occurrence of cardiac arrest that has not been caused by acute myocardial infarction, antiarrhythmic or other drug toxicity or severe electrolyte disturbance, or recurrent sustained life-threatening ventricular tachycardia (VT). Smaller numbers of patients receive the device because of syncopal episodes of undetermined cause and induction of nonsustained ventricular tachycardia at electrophysiological study or because of the existence of a familial syndrome of sudden death associated with inducible sustained VT. The 'ideal' candidate for management with an ICD would have infrequent episodes of ventricular arrhythmia associated with syncope. There is also a role for the ICD as part of combination therapy in patients whose frequency of arrhythmias has been reduced by drug therapy or surgery, but who still continue to experience infrequent episodes of ventricular arrhythmia or who remain inducible at electrophysiological study (EPS).

Currently available implantable cardioverter-defibrillators

The pace of technical developments in this field is such that each of the companies which are manufacturing ICD's are likely to produce a new model every nine months or so. The latest generation of devices are able to distinguish two, and sometimes more, tachycardias using a number of tachycardia detection criteria, and can respond in a number of preprogrammed ways. These include antitachycardia pacing modalities, low energy cardioversion and higher energy cardioversion-defibrillation. They also offer bradycardia support pacing, and have in-built Holter and/or telemetry facilities.

Tachycardia detection is possible using a number of programmable variables. These include heart rate, rate of onset of tachycardia, tachycardia duration and tachycardia 'stability'. The latter can be defined in terms of the variation in successive R-R intervals over a predetermined period of time, or as a series of R-R intervals of which the majority are less than the programmed detection interval. The Ventak devices (CPI) also incorporate an optional non-rate dependent criterion referred to as the 'probability density function' which is an index of the proportion of time that the electrocardiogram remains on the isoelectric line. The programmability of these devices in such that different criteria can be selected to define 'ventricular tachycardia' and 'ventricular fibrillation'; the triggered response of the device depends on how the tachyarrhythmia is interpreted. If cardioversion is the selected treatment, the device takes some time to charge up. To avoid inappropriate delivery of the stored energy to the patient in the case of a non-sustained tachycardia some of the devices require confirmation of continuing tachycardia before discharging.

Tachycardia termination can be achieved in a number of ways [2, 3]. In general, pacing techniques are better tolerated than low-energy cardioversion, which itself is better tolerated than high-energy cardioversion. Most of the latest devices incorporate sophisticated tachycardia termination pacing modalities. Although simple extrastimulation techniques are possible, it is clear that rate-related and/or decremental extrastimulus or burst pacing, together with the capacity to adapt the pacing sequence between one attempt at termination and another, provide effective and safe means of tachycardia termination. They also enable the device to cope with spontaneous changes in the characteristics of the target tachycardia and to treat two or more different tachycardias in the same patient. If pacing sequences fail to terminate the tachycardia, or, more disastrously, cause the tachycardia to accelerate or degenerate into ventricular fibrillation, then the device is triggered to deliver a cardioverting or defibrillating shock. Many of the devices now offer the capacity to deliver a sequence of responses depending on the characteristics of the tachycardia(s) suffered by the patient.

If, for example, a relatively slow sustained ventricular tachycardia is detected, the first response of the device might be an autodecrementing pacing sequence; if this fails, the second response could be similar, but after a preprogrammed change in the number, or coupling intervals, of the extra-stimuli in the pacing sequence; if tachycardia persists, the third attempt at termination could be low-energy cardioversion, and the fourth high-energy cardioversion. If a fast tachycardia is detected, the initial response of the device could be high-energy cardioversion.

Clinical experience has shown that the energy needed for successful defibrillation is often greater than 20 J, whereas monomorphic ventricular tachycardia can be terminated with much lower energies. Most devices deliver a maximal shock of 30–40 J, with lowest cardioverting energies of 0.1–3 J.

Unfortunately, tachycardia acceleration and degeneration can occur with cardioversion as well as pacing techniques. These will possibly be less of a problem with low-energy cardioversion. In addition, the use of different shock waveforms such as bidirectional and biphasic shocks or sequential shockwave therapy may enhance the efficacy and safety of tachycardia termination.

Electrode systems. At present, all devices use epicardial patch electrodes in addition to myocardial lead electrodes. Rate sensing is usually achieved with two myocardial unipolar electrodes. An option for a transvenous bipolar electrode which replaces these unipolar leads is available in the newest devices. If tachycardia detection in the Ventak series utilises the probability density function, then one of the patch electrodes is also used for sensing. Cardioversion is performed with two patch electrodes in all of the devices, although the PCD series (Medtronic) has an option for three patches, thus allowing for bidirectional shocks. An option for a vena caval spring electrode is now available in the Ventak series, and is becoming available with other manufacturer's devices. Transvenous cardioversion is thus possible, and in combination with patch electrodes, whether positioned epicardially, subcutaneously or submuscularly, this system can also be used to deliver bidirectional or (in some devices) sequential shocks.

Other facilities. All of the latest devices incorporate bradycardia support pacing. This is desirable because patients receiving these devices may sometimes suffer from significant bradycardias, and, in addition, successful tachycardia termination may be followed by temporary bradycardia. A range of Holter and telemetry facilities enable the physician to interrogate the device for details concerning the number of tachycardias detected and successfully (or unsuccessfully) terminated. Such facilities will improve the clinical follow-up of the patient.

The basic details of the latest devices available from the manufacturers are described in Table 1. The life-span of these newest devices is not yet known, but the manufacturers quote a maximum expected period (of the order of 4–5 years), which is then reduced by a period of 7–10 days for every higher energy shock delivered to the patient.

Table 1. The latest generation of ICD's

Manufacturer	CPI	Telectronics pacing systems	Medtronic	Intermedics	Ventritex	Siemens-pacesetter
Device	Ventak PRX	Guardian 4210	PCD 7217	The Res-Q	Cadence	Thor
Tachycardia detection criteria						
Trigger rate	+	+	+	+	+	+
Rate of onset	+	+	+	+	+	+
Duration	+	+	+	+	+	+
Stability	+	+	+	+	+	+
Other	PDF	–	–	–	–	–
Confirmation before discharge	+	+	– (VF) + (VT)	–	–	–
Differentiation of different tachycardias	+	+	+	+	+	+
Bradycardia pacing	+	+	+	+	+	+
Antitachycardia pacing	+	+	+	+	+	+
Programmable sequence of treatments	+	+	+	+	+	+
Highest stored energy	30 J	30 J	34 J	40 J	35 J	40 J
Minimal cardioversion energy	3 J	0.5 J	0.2 J	0.1 J	0.1 J	2.5J
Transvenous defibrillator electrodes	+	–	+	–	–	?
Weight	220 g	?	200 g	220 g	240 g	200 g

Key: PDF = probability density function; VF = ventricular fibrillation; VT = ventricular tachycardia ? = data not known.

Clinical outcome

The efficacy of implantable cardioverter-defibrillators in the treatment of ventricular tachyarrhythmias is now well established [3]. An estimated arrhythmic mortality rate of 2% or less at one year and 6% at 4 years is reported in the highly selected patients who have received a device. Total mortality is somewhat higher, with rates of about 8% at 1 year and 26% at 5 years (see Figure 1) [8]. Although a direct comparison with other studies is not valid because of different patient characteristics, these figures represent a major advance in the management of ventricular tachyarrhythmias. The sudden cardiac death rates after successful suppression of inducible ventricular tachycardia in survivors of cardiac arrest are 6% at 1 year, and 19% at 4 years. The same figures for patients treated empirically with amiodarone are 9% and 21% respectively. More recent evidence, however, suggests that the improved survival of patients with these devices diminishes after 3–4 years, with mortality rates after this time approaching those of similar

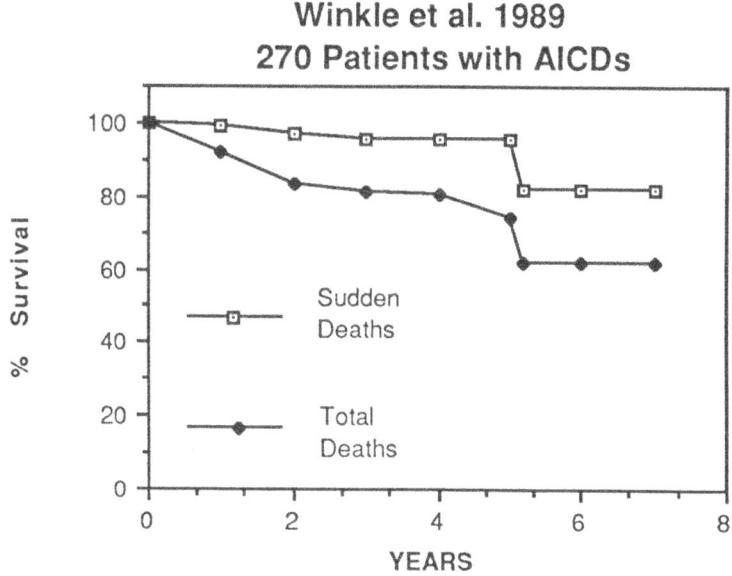

Figure 1.   Overall survival and incidence of sudden death after AICD implantation.

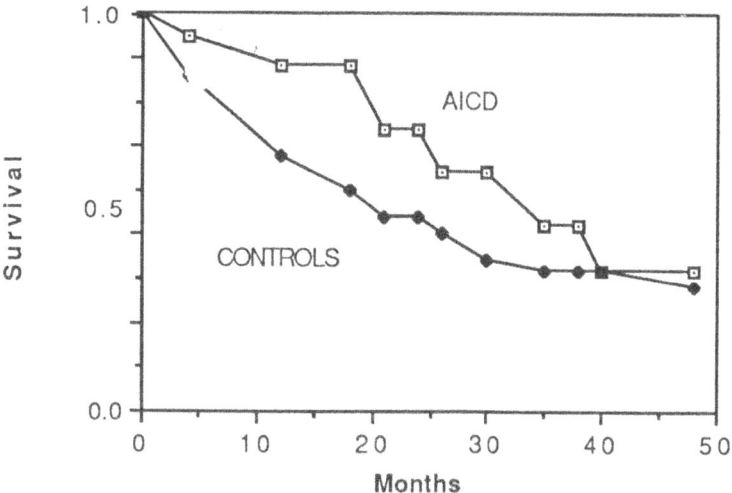

Figure 2.   Survival after AICD implantation compared with controls.

patients who have not received a device (Figure 2) [7]. It is also clear that the efficacy of these devices will depend largely on patient selection. Well-tolerated but recurrent sustained monomorphic tachycardia can be reliably terminated with pacing techniques in 60% of patients, but this is the same group for whom electrophysiologically guided drug therapy or surgery is effective. Patient and physician preference might then be a factor in the selection of treatment. Implantable devices would be expected to be highly effective in this group. In other patients, drug therapy may be ineffective or poorly tolerated, and the selection criteria for surgery excludes many higher risk patients from gaining benefit from a surgical option. In these patients, these devices may well be the only therapy that effectively improves prognosis as well as quality of life. Because of their high-risk nature, however, one must be guarded in forecasting the overall efficacy of implantable devices in this group. Recently (McAlister et al. *JACC* 1989; 13: 66A) [5], it has been demonstrated that those patients receiving the most shocks have the worst prognosis.

References

1. de Belder MA, Camm AJ (1989) Implantable cardioverter-defibrillators (ICDs) 1989: how close are we to the ideal device? *Clin Cardiol* 12: 339–345.
2. Fisher JD, Kim SG, Mercando AD (1988) Electrical devices for treatment of arrhythmias. *Am J Cardiol* 61: 45A–57A.
3. Kelly PA, Cannom DS, Garan H et al. (1988) The automatic implantable cardioverter-defibrillator: efficacy, complications and survival in patients with malignant ventricular arrhythmias. *JACC* 11: 1278.
4. Lehman MH, Steinman RT, Schuger CD, Jackson K (1988) The automatic implantable cardioverter defibrillator as antiarrhythmic modality of choice for survivors of cardiac arrest unrelated to acute myocardial infarction. *Am J Cardiol* 62: 803–805.
5. McAlister HF, Gross J, Castle LW et al. (1989) Automatic implantable cardioverter defibrillator: analysis of spontaneous shocks. *JACC* 13: 66A (abstr).
6. Mirowski M, Mower MM, Reid PR (1985) Management of sustained ventricular tachycardia. *JACC* 6: 213–214.
7. Newman D, Herre J, Sauve MJ et al. (1989) The automatic implantable cardioverter-defibrillator and patient survival: a case control study. *JACC* 13: 65A (abstr).
8. Winkle RA, Mead RH, Ruder MA et al. (1989) Long-term outcome with the automatic implantable cardioverter-defibrillator. *JACC* 13: 1353–1361.

37. Surgical ablation of ventricular tachycardias

A. HANNEKUM

Summary

Summarizing the hospital mortality and the long-term results of antitachy-cardiac surgery by regarding the actuarial long-term survival after onset of disease or operation (Figure 11) antitachycardiac surgery has a beneficial effect in this highly problematic patient population with drug refractory VT, comparing the outcome with the above mentioned natural history. After an initially high early hospital mortality rate of about 14% the direct endo-cardial operations for ablating or isolating the underlying arrhythmogenic tissue can improve the prognosis significantly. Regarding the initially high operative risk we have to be aware, that this data are including the learning curves and that future results can be improved by considering the risk factors for mortality and recurrence of VT in the selection of appropriate candidates.

For patients with a predictable high risk of operation alternative pro-cedures to the direct endocardial surgery such as the AICD, ablation techniques or cardiac transplantation should be discussed.

In case of an ischemic cause of VT, well defined inducible monomorphic VT, a discret area of dyskinesis or well demarked aneurysm and in case of a well preserved function of non aneurysmal ventricular wall the direct endomyocardial electrophysiological guided operation is at present still the therapy of choice with encouraging short- and long-term results compared with alternative therapies.

Introduction

With clinical evaluation of interventional ablative techniques for the treat-ment of supraventricular and ventricular tachycardias and extending indi-cations for implantation of antitachycardic devices, especially the automatic implantable cardioverter defibrillator, the indications for direct antitachy-cardic surgical operations are discussed more controversial. In contrast to

V. Hombach et al. (eds), Interventional Techniques in Cardiovascular Medicine, 319–332.
© 1991 *Kluwer Academic Publishers.*

some indications for ablation techniques the role of antitachycardic surgery concentrates on the treatment of *ischemic* recurrent sustained ventricular tachycardia with a *morphologic* arrhythmogenic substrate, predisposing electrophysiologic reentrant phenomena.

After the first antiarrhythmic operation in 1956 by Dr. Bailey[1]—resection of a left ventricular aneurysm with postoperative stabilized pre-existent ventricular tachycardia—a lot of indirect surgical approaches as revascularisation, sympathectomy and ventricular wall resection were proposed for the treatment of VT with at least disappointing short and long term results. With introduction of the mapping guided intraoperative electrophysiologic studies direct endocardial surgical ablating or isolating procedures, the *complete* encircling endocardial ventriculotomy, inaugurated by Giraudon [2] in 1978 and the endocardial resection by Harken [3] even in 1978 became standard in some specialized institutions. Several modifications of these techniques as the *partial* encircling ventriculotomy or the moderate endomyocardial incision are concentrating on a more limited circumscript intervention to avoid damage to the non arrhythmogenic and still contracting myocardium and therefore to reduce the initially high operative mortality caused by further deterioration of the mostly poor left ventricular function. This requires an intelligent intraoperative left ventricular endocardial activation mapping with identification of the arrhythmogenic area, showing the earliest endocardial activation during VT. If ventricular tachycardia is not inducible intraoperatively (in 25% of our patients), mostly because of the influence of general anesthesia, hypothermia or extracorporeal circulation, a pace-mapping can be helpfull. Furthermore even delayed fragmented and low amplitude signals during sinus rhythm can indicate the arrhythmogenic area. In this case a more extended operative procedure may be necessary to warrant the antiarrhythmic success.

In this book section it's our task to discuss the appropriate role of each therapeutic method in well defined patients. The challenge will remain to elucidate the specific variables, related to the details of the tachyarrhythmia and underlying derangements of cardiac structure and function, which influence the early and late overcome after each procedure. The review and comparison of all published data of individual institutions becomes more difficult because of the difference in the characteristics of the patient populations, the indications for the chosen procedures, the different surgical approaches, the different additional drug regimes and at least the different protocols during the electrophysiologic studies to control the antiarrhythmic success.

Therefore the comparison of the published data of antiarrhythmic operations have to be regarded restrictively. Furthermore in the past many inappropriate patients have been recommended to direct surgery, responsible for initially disastrous results.

Indications for antiarrhythmic surgery

The leading and up to now generally accepted indication for mapping guided surgery is the drug refractory life threatening ventricular tachycardia on the base of an ischemic disease with a morphologic arrhythmogenic substrate. Next even the controlled arrhythmia can indicate a surgical procedure in case of severe side effects of drugs, which force the withdrawal of medication. Furthermore antiarrhythmic surgery can be indicated as an additional procedure in case of primary indication for aortocoronary bypass grafting and/or ventricular wall resection and/or valve replacement. At least the patient with very frequent occurrences of VT, therefore an inappropriate candidate for the automatic implantible cardioverter defibrillator (AICD) and the patient in whom an ablation procedure was unsuccessful, should be treated surgically (Table 1).

Table 1. Indications for antitachycardiac surgery

1. Drug Refractory VT
2. Severe Side Effects of Drugs
3. Additional Indication for Revascularisation etc.
4. Frequence of VT (Contraindication for AICD)
5. Failure of Ablation Procedures

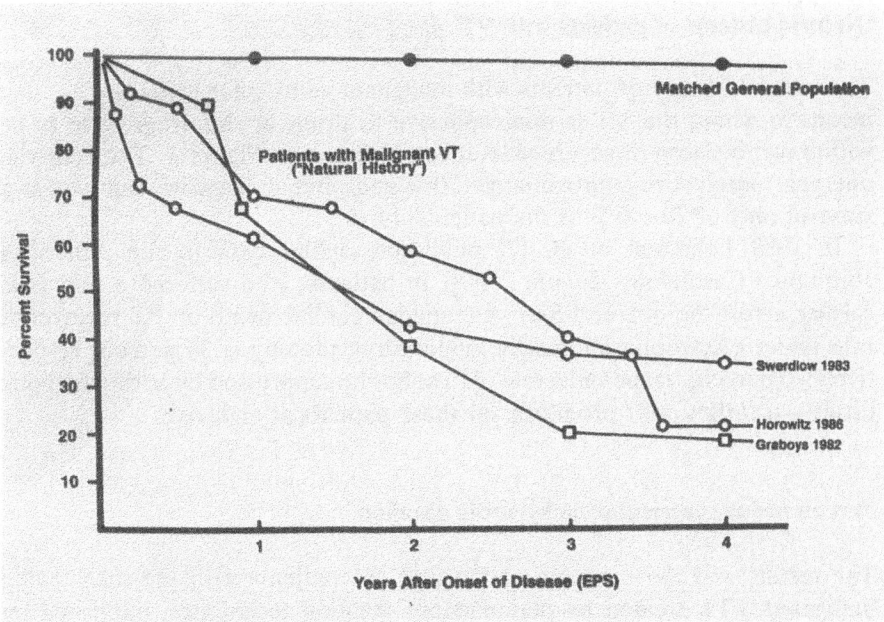

Figure 1. Long-term survival of patients with malignant VT ('natural history').

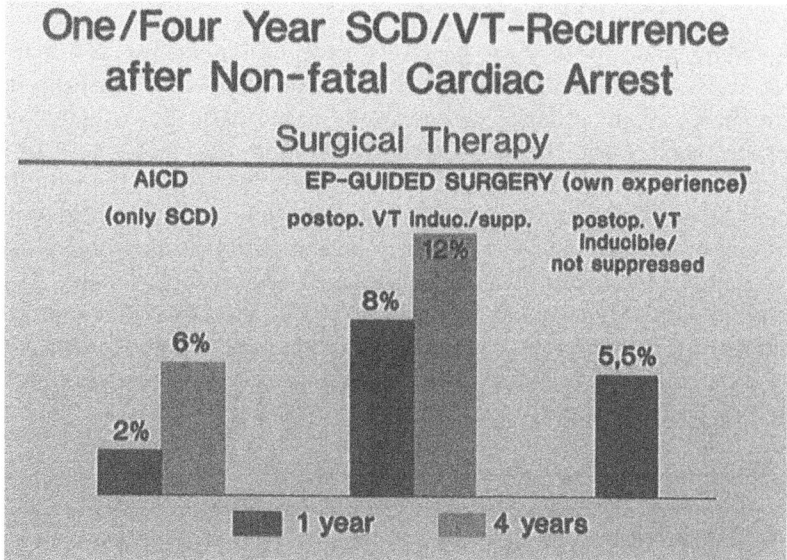

Figure 2. Influence of electrophysiologically guided drug therapy (Lehmann, American Journal of Cardiology, 1989).

'Natural history' of patients with VT

The natural history of patients with malignant ventricular tachycardias, that means in whom the VT is nonresponsive to drugs or the drugs have to be withdrawn because of severe side effects is shown in Figure 1. The actuarial one year survival is approximately 70% and after 4 years we can expect a survival only of 20–40% of the patients. [4–6].

In 1988 Lehmann et al. [7] published similar data in the American Journal of Cardiology (Figure 2) [7]. In patients, who suffered a non fatal cardiac arrest the one and four year sudden cardiac death or VT recurrence rate under electrophysiologically guided drug therapy is 34 percent respectively 70 percent, if the inducible VT cannot be suppressed by antiarrhythmic drugs—a rather poor prognosis for these patients at high risk.

Percutaneous ventricular tachycardia ablation

The results and the outcome of the first 141 patients with life threatening malignant VTs, treated by percutaneous ablation techniques, published by the percutaneous cardiac mapping and ablation registry in 1986 are as well discouraging (Figure 3) [8]. In the patients with an underlying ischemic disease the arrhythmocenic area was located in the left ventricle or the

Percutaneous Cardiac Mapping and Ablation Registry (1986)

Ventricular Tachycardia Ablation
in 141 Patients (89 CHD)

70%	single morphology	
22%	multiple unimorphic morphologies	
8%	polymorphic VT or VF	
localization RV		35%
localization LV		36%
localization septum		29%

Figure 3.

interventricular septum in more than 80%. This coincides with the intraoperative findings in our own experience. The response of therapy did not depend on the number and the different morphologies of the VT.

The mortality within a mean follow up period of 12 months was nearly 25% with 7 procedure related early deaths, 14 sudden deaths, 3 non cardiac deaths and 7 deaths caused by congestive heart failure (Figure 4).

The clinical response of 117 patients with a mean follow up of 12 months is not very encouraging as well. Only 33 patients remained asymptomatic without drugs and 35 patients showed no response to ablation (Figure 5).

With this in mind the surgical results have to be reviewed, especially the hospital mortality, the long term survival and the recurrence of VT or sudden cardiac death. Furthermore the factors influencing the success or failure of antitachycardiac surgery have to be evaluated.

Percutaneous Cardiac Mapping and Ablation Registry (1986)
Results of Ventricular Tachycardia Ablation

Mortality (mean follow up 12 months)

• procedure related early deaths	7
• sudden deaths (9 with documented VT)	14
• congestive heart failure	7
• noncardiac deaths	3
	31 patients

Figure 4.

Percutaneous Cardiac Mapping and Ablation Registry (1986)
Results of Ventricular Tachycardia Ablation

Clinical Response (mean follow up 12 months)

● asymptomatic without drugs	33 (28%)
● arrhythmia, controlled with drugs	49 (42%)
● no response	35 (30%)
	117 patients

Figure 5.

Concept for operative procedures in VT surgery

The operative technique in antitachycardiac operations requires an intelligent procedure, considering the intraoperative mapping findings as well as the anatomical and macroscopic morphology. Figure 6 represents the surgical concept of the authors working group in the first 42 patients (University of Cologne and Göttingen) [9]. As mentioned before the surgical technique should be kept as limited as possible to encompas and ablate exclusively the arrhythmogenic substrate and not to cause a deterioration of left ventricular function. On the other hand the more extensive the ablation procedure,

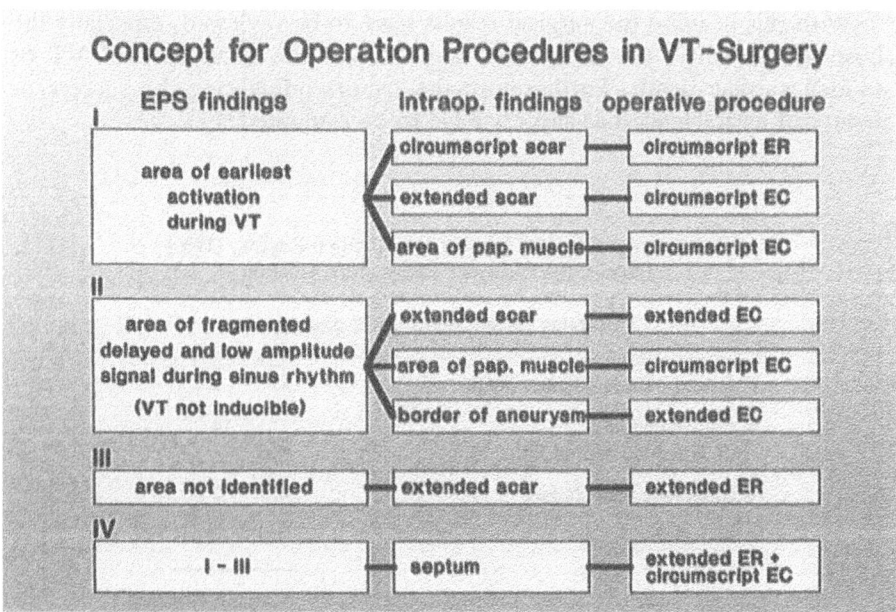

Figure 6.   ER = endocardial resection; EC = endomyocardial incision.

especially regarding the extended encircling endomyocardial ventriculotomy, the better the antiarrhythmic results.

In 70% of the patients a VT was inducible intraoperatively and the area of earliest activation could be identified (group I). Depending on the macroscopic findings a circumscript endocardial resection (ER)—first choice—was carried out. In case of VT origin in the vicinity of the papillary muscles or inside of an extended scar the area was isolated by a circumscript endomyocardial incision (EC).

In 30% the VT was not inducible and the arrhythmogenic area was indicated only by fragmented, delayed or low amplitude signals during sinus rhythm or the area could not be identified clearly (group II and III). With exception of the papillary muscle an extended resection or incision was carried out depending on the anatomical situation.

Up to 80% of the arrhythmogenic areas were found in the high inter-ventricular septum. The angiographic correlate of these patients was a proximal total occlusion of the left anterior descending artery in all cases. In most of the patients the anterior wall of the left ventricle suffered a transmural infarction, while the interventricular septal scar did not extend *transmurally*. Probably a remaining perfusion of the septum via the posterior branches of the right coronary artery prevented the *transmural* infarction. In some of these patients a combined procedure was carried out: After extended

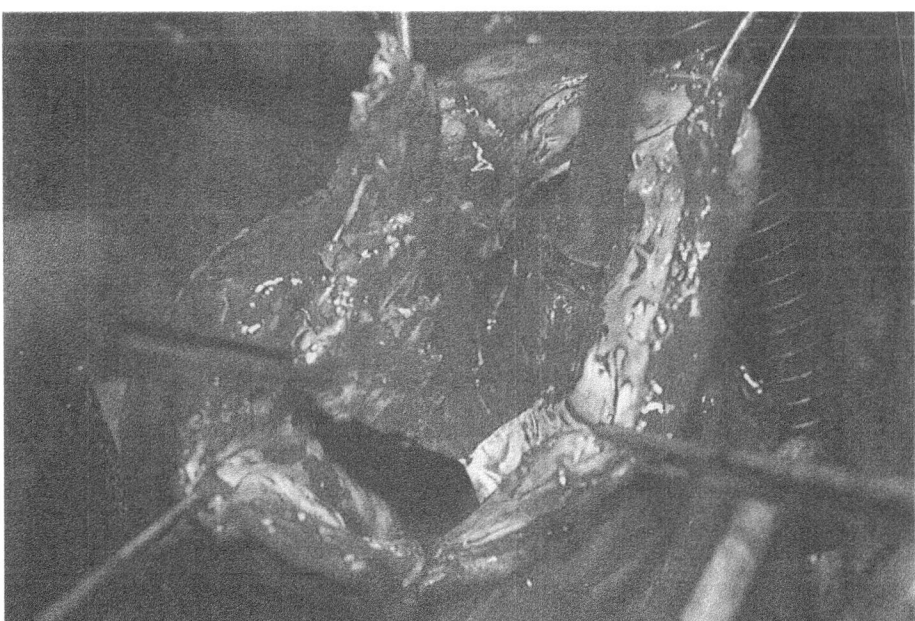

Figure 7. Resection of an extended fibrotic endomyocardial scar (interventricular septum) with underlying vital myocardium.

resection of the endocardial fibrotic tissue an additional circumscript incision of the underlying partially vital tissue was carried out in the region of interest.

Figure 7 demonstrates the intraoperative finding in one of this patients: After an extended endocardial resection the underlying vital contractile myocardium is visible.

Material and methods

In our own experience antitachycardiac electrophysiologically guided operations for malignant ventricular tachycardia were carried out in 42 patients. In 29 patients (Table 2) the ventricular tachycardia was the primary indication for operation. In 13 patients the tachyarrhythmia was suppressed by drugs, but additional leasons indicated the operation. 26 patients suffered up to 4 cardiac arrests with subsequent resuscitation before surgery. The interval between onset of disease or infarction and the antiarrhythmic operation ranged between two days and 248 months. The hospital mortality in this group of patients was 14%.

Table 2. Indications for electrophysiologically guided operations for ventricular tachycardia (Cologne-Göttingen 1983–1988)

Primary indication for VT-surgery	n = 29	
Additional indication for VT-Surgery		42
(associated procedure during ACVB	n = 13	
or VWR)		
Previous non-fatal cardiac arrest		
with resuscitation (1-4)	n = 26	
Interval infarction – operation	2 days – 248 months	

Table 3. Electrophysiologically guided operations for ventricular tachycardia (Cologne/Göttingen 1983–1988) n = 42 (+ 6)

Surgical techniques		Associated procedures	
ER	15	* VAR	37
ER + EC	11	ACBG	22
EC	14	** AICD-EI.	9
		MVR	4 (+ 3)
VWR	2	VSD-Closure	2 (+ 1)

*   Endoventricular circular plasty (DOR) in 2 pts.
** AICD Implantation after postop. PVS in 2 pts.

In 15 patients an endocardial resection was carried out, in 14 patients a circumscript endocardial incision and in another 11 patients a combined procedure of ER and EC was necessary. In two patients the ventricular wall resection was sufficient to ablate or isolate the arrhythmogenic tissue (Table 3). The VT was not inducible intraoperatively, early and late postoperatively the VT was not inducible without any additional antiarrhythmic drugs. In most of the patients associated procedures as resection of ventricular aneurysm, aortocoronary bypass grafting, mitral valve replacement or closure of a ventricular septum defect where necessary. Four of the 6 early postoperative deaths occurred in patients with additional mitral valve replacement or ventricular septum defect. The associated implantation of defibrillator electrodes occurred in 9 patients in whom the intraoperative mapping findings could not identify the tachycardia origin clearly. The implantation of an AICD was necessary in two cases two weeks postoperatively because of inducibility of VT.

Hospital mortality after antitachycardiac surgery for ischemic VT

Table 4 represents the data of the main centers performing antiarrhythmic surgery. The operative mortality ranges between 5 and 23% (13. 9) [10]. Analyzing the reasons for this wide spreading results Ostermeyer et al. found the following predictable risk factors for antitachycardiac surgery for ischemic VT by collecting the data of a combined study of the University of Düsseldorf and Alabama and of a collaborative registry of 8 European and North American Institutions (Table 5): The most sufficient predictive factors, determining hospital mortality, are the severity of the underlying ischemic heart disease, the presence and severity of congestive heart failure and the presence or absence of left ventricular aneurysm [10]. These factors

Table 4. Hospital mortality after antitachycardiac surgery for ischemic VT

	n	t	%
Birmingham (UAB)	123	28	23
Boston	36	6	17
Durham	65	9	14
Düsseldorf	93	5 5	
Hannover	74	6	8
Philadelphia	206	29	14
Stanford	105	17	17
Cologne/Göttingen	42	6	14
TOTAL	744	106	13.9

Table 5.   Antitachycardiac surgery for VT – influencing factors for hospital mortali

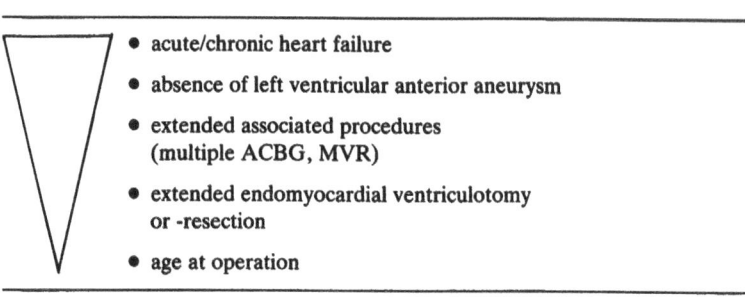

- acute/chronic heart failure
- absence of left ventricular anterior aneurysm
- extended associated procedures (multiple ACBG, MVR)
- extended endomyocardial ventriculotomy or -resection
- age at operation

are more powerful in predicting the postoperative survival than the type of surgical technique, when carried out as limited as possible, or the age at operation.

Figure 8 demonstrates impressively the influence of a ventricular aneurysm on the probability of survival after antitachycardiac operation [10]. In case of absence of well demarked aneurysm the ventriculotomy can lead to a deleterious impairment of the ventricular function, associated with a high operative and late postoperative mortality.

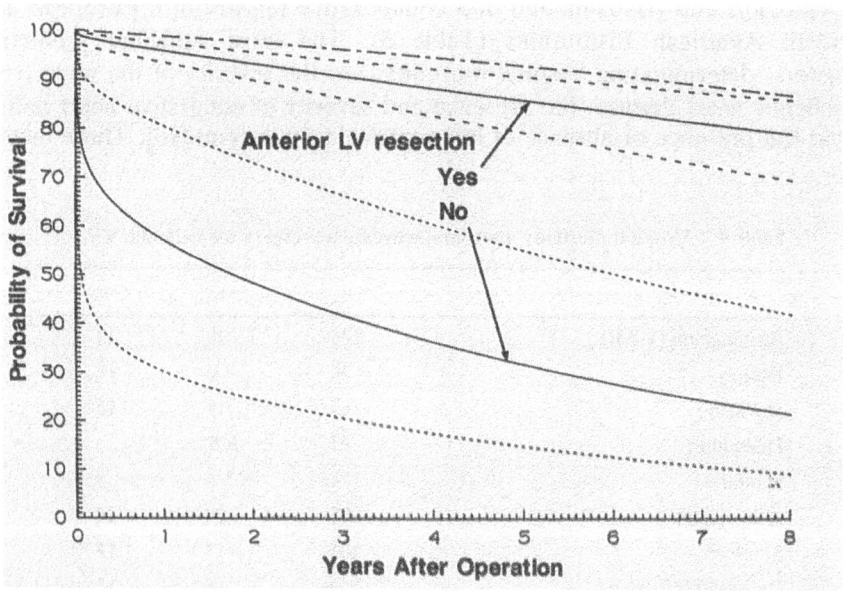

Figure 8.   Influence of presence or absence of a well demarked left ventricular aneurysm on the long-term survival after antitachycardiac operations.

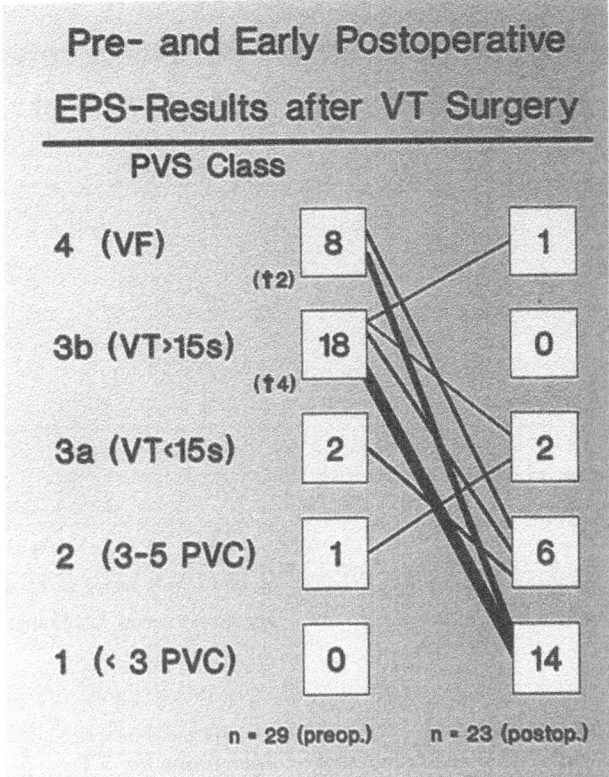

Figure 9.

Recurrence of VT after antiarrhythmic operations

Referring to the experience in the treatment of recurrent VT by anti-arrhythmic drugs the efficiency and quality of the operative therapy can be assessed and predicted by the programmed stimulation as well.

Figure 9 represents the early postoperative electrophysiological findings in 23 patients in our own group [9]. Malignant ventricular tachyarrythmias and/or recurrent non fatal cardiac arrests were primary indication for operation in these patients. The programmed ventricular stimulation was carried out within 2 or 3 weeks postoperatively. The one patient in PVS class 2, with inducible premature ventricular contractions but no inducible VT preoperatively had suffered 3 non fatal cardiac arrests with resuscitations. The VT, inducible after surgery could be suppressed by drugs.

The actuarial one and four year recurrence rate for VT with inducible but drug responsive ventricular arrhythmias after surgery is 8 and 12 percent in our own experience. One patient with inducible drug refractory VT died before the additional implantation of an automatic defribrillator (Figure 10).

330   A. Hannekum

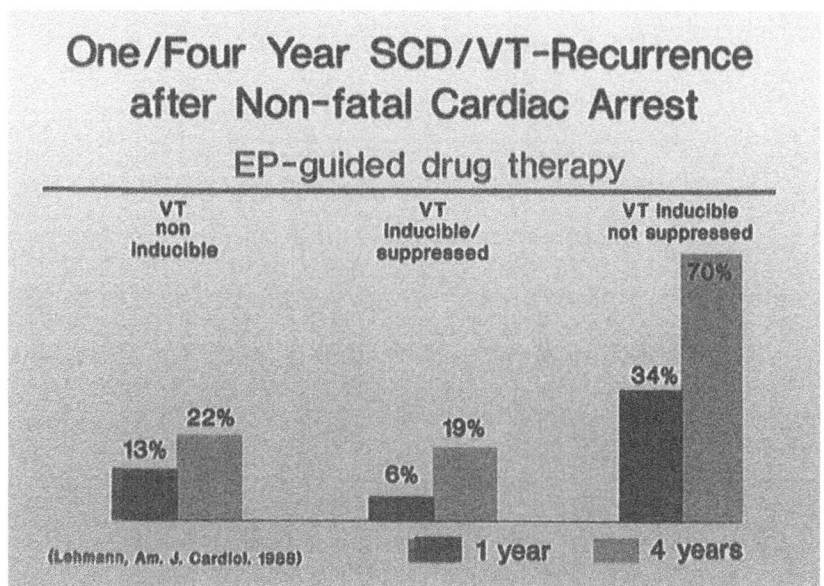

Figure 10. Results of EP guided surgery (own experience) versus AICD therapy (results of the literature).

Long-term results after antitachycardiac operations for VT

Regarding the long term results of antitachycardiac surgery, especially the antiarrhythmic effect of the endomyocardial procedure of the main institutions, again we have to consider the above mentioned difficulties in comparing different procedures, different patient populations, different pre- and postoperative electrophysiologic protocols with or without concomitant

Table 6. Long term results after antitachycardiac operations for VT

	Survivor (n)	SCD+ VT-Rec.	Long Term Survivor	Induc. VT	Antiarr. Drugs
Philadelphia	(126)89	16	60	37	37
Stanford	(89)84	60	62	32	?
Birmingham	(95)77	22	54	33	?
Dusseldorf	(88)94	20	78	40	?
Hannover	(63)86	13	75	14	22
Cologne/ Gottingen	(42)86	8	75	12	22

in percent

Table 7. Antitachycardic surgery for VT – influencing factors for return of VT/SCD

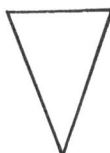

- impairment of left ventricular function
- absence of left ventricular aneurysm
- postoperative inducibility of VT
- multiple sites of VT

drug therapy. Therefore an overview of the results in the literature has to be interpreted with caution (Table 6) [11–14]. The most important predictors for return of VT or sudden cardiac death again seem to be the impairment of left ventricular function and the absence of a left ventricular aneurysm as Ostermeyer pointed out in his retrospective multicenter analysis [10]. Furthermore, in a decreasing range the postoperative inducibility of VT and multiple sites of VT origin are important factors for predicting the recurrence of VT and long-term prognosis (Table 7).

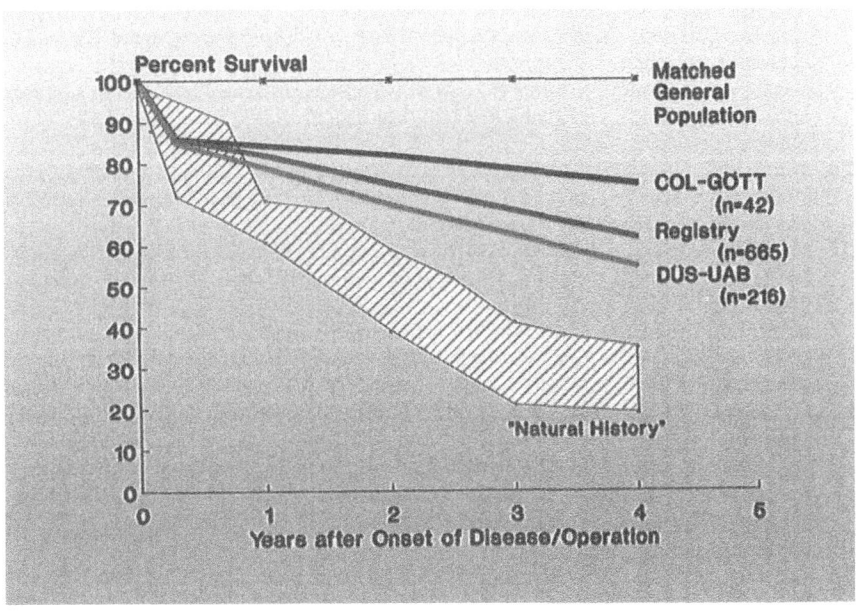

Figure 11. Long-term survival after antiarrhythmic surgery/'natural history'.

References

1. Couch OA (1959) Cardiac aneurysm with ventricular tachycardia and subsequent excision of aneurysm. *Circulation* 20: 251.
2. Guiraudon G, Fontaine G, Frank R, Escaude G, Etievent P, Cabrol C (1978) Encircling endocardial ventriculotomy: a new surgical treatment for life-threatening ventricular tachy-cardias resistant to medical treatment following myocardial infarction. *Ann Thorac Surg* 26: 438.
3. Josephson ME, Horowitz LN, Spielmann SR, Greenspan AM (1980) Electrophysiologic and hemodynamic studies in patients resuscitated from cardiac arrest. *Am J Cardiol* 46: 948.
4. Swerdlow CD, Winkle RA, Mason JW (1983) Determinants of survival in patients with ventricular tachycardia. *N Engl J Med* 308: 1436.
5. Horowitz LN (1988) Sudden arrhythmic death: prediction and prevention in: Iwa T, Fontaine G (eds), *Cardiac Arrhythmias: Recent Progress in Investigation and Management*. Elsevier Science Publishers BV.
6. Graboys TB, Lown B, Podrid PJ and DeSilva (1982) Long-term survival of patients with malignant ventricular arrhythmia treated with antiarrhythmic drugs. *Am J Cardiol* 50: 437.
7. Lehmann MH et al. (1988) The automatic implantable cardioverter defibrillator as anti-arrhythmic treatment modality of choice for survivor of cardiac arrest unrelated to acute myocardial infarction. *Am J Cardiol* 62: 803.
8. Scheinman MM, Evans jr GT (1987) Catheter electrical ablation of cardiac arrhythmias: a summary report of the percutaneous cardiac mapping and ablation registry, in: Brugada P, Wellens HJJ (eds), *Cardiac Arrhythmias: Where to Go from Here?* Mount Kisco: Futura Publishing Company.
9. Hannekum A, Hoffer H, Beyer M, Laß M (1990) Chirurgische Therapie von supraventri-kulären Arrhythmien, in: Hombach V (ed), *Kardiologie, Bd. 3, Kardiovaskuläre Chirurgie*. Stuttgart: Schattauer Verlag.
10. Ostermeyer J, Kirklin JK, Borggrefe M, Cox JL, Breithardt G, Bircks W (1989) Ten years electrophysiologically guided direct operations for malignant ischemic ventricular tachycardia — results. *Thorac Cardiovasc Surg* 37: 20.
11. McGiffin DC, Kirklin JK, Plumb VJ, Blackstone EH, Waldo AL, Kirklin JW, Karp RB (1987) Relief of life-threatening ventricular tachycardia and survival after direct operations. *Circulation* 76: 93.
12. Borggrefe M, Podczek A, Ostermeyer J, Breithardt G and the Surgical Ablation Registry (1987) Long-term results of electrophysiologically guided antitachycardia surgery in ventri-cular tachyarrhythmias: A collaborative report on 665 patients. In: Breithardt G, Borggrefe M, Zipes DP (eds), *Nonpharmacological Therapy of Tachyarrhythmias*. Futura Publishing Company.
13. Ostermeyer J, Borggrefe M, Breithardt G, Podozek A, Goldman A, Schoenen JD, Kolvenbach R, Godehardt E, Kirklin JW, Blackstone H, Bricks W (1987) Direct opera-tions for the management of life-threatening ischemic ventricular tachycardia. *J Thorac Cardiovasc Surg* 94: 848.
14. Swerdlow CD, Mason JW, Stinson EB, Oyer PE, Winkle RA, Derby GC (1986) Results of operations for ventricular tachycardia in 105 patients. *J Thorac Cardiovasc Surg* 92: 105.

Developments in Cardiovascular Medicine

Developments in Cardiovascular Medicine

Developments in Cardiovascular Medicine

Developments in Cardiovascular Medicine

Developments in Cardiovascular Medicine

Developments in Cardiovascular Medicine

Developments in Cardiovascular Medicine

Previous volumes are still available

KLUWER ACADEMIC PUBLISHERS – DORDRECHT / BOSTON / LONDON

The manufacturer's authorised representative in the EU is Springer
Nature Customer Service Centre GmbH, Europaplatz 3, 69115 Heidelberg,
Germany. If you have any concerns regarding our products, please
contact ProductSafety@springernature.com

Printed and bound by CPI Group (UK) Ltd, Croydon, CR0 4YY
23/04/2026
02095624-0004